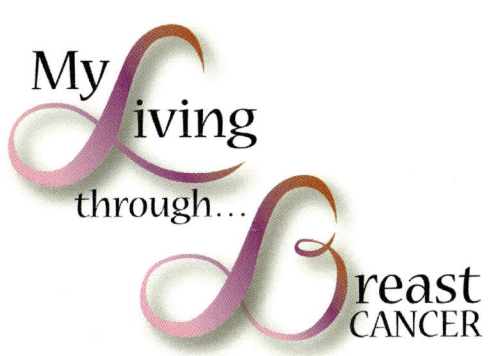

The brave journey of 44 survivors.

Tom Denlick and
Joanna Herr

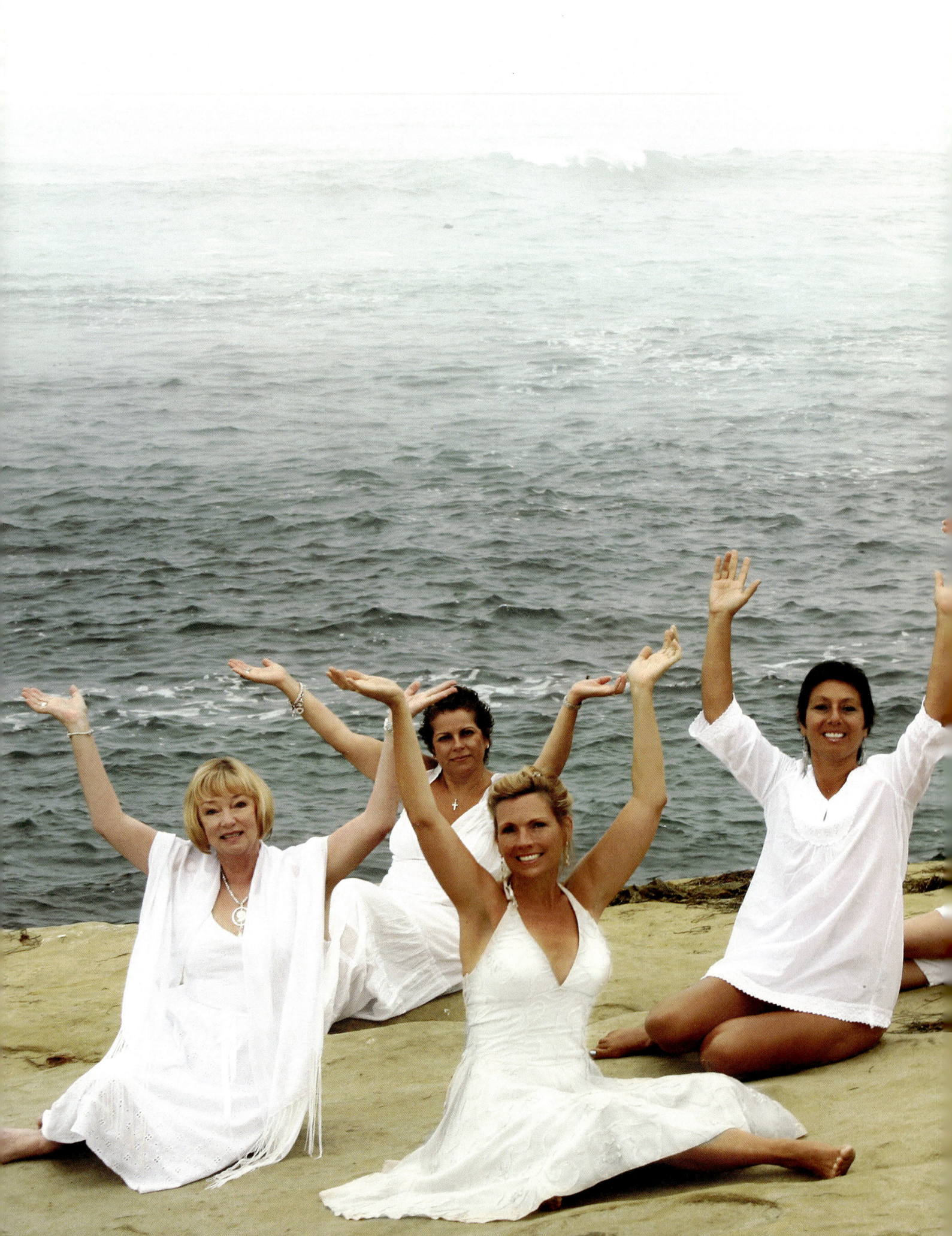

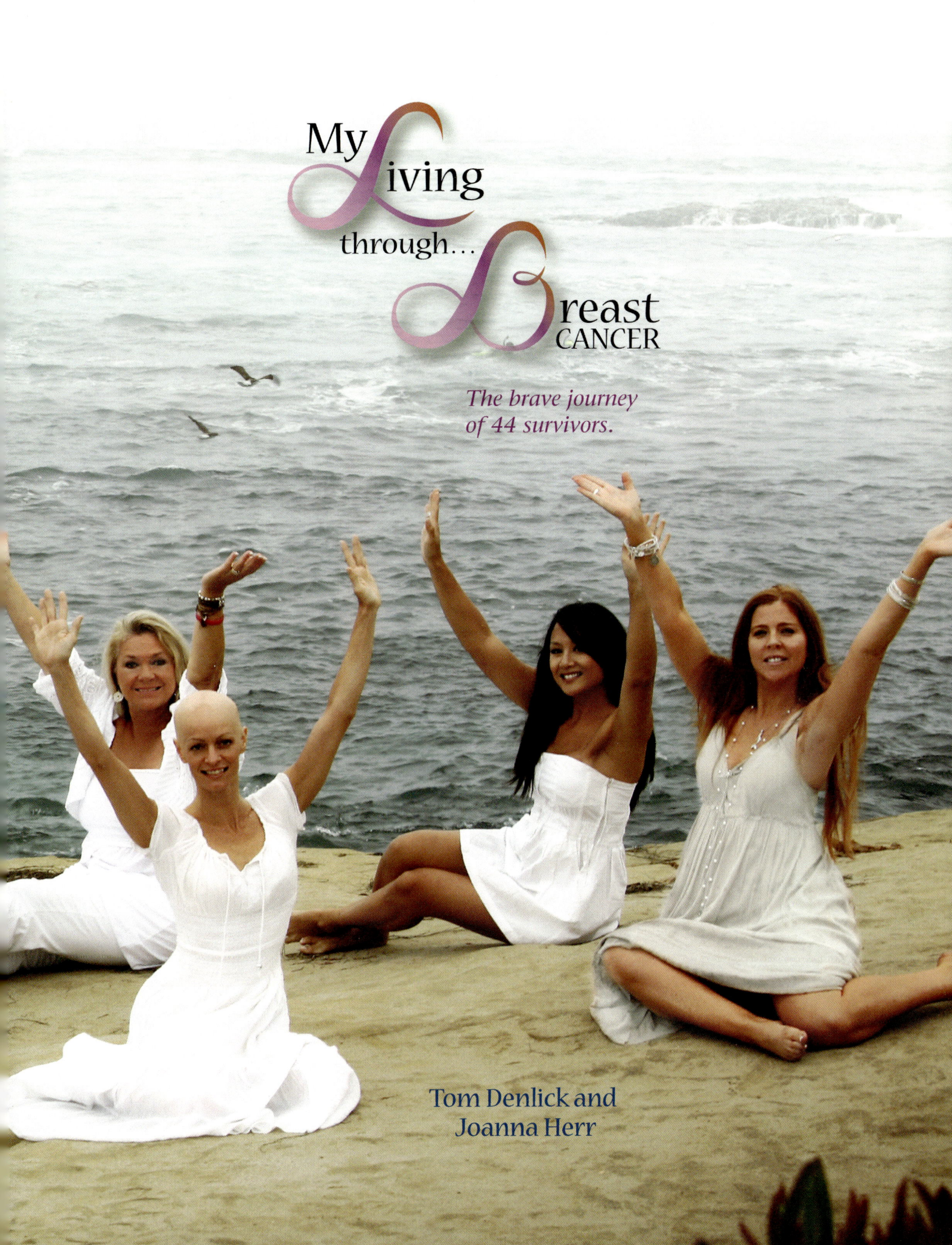

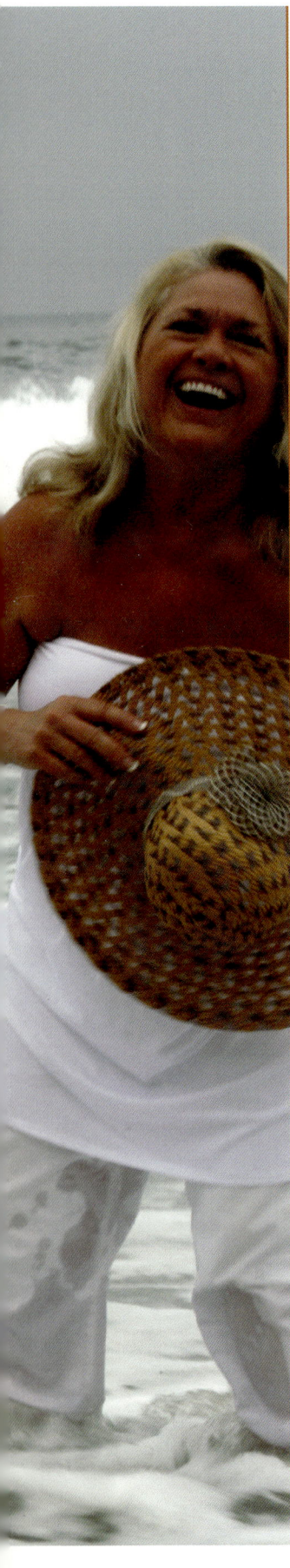

Copyright © 2012 by Tom Denlick;
3rd Edition
Photographs © 2011 by:
Tom Denlick, Joanna Herr and other
photographers as credited.

"My Living Through" a book series
and "My Living Through" brand and logo
have trademarks pending with the
United States Patent and Trademark Office.

All rights reserved. No part of this work
may be reproduced or used in any form or
by any means—graphic, electronic, or mechanical,
including photocopying or information storage
and retrieval systems—without written
permission from the publisher.

The scanning, uploading and distribution
of this book or any part thereof via the Internet or
via any other means without the permission
of the publisher is illegal and punishable by law.
Please purchase only authorized editions
and do not participate in or encourage
the electronic piracy of copyrighted materials.

ISBN: 978-0-615-56480-7
Printed in United States of America

Book, cover & custom font designer:
Olivia V. Francis

Type set in: Nueva Standard and
ITC Stone Serif.

Book printer: Peggy Sauer, L&L Printers

Published by:

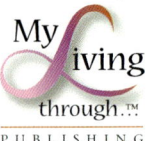

My Living through.™
PUBLISHING

P.O. Box 710250, Santee, California 92072
Phone: (619) 851-7608
E-mail: thomasdenlick@yahoo.com

For more information about this book,
the "Tree of Life" in La Jolla, California,
how you may participate in upcoming books,
or how you may distribute books in your area,
please visit our website at:

www.mylivingthrough.com

My Living Through™ Books are available
at special discounts for bulk purchases
for sales promotions or premiums.
Special editions, including personalized covers,
corporate imprints, and excerpts can be
created in large quantities for special needs.
Contact the publisher for more information.

This book may be purchased from
the publisher for $29.99. Please include an
additional $5.00 for shipping & handling.

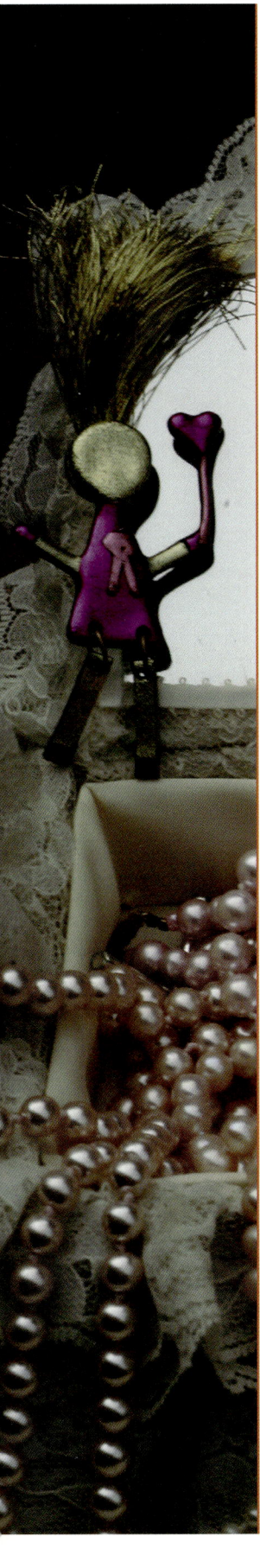

Table of Contents

The Authors 7
Behind the Scenes: *Acknowledgements & Credits* 8
Introduction: Survivor or Supporter 9
1. From War Orphan to Cheerleader – Lyly Thanh Koenig 10
2. The Blues Brothers – Jake & Elwood – Andi Bird 13
MammoSite Radiation Therapy 13
3. My Mom, My Sister and Me – Sharon Stephens 14
Breast Cancer Prevention 15
4. When I Think Cancer, I Think About Healing – Cynthia Paulo 16
Lipoma 17
5. My Severe Mercy – Laura Farmer 18
6. Nine Years and Counting Many More… – Dikla Benzeevi 20
Humorous Tales 25
7. One Way to Really Live… Beat Cancer Twice!!! – Julie Goiset 26
8. Getting to the Other Side of Breast Cancer – Sandy Lee Rabourne 28
9. You Talkin' to Me? You Talkin' to My Mama? – Rosalie Huntley 30
10. Not Too Young – Jennifer Tullis 33
Love…No Matter What 34
11. I'll Never Win the 'OWIE' Game – Sonia Encinias 36
   (Nunca Ganaré en el Juego de el Moretón) 37
12. Tradin' Chevys for Ferraris – Sherry Bittner 39
13. A Breast Is Just That…a Breast. – Nancy Barnes 40
14. Don't Sweat the Small Stuff – Jean Stringer 44
15. Get a 2nd, 3rd or 4th Opinion – Sara Klinzman 46
16. Honor Your Intuition – Nataly Pluta 48
17. Cancer Taught Me How to Live – Crystal Crawford 50
Team Survivor San Diego 52
18. Just a Bump in the Road – Eleanor Girard 56
19. Twenty-Seven Extra Years – Angie Bagnas 57
20. Quench My Spirit—No Way – Pam McGregor 58
21. Hidden Beauty – Laura Sutton 60
22. Next to Flossing – Lisa Alexander 62
23. 1 in 8 Isn't Just a Statistic – Lucy Cafiero 64

One in Eight: *A Teen's Guide to Understanding Breast Cancer* 67

24. *Don't Fight It Alone* – Melanie Hansen 68

The 4 Stages of Cancer 70

25. *Has Anyone Seen My Basket?* – Heather Veirs 71
26. *From Moccasins to Stilettos* – Denise Lindstrom 72
27. *You Just Know* – Nancy Robinson 76
28. *One in a Hundred* – Laura Downing 79
29. *A Journey to Remember* – Christina David-Falls 82

The Brighter Side 87

30. *Turning 60 Is Better Than the Alternative* – Chris Eberhardt 88
31. *A New Chapter Begins* – Julie Heimburge 91
32. *My Cancer is a Gift* – Sammi McDonald 94
33. *My Daily Journal* – Cindy Matranga 96
34. *Never, Ever, Give Up* – Melissa Maki 99
35. *Case of the Flying Prostheses* – Ana Maria Montes de Oca 100
36. *The Delivery* – Grace Bernal 102
37. *I Will Survive!!!* – Mary Brewer 108
38. *3-Time Survivor* – Gail Bishop 110

The Emotional Stages of Breast Cancer 112

39. *No Return Policy* – Tina Poirier 113

Survivors Park 114

40. *Cancer and the Husband* – Sue LaVoie 116
41. *The Angel Nurse* – Virginia Laffey 118
42. *To the Point* – Shirley Rogers 119
43. *Life's Biggest Disappointments Become God's Biggest Appointments* – Maria Delis 120
44. *Power to Be* – Regina Savage 122

Links & Groups 126

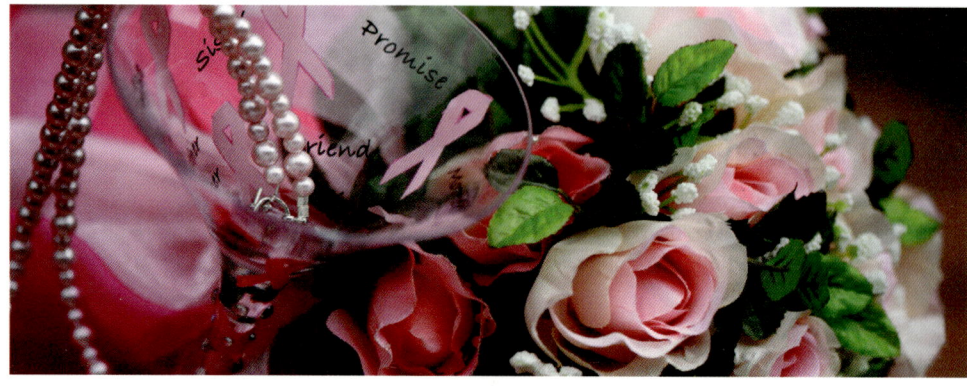

The Authors

Tom Denlick
Photographer & PhotoTherapist

Following a 20-year career as a licensed marriage and family therapist, I was fortunate to be able to make a profession from my photography hobby. This is my third book. I started out doing mainly architectural photography, but quickly turned to what I truly love—photographing people.

There is nothing like getting behind a camera and just watching for that magical moment when the expression, the pose, the gleam in the eyes meet the smile of the lips and wow you just see it. After doing hundreds of photo shoots of every imaginable genre you begin to see things differently. You see life differently.

I have had the privilege of photographing many of the women in this book. These ladies are truly beautiful. They are the most beautiful women that I have ever photographed. Part of it is the smiling eyes. I know, I know, what in the world are smiling eyes? I believe it's a gift given to those who are incredibly grateful to be alive. I see it through my lens as pure joy. And when it happens you know that you have been joined by a third party, because it is heavenly and you can just feel the spirit come alive.

It doesn't happen all the time but when it does it is unforgettable. I live for these moments.

"OMG! I have never and I mean never seen myself like this before…these pictures brought tears to my eyes. I now see that it was not my hair…not my brows or eyelashes…not my boobs that made me beautiful…it was just me." ~ Sonia

Getting involved with the women in this book has been one of the most rewarding experiences of my lifetime. "Until you know that life is interesting—and find it so—you haven't found your soul." Geoffrey Fisher

The ladies in this book have given me the opportunity to find my soul. Thank you, thank you, thank you.

Tom Denlick
thephototherapist@yahoo.com
www.mylivingthrough.com

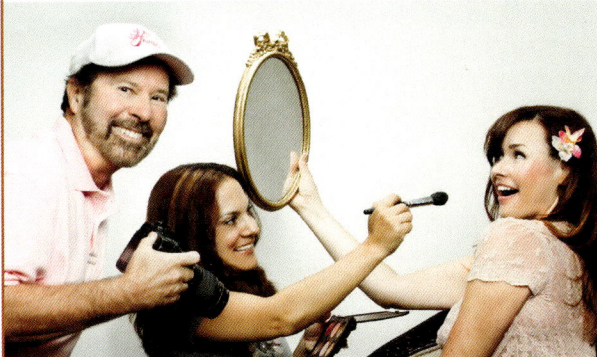

Photo by Eric Denlick: (from left to right) Tom Denlick–Photographer; Olga Villarreal–Hair & Makeup; Michelle Snyder–Set Coordinator

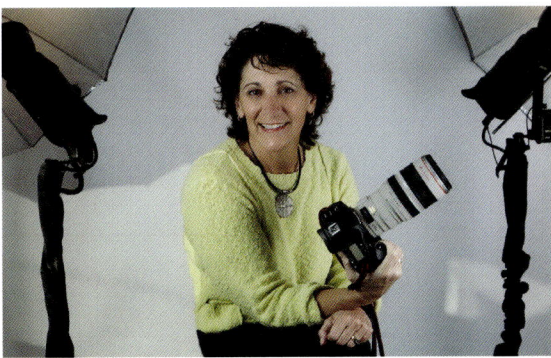

Joanna Herr-Hanks
Photographer & Entrepreneur

My Aunt Anna was a big woman with a big heart. Always smiling and reaching out to others to lend a hand…never complaining. I watched her take care of her sister with Down syndrome and her husband blinded by diabetes. When she was diagnosed with breast cancer, her life dramatically changed. I helplessly witnessed her shrivel away—her image at 95 pounds will forever be etched in my memory. Doctors warned all the girls in our family to get annual check-ups, but at 30 years old, I doubted that meant me.

I had multiple surgeries to remove large cysts from both breasts and had a breast reduction to remove some dense breast tissue. Scars from my multiple surgeries looked like shark bites—both unsettling and unattractive. The thought of even more surgeries in the future was unnerving, so at age 33, after discussing my options with my doctor, I made the decision to have a double mastectomy rather than face more surgeries.

Dealing with scars was not easy and I did everything I could to hide them. One day a photographer asked me to model a tank top for a photo shoot he was doing. My immediate response was 'No, my scars will show.' With some coaxing, I reluctantly agreed. Even though I was uncomfortable, I was pleased with the images. It got me thinking that there must be other women who feel self-conscious about their bodies after undergoing surgery. Wouldn't it be great to capture their images and show them their beauty? I started offering photography to women who had undergone mastectomies. At the same time, my friend Francine Zorehkey was working towards her Ph.D. in Psychotherapy and together we came up with the idea of a special retreat—*AWOL—A Way of Life After Cancer Diagnosis*—to pamper women who have or have had breast cancer.

I currently serve on the Board of 'From Chrysalis to Wings' and donate my time and materials to provide glamour photography to women fighting breast cancer. I frequently offer portrait packages as fundraiser prizes, and work with military families and personnel to provide low-cost family and newborn portraits.

The philosophy of "giving back" is vitally important to me, and led me to collaborate with Tom on this amazing book, "My Living Through Breast Cancer."

Joanna Herr
photog@herrphotography.com
www.herrphotography.com

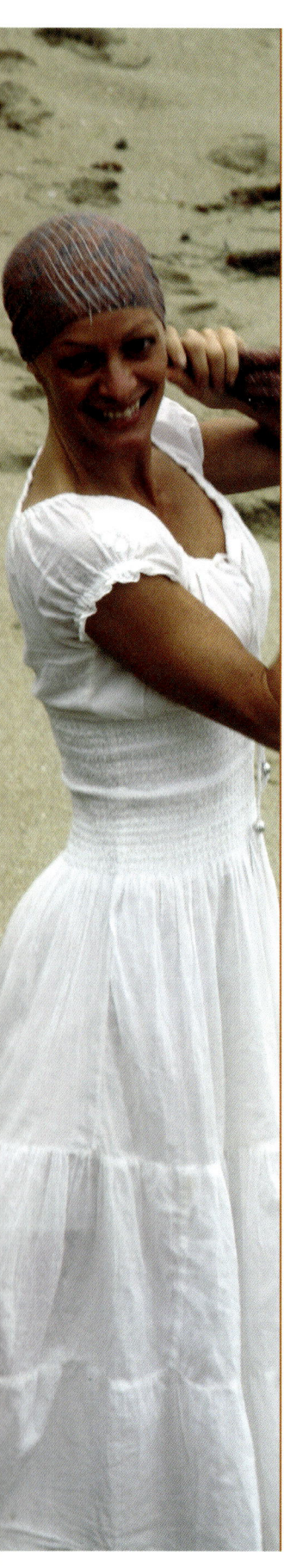

Behind the Scenes
Acknowledgments & Credits

Olga Villarreal is a Professional Makeup Artist, Master Esthetician and ITEC beauty specialist. Olga is the best. We've worked together on photo shoots for many years. She provided the excellent hair and makeup for most of the women in this book.

> *Olga Villarreal*
> *Hair & Makeup Stylist*
> olgapvilla@gmail.com
> www.allaboutbeautyandspa.com

Michelle Snyder, my all time favorite photography assistant, takes over from there. She has such an eye for detail whether she's helping with the outfit changes or getting the set to look just right.

> *Michelle Snyder*
> *Set Coordinator & Photography Assistant*

Thanks also to **Sarah Baldino** at Yardage Town for her expertise in choosing fabric and colors that are perfect every time.

> *Sarah Baldino*
> *Fabric & Color Coordinator*
> Yardage Town
> www.yardagetown.com

After a photo shoot we deliver the CD's and memory cards to the very best photo editor ever and that is **Sarah Soto**. She will make any photo look great. She will make any photographer look great. All the women love her. Hey, a little tuck here or there can make all the difference, right? Thanks for the many years and thousands of photos that you've enhanced for me.

> *Sarah Soto*
> *Sarah Soto Photographics*
> sarahsotophoto@gmail.com
> www.sarahsoto.com

Can't give enough kudos to **Olivia Francis**. She has done such a masterful job of creating this book. She gathered up all the photos and stories and put them together seamlessly. She designed front and back covers, logos, the ribbon lettering for each of the 44 names, and the entire book layout. What a talented artist!

> *Olivia V. Francis*
> *Graphic Designer*
> ofrancis@san.rr.com
> www.ofrancisdesign.com

Peggy Sauer has been instrumental in bringing this project to print. What a group of wonderful folks at L+L Printers.

> *Peggy Sauer*
> *L+L Printers*
> 7270 Engineer Road, San Diego, CA 92111
> www.llprinters.com

Thanks to my wife, **Paula**, whose technical and proofreading skills as well as support has been invaluable. After learning that I was unable to locate the songwriter who holds the copyright to Celine Dion's "I'm Alive", my daughter, **Jennifer**, wrote her own poem "Grateful to be Alive." Is that precious, or what? And thank you to my son, **Eric**, my best friend. His ability to hear beyond words provided a constant source of wisdom and encouragement.

"GRATEFUL TO BE ALIVE"

We face many challenges each day
Keeping in mind what we live for

Our scars will never vanish
As we go on searching for so much more

Blissful moments make us want to fly
As freely as a soaring dove

We continue on realizing we need to be here
For the ones we love

Every human being faces times
Where they barely make it through

As we feel weaker than ever
We then discover our hopeful rescue

Remember your talents, treasures,
The reasons for your existence

Moving forward after these trials
Will show your true persistence

Years will fade as you look back
On what you were able to endure

The medicine, the prayers,
The support was not your only cure

You as a whole got yourself past
All of this trauma in your life

As you look up to the sky you whisper to yourself,
"I'm so grateful to be alive"

> ~ *Jennifer Denlick*
> *Songwriter, Age 19*

Joanna Herr and I met some nine months ago to discuss publishing a book that would give a voice to women who have journeyed through the rigors of breast cancer. We proudly present the incredible real life stories of 44 of the most courageous women you will ever meet.

Enjoy! **Tom Denlick**

Survivor or Supporter

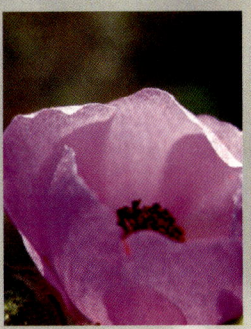

This book is written by survivors for survivors. It is also written for supporters. You are either a survivor or a supporter. You could be just recently diagnosed or a twenty-year survivor. You could be one of the 230,480 who will be diagnosed with breast cancer this year. Or, you could know a survivor. We all do. It could be your mother, your sister, your aunt, cousin, wife, or best friend.

One way or another we are all affected by breast cancer. We are either going through breast cancer or we know someone who is. Excluding cancer of the skin, breast cancer is the most frequently diagnosed cancer in women.

Yet, despite these overwhelming statistics, women with breast cancer are drawing on early detection and treatment breakthroughs, along with their own strength and resilience, to survive this deadly disease. They are also drawing on the strength, wisdom, and guidance of the community of survivors who are willing to share the most intimate details of their lives.

"If you have cancer, cry about it, pray about it, and talk about it. Otherwise no one will benefit from your experience and your knowledge." ~ Cynthia, Chapter 12

That's the cornerstone of **My Living Through Breast Cancer**. Courageous real life stories are told by 44 female breast cancer survivors. You will be touched… inspired. These stories are not sugar-coated. They are real life in real time. In order to preserve each survivor's unique, individual voice, these stories have been minimally edited.

Flower Photos: "LoveNoMatterWhat.com" by Petra

"If you want to live, here's how. You can do it. We all did, in our own way. And so can you."

This is their message. It's intended for all survivors and all supporters, and that means each and every one of us.

Our Goal

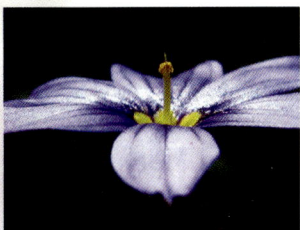

Our intent is to provide information and guidance about dealing with breast cancer by means of our survivors' personal stories. Our mission is to distribute this book to the waiting rooms of each of the 800,000 physicians practicing nationwide. It's a huge goal and we're going to give it our all.

How can you help? By placing a book in the waiting room of your physician. Don't worry. They won't mind!

The FABulous 44 will thank you and we thank you, too, from the bottom of our hearts, for helping our goal become a reality.

Tom Denlick and *Joanna Herr*

DEDICATION

This amazing team of 44 survivors represent the thousands of women that are fighting this insidious disease. Unfortunately, the team has lost one of their own just two weeks before the publication of this book.

We regret to announce the passing of Melanie Hansen, who fought with incredible courage for most of her young life. We would like to extend our prayers and support to her family and dedicate this book in Melanie's name.

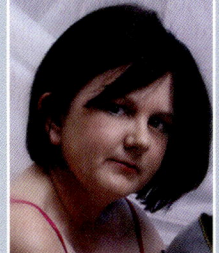

Photo by Joanna Herr

Lyly

"From War Orphan to Cheerleader"

Hi! My name is Lyly Thanh Koenig, I am a former Vietnamese war orphan, a former 2-Team NFL Cheerleader for the St. Louis Rams, and the San Diego Chargers, an actress and model, the owner of two clothing lines, Chickie & Smoove and LylyThanh, and at just 36 years old, my most prized title is, 2-time breast cancer survivor.

I am enormously proud to be a part of this book. When I was approached about being a part of it, I thought, "Who me!? Why!? I didn't do anything!" Then I thought, "I did beat breast cancer. I guess I am a survivor." So that got me thinking about this new title of SURVIVOR. It's not a title that should only be given after one beats cancer.

I'd found the pea-sized lump myself while putting on lotion after a shower. My first diagnosis came the week of my 32nd birthday. It was early November in San Diego, California. The Santa Ana's were blowing in from the desert keeping it warm out. It was an ordinary afternoon at work.

I was anxious for the week to end; my friends were whisking me away to Scottsdale, Arizona for a girl's celebration weekend. While working away at my desk I received a call from my breast surgeon. I hurried out to the parking lot to take the call. "I'm afraid that some of the cells we tested were cancerous". Just like that. I couldn't believe how calm he was. I had cancer after all! I stood frozen like a statue out on the empty black asphalt parking lot. Suddenly the warm breeze disappeared and extreme heat pounded down on me. I thought, "SOME?! You have cancer or you don't! Wait! I'm a former NFL Cheerleader and I have cancer… WHAT!? I cheered in a Super Bowl… and we won… and I HAVE CANCER!? No way." Like a robot, he began emitting medical terminology for everything I had. At this point in the game, I knew nothing of medical lingo, the only thing I heard was… CANCER. I'd received a gift of Stage I invasive ductal carcinoma and a BRCA II gene mutation! Happy Birthday to me! Surprisingly, there were no tears. My mind went blank.

I had two options, totally fall apart and let this disease kick my butt. Or fight. I took what my docs called, "the Lance Armstrong approach" to beating cancer. Excuse the cliché, but I began to LIVE STRONG.

So my 15 girlfriends and I headed off to Arizona. It was the best birthday ever. The possibility of never getting to party like this again, was very evident, so I partied with reckless abandon, all the while…with cancer.

Upon returning from Arizona, I packed up my condo and moved back to my home state of Missouri, where I'd undergo treatment. I endured bilateral mastectomies, 3 reconstruction surgeries, chemotherapy, followed by 1 year of an IV drip called Herceptin, 28 doses of radiation therapy, and about 3 years worth of tamoxifen to become cancer free. The first time.

I realize now, that prior to my diagnosis, I wasn't fully living life. I laughed and loved, but not like I do now. Now, I truly live in every moment. I revel in every aspect of an experience, a person, a day. I also learned I wanted to be fulfilled in my work. Which is what motivated me to pursue a career change.

> *Wait! I'm a former NFL Cheerleader and I have cancer… WHAT!? I cheered in a Super Bowl… and we won… and I HAVE CANCER!? No way."*

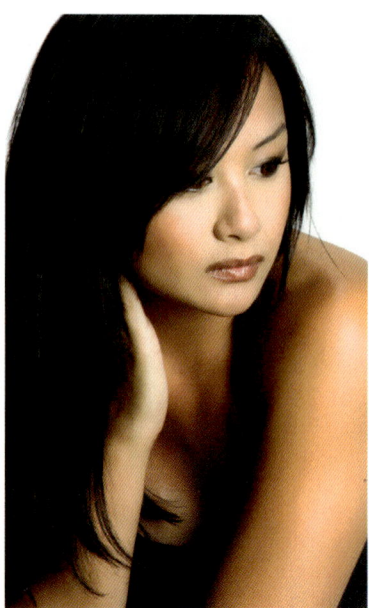

During that time of my life, my sister, brother, and all my friends were getting married, having babies, and their careers were in full bloom. Me, on the other hand, was forced to put all that on hold for cancer. Cancer stole that time from me. As a result, I began to think about

> *I realize now, that prior to my diagnosis, I wasn't fully living life. I laughed and loved, but not like I do now. Now, I truly live in every moment.*

the things that mattered. What can I be doing with my life that would make a difference in another's life, and what could I be doing to make changes in my own life, changes that would make my life more fulfilling. My livelihood had to be something I actually loved to do, something that, in a way, filled the void left behind from that stolen time.

As soon as I finished my last radiation treatment, I packed up my car and moved to Miami, Florida. I was going to help one of my oldest friends with my Godchildren while her husband was stationed in Haiti and I was going back to school. Miami was a blessing for two reasons, one, because I was able to spend the first 3 years of my Godchildren's lives with them, and, two, because it took me less than 2 years to complete my second degree, a degree in Fashion Design. I was there when my godchildren took their first steps and I was there when they said their first words. Blessed. I spent my entire time at the Miami International University of Art & Design on the Dean's List, and I graduated Cum Laude! Blessed. Following graduation, I was fired up! I was a newly minted fashion designer, cancer free, and ready to pick up my life where I'd left off. So, I packed up my car again and headed back to California to kick off my new career.

Not again.

Over the final few months of school I'd noticed a small lump forming in the middle of my chest. I did exactly what I tell others not to do… I ignored it. "It's just the bone that's exposed from the mastectomies" I tried to convince myself. My intuition skills are through the roof now. I knew it. I had cancer… again. Multiple tests and scans revealed nothing. Only after full biopsy surgery did I learn, officially, I had cancer again.

This time it was serious.

As it turns out, they'd cured my first cancer and this one was a new one. This time I had stage 4 invasive carcinoma that was attached to two of my ribs, my sternum, and invading the skeletal muscle. To save my life I'd have to have the whole kitchen sink all over again including a major thoracic surgery.

I began treatment for a second time in St. Louis, Missouri at St. Louis Cancer and Breast Institute, and finished my treatments at MD Anderson Cancer Center in Houston, Texas. I had major thoracic surgery to remove portions of two ribs and to insert a bioprosthetic mesh implant to fill the deficit left behind, chemotherapy again, 28 doses of radiation again, and after I have my family, I will eventually start taking femara, a pill I will take for 5 years that will throw me into early menopause, and I'll get a zolodex shot to shut down my ovaries until I have to have my ovaries removed to help prevent ovarian cancer. And to wrap it all up, I will need at least two more reconstruction surgeries.

Surviving.
Happy Birthday to Me!

When people hear that I've fought breast cancer twice and beat it twice, their first reaction is, "I'm so sorry!" Their compassion is comforting. But I am not sorry I got sick, believe it or not! I am grateful for my burden turned blessing! Battling cancer was the hardest thing I've ever done. It was painful… emotionally and physically. It was TRULY life changing. However now, looking

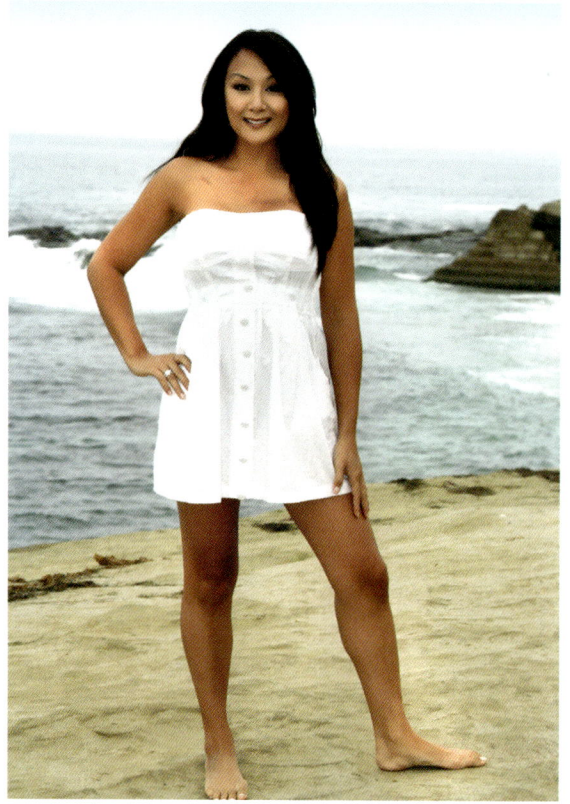

back, it wasn't so hard after all. It was never a death sentence for me.

I hold fast to something my Mom said to me upon getting my first diagnosis, "This is just a medical situation. We will take care of it, and we'll move on!" Which is exactly what I did. I dug in and became a survivor. I approached every appointment, every chemo treatment, every surgery, as a step closer to "taking care of it".

Countless Dr. appointments, numerous tests, scans, biopsies, a bilateral mastectomy, multiple reconstructive surgeries, chemo-TWICE, radiation-TWICE, LOSING ALL MY HAIR… TWICE!!! I am SURVIVING…

> **I was not getting voted off of this island…twice. Now, I'm cancer free…twice! I took care of it, mom! I'M A SURVIVOR!**

Today I am focused on picking up where I left off before my cancer diagnoses. I'm back in Southern California where I'm building my clothing companies. I spend lots of time with family. I especially love watching my 3 nephews and niece experience the world. Their curious innocence is something I believe I relearned through cancer. Good friends and their growing families surround me and bring me joy. The possibility of having a family of my own one-day enlivens me.

I'd like to say a special thank you to my Mom, Karen Koenig. Thank you for being my rock. If you're a mother of a cancer survivor, or to someone currently in the fight, your love and support is better than any medicine.

Cancer is like a black and white photograph. Instantly stripped away is all that is not essential, leaving behind the framework of what is. Having cancer takes you to the heart of what really matters—family, friends and humankind. The sadness in my world is cancer, but despite that, I live every day in joy and abundance. At the moment I am cancer free, but death still looms in the background. Hope overrides that reality and I stand resolute bolstered by the words of Ralph Waldo Emerson, "What lies behind us and what lies before us are tiny matters compared to what lies within us."

You can do your part for breast cancer. Sit with your Mom, your aunt, friend, sister, and your coworker during her treatments. Walk in a 3-Day, Run in a 5k. Most importantly, support funding. Increase your Impact. Do whatever you can to get in the fight. Ladies, do your self-exams. Remember, early detection saves lives. We can beat this!

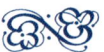

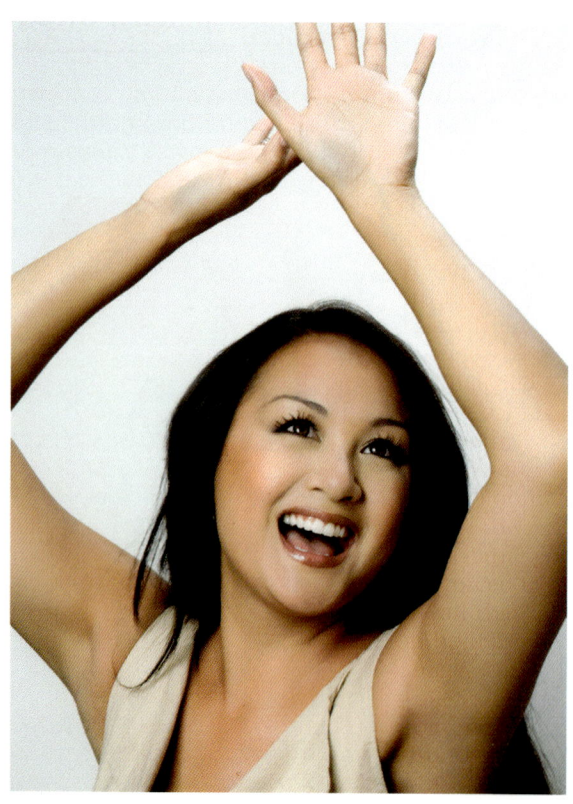

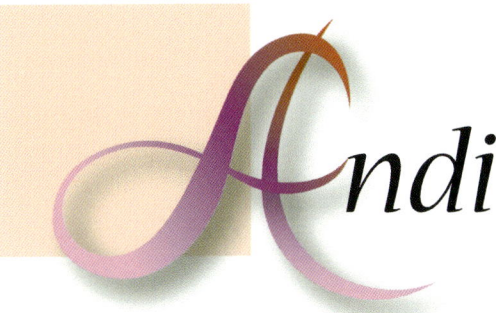

Andi

"The Blues Brothers– Jake & Elwood"

I am Andy Bird and was 47 when I was diagnosed with Breast Cancer. I had a large non-malignant tumor (in my uterus) that was so annoying that I named it Elwood. I joked that if I ever had another tumor I would name it Jake. So I could have the "Blues Brothers" with me... Little did I know that Jake had already taken residence in my left breast.

My Diagnosis was Ducal Carcinoma in Situ (DCIS), stage 0 (0-4 scale). I remembered I cried a lot. I felt like my body had betrayed me.

But I took comfort in Matthew 5:45, *"He causes his sun to rise on the evil and the good, and sends rain on the righteous and the unrighteous"*. God is in control...

I had **MammoSite radiation**, which takes 5 days (twice a day) instead of 6 weeks. It does mean two surgeries and several hours a day of treatment. I slept a lot and was very HOT.

I found relief at weekend retreats that are designed to meet the needs of breast cancer survivors regardless of the stage they are in their journey. It is wonderful to share with other women who come from a variety of backgrounds.

Living as a survivor sometimes feels like a timer ready to go off. Each mammogram could change everything.

I have met several people who I now call my friends. Not all have

> *Living as a survivor sometimes feels like a timer ready to go off. Each mammogram could change everything.*

been survivors... I would like Breast Cancer to be something that is read in a book and no one has to know what it feels like.

Today I am a 4½ year survivor. Both Elwood and Jake are gone. Hopefully to never return. But that is what annual (or quarterly or semiannual) testing is for.

What is MammoSite 5-Day Targeted Radiation Therapy?

The MammoSite® Radiation Therapy System received FDA clearance in 2002. Since then, over 50,000 women have been treated. MammoSite Targeted Radiation Therapy works from the inside, meaning that a higher daily dose can be used for a shorter period of time—5 days vs. 5-7 weeks.

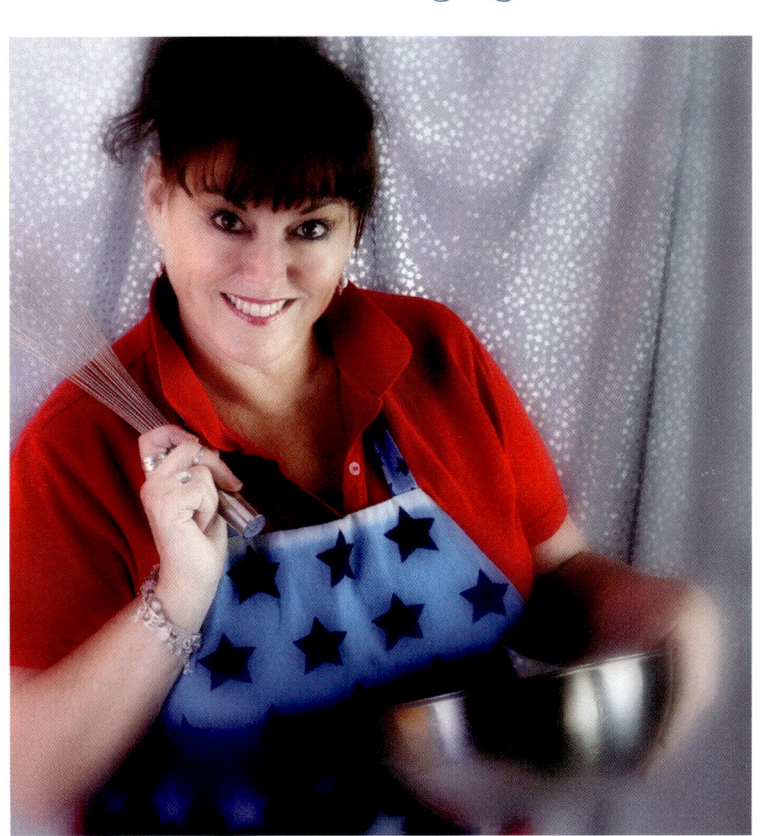

Photography by Joanna Herr

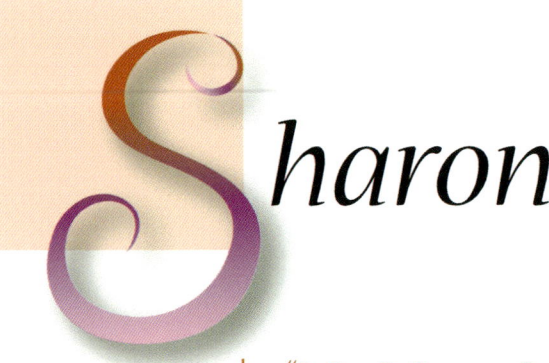

Sharon

"My Mom, My Sister and Me"

On October 4, 2007 I got "the call". The call that would dramatically change my life forever. However, my breast cancer story actually starts in June of 2000 when my 33 year old sister was diagnosed.

That experience was a whirlwind of technical speak and treatments we did not understand. As a family we pulled together and helped my sister through surgeries, chemo and radiation, which is something that nobody in their 30's should experience. Then 8 years later after a routine mammogram my world changed again.

Even though my sister had been diagnosed, I honestly never thought that I would get breast cancer. So on that day in October, at age 37, I got the call less than 24 hours after my biopsy

> …three of my friends decorated my bedroom with balloons & flowers topped off with a sign on the toilet that read "worship me no longer".

that it was cancer, but "good news", it was DCIS (non-invasive breast cancer). From there started a journey of surprises. First my sister and I immediately decided to get genetic testing. While waiting for the results my mother was diagnosed with DCIS Breast Cancer on October 24th. Needless to say it was a very eventful Breast Cancer Awareness Month. In November, my sister and I both got our positive results for BRCA II breast cancer gene. That prompted my decision to have a bilateral mastectomy.

My surgery which included a sentinel node biopsy on both sides just for precaution, was long and ended up being another eventful part of my journey. I went in to surgery knowing that after that I would be done and would not need to do any follow up treatment. Little did I know that there was a 1.3 cm tumor and a positive lymph node hiding. So I came out of surgery needing 8 rounds of chemo. Remarkably, I was not angry or disappointed but relieved

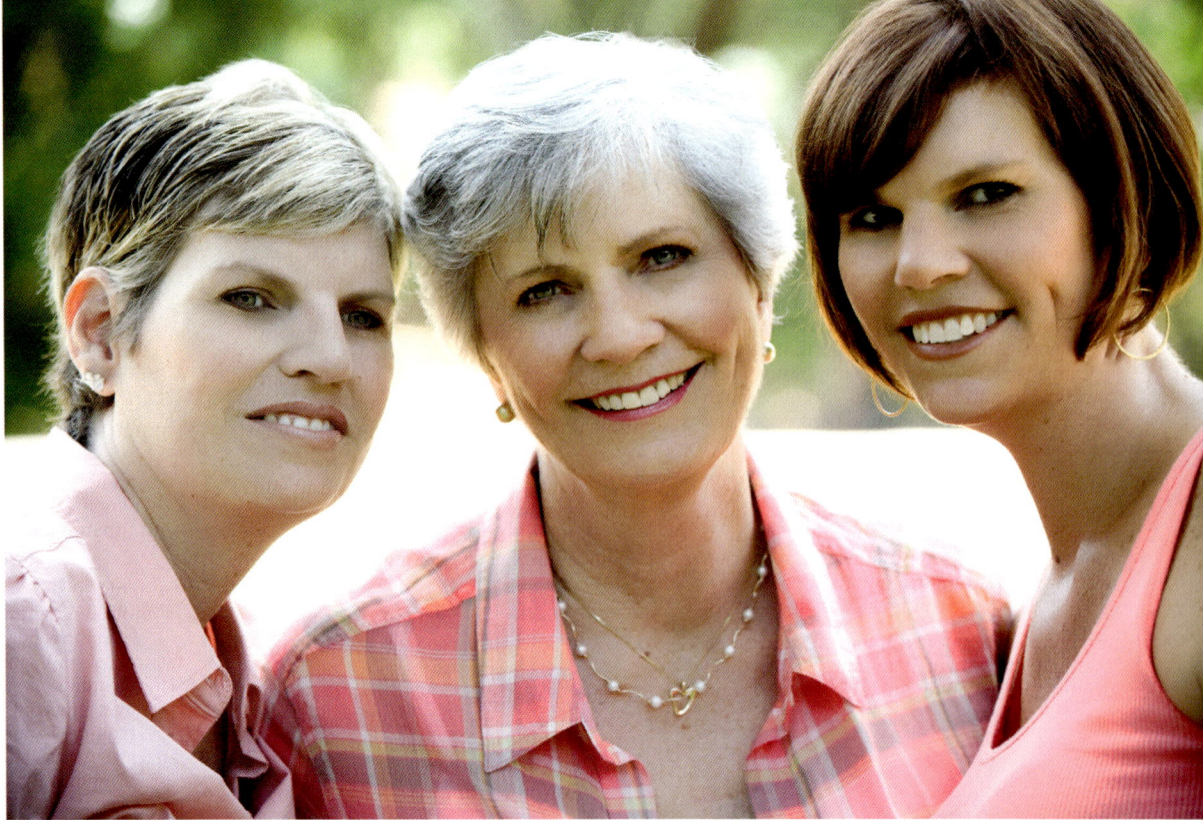

because had I not made the decision to have a bilateral mastectomy they may not have found the tumor. The following months brought dose dense chemo and well, chemo is chemo, but I got through it with the help of my family and many phenomenal friends. In fact the day I got home from my last chemo three of my friends decorated my bedroom with balloons & flowers topped off with a sign on the toilet that read "worship me no longer".

Our surprises were not over yet though. My mother was scheduled to have a lumpectomy and because her cancer was non-invasive, she just had follow up radiation. She had another biopsy on another "hot spot" that came up on an MRI. Fortunately it came back negative for breast cancer but don't get relieved just yet. Dr. Comstock, the UCSD radiologist, did not like the look of the spot and even though it was negative, he was adamant that Dr. Wallace, our now family breast surgeon, take it out.

> *Fortunately it came back negative for breast cancer but don't get relieved just yet.*

Well, Thank God for Dr. Comstock. The spot ended up being invasive breast cancer and had it been left alone would probably have resulted in my mother doing chemo a year later. Since it was caught so early it had not spread and she did not have to do chemo.

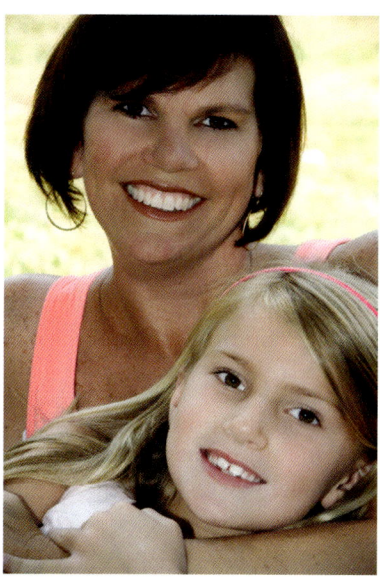

My sister celebrates her 11-year survivor mark in June of this year. My mom and I are coming upon 4 years as survivors. Since I finished my treatment in May of 2008 I have become involved with the San Diego affiliate of Susan G. Komen for the Cure because I feel that by sharing my story and experience I can help women, young & old, through this journey. I also feel I need to do everything I can so that my 7 year old daughter never has to experience this life altering disease. Friends and family carried me through this last year & I can never thank them enough.

BREAST CANCER PREVENTION
By Mayo Clinic staff

If you're concerned about breast cancer, you may be wondering if there are steps you can take toward breast cancer prevention. Understand the lifestyle factors that may affect your risk of breast cancer and what you can do to stay healthy.

What can I do to reduce my risk of breast cancer?

Breast cancer prevention begins with various factors you can control. For example:

Limit alcohol. The more alcohol you drink, the greater your risk of developing breast cancer. If you choose to drink alcohol—including beer, wine or liquor—limit yourself to no more than one drink a day.

Control your weight. Being overweight or obese increases the risk of breast cancer. This is especially true if obesity occurs later in life, particularly after menopause.

Get plenty of physical activity. Being physically active can help you maintain a healthy weight, which, in turn, helps prevent breast cancer. For most healthy adults, the Department of Health and Human Services recommends at least 150 minutes a week of moderate aerobic activity (think brisk walking or swimming) or 75 minutes of vigorous aerobic activity (such as running), in addition to strength training exercises at least twice a week. If you're just starting a physical activity program, start slowly and build intensity gradually.

Breast-feed. Breast-feeding may also play a role in breast cancer prevention. The longer you breast-feed, the greater the protective effect.

Discontinue hormone therapy. Long-term combination hormone therapy increases the risk of breast cancer. If you're taking hormone therapy for menopausal symptoms, ask your doctor about other options. You may be able to manage your symptoms with non-hormonal therapies, such as physical activity. If you decide that the benefits of short-term hormone therapy outweigh the risks, consider using the lowest dose that's effective for your symptoms, and plan to use it only temporarily.

Avoid exposure to environmental pollution. While further studies are needed, some research suggests a link between breast cancer and exposure to the polycyclic aromatic hydrocarbons found in vehicle exhaust and air pollution.

Can a healthy diet prevent breast cancer?

Research shows that eating a diet rich in fruits and vegetables doesn't offer direct protection from breast cancer. In addition, a recent study of dietary fat and breast cancer showed only a slight decrease in the risk of invasive breast cancer for women who ate a low-fat diet. However, eating a healthy diet may decrease your risk of other diseases, such as diabetes, cardiovascular disease and stroke. A healthy diet can also help you maintain a healthy weight—a key factor in breast cancer prevention.

Is there a link between birth control pills and breast cancer?

Current evidence suggests that use of oral contraceptives doesn't increase the risk of breast cancer. While older research showed a slight increase in risk, those studies included pills with higher estrogen doses than what's available today. In addition, the older research showed that 10 or more years after stopping oral contraceptives, the risk of breast cancer returned to the same level as that of women who never used oral contraceptives.

What else can I do?

Be vigilant about breast cancer detection. If you notice any changes in your breasts, such as a new lump or skin changes, consult your doctor for an evaluation. Also, ask your doctor when to begin mammograms and other screening procedures to detect breast cancer.

Remember, it's not always possible to prevent breast cancer. By practicing healthy habits, however, you're taking an active role in breast cancer prevention.

Reprinted from the Mayo Clinic website: www.mayoclinic.com/health/breast-cancer-prevention/WO00091

Cynthia

"When I Think Cancer, I Think About Healing"

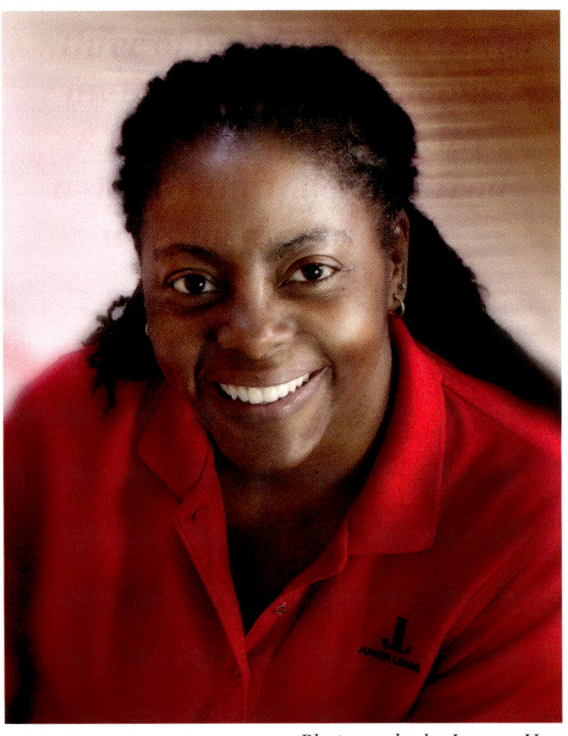
Photography by Joanna Herr

My name is Cynthia Paulo. I am 54 years old and was diagnosed at age 42. I had a burning sensation in my left breast and went in to have it checked. My doctor, Dr. G., sent me to have a mammogram, and followed that up with ultrasonic imaging. The ultra sound only showed "something" in the field of concern. I then had a needle biopsy followed by a lumpectomy in September of 1999.

During the lumpectomy my doctor said he thought I had lipoma but he wanted to get everything to the lab. The 30-minute lumpectomy lasted 90 minutes because he wanted to remove as much questionable tissue as possible. He called me 2 weeks later and explained that I had a non-invasive breast cancer, Ductal Carcinoma in Situ (DCIS). Since he had seen the breast he was comfortable scheduling surgery in late January or early February of 2000. I had surgery in early 2000, which included removal of left breast tissue and several lymph nodes in the left armpit. I did not have radiation, but took oral medications for 5 years. Doctor G ordered my meds and mammograms, and followed me for 4 years until my current doctor took over. I have been cancer free for 11 years!

I was relieved to hear it was non-invasive, but it was still cancer. I did as much research as I could on DCIS, and found that there were two schools of thought: one school said it was cancer, the other said it was not. So what was I to think? Most of the research was in the non-invasive cancer camp, and my doctor agreed. I wasn't terribly worried for myself, but for my family. I had had a number of other surgeries, but this wasn't just another. My daughter, who was 10 at the time, wanted to know everything. So I told her. My twin sister was supportive, as were my husband's parents. I waited a while before I told my parents, who told me about their siblings who also had cancer. They turned out to be not too worried, and supportive. The pastor I knew at the church I attended had a prayer session for me. She phoned me and asked how I was every time she saw me. She is a kind and wonderful person.

> ...found that there were two schools of thought: one...said it was cancer, the other said it was not. So what was I to think?

The medication didn't make all my hair fall out, but I had bare spots on my head where the hair wasn't growing. I talked to my hair dresser about shaving my head. She said I'd look funny because the bare spots would look different from the shaved spots. So she kept me looking good through the drug treatment. My daughter would let me know when my bald spots were showing; we'd move my hair around to cover them up. She also let me know when my bra wasn't properly adjusted, showing the larger right breast not positioned to de-emphasize the smaller left breast. She was a great help, and she is still my fashion police to this day! I am proud of my daughter for standing up for me, being my friend, and helping me through every day.

I received a lot of support from friends who knew. My husband drove me to and from surgeries, and did all the cooking and cleaning when I couldn't. He is a breast cancer research advocate, and I am proud of the support he gave me, and still does.

In 2007, I attended a retreat for breast cancer survivors put on by Chrysalis to Wings and learned a lot about my feelings and how others felt about cancer. This retreat, A Way of Life After Breast Cancer, AWOL for short, was good for me in so many ways. This retreat inspired me to be the breast cancer research and prevention advocate I am today. I donate to breast cancer organizations and other cancer organizations. I have walked many miles for breast cancer. I have golfed for breast cancer. I have even spoken about breast cancer advocacy to groups. When a friend or acquaintance tells me they've been diagnosed with cancer, I tell them how I felt and what I went through, and I offer them my ear whenever they want to talk about it. Prior to the retreat, I was a closet breast cancer survivor. Now I'm open and honest about what my being a breast cancer survivor is all about. If I could talk to new patients I would tell them to not be afraid of talking about their cancer with family and friends. I would also tell them to do their homework! Learn what you can, and ask questions of your doctors and health care providers. They don't know what you're thinking, so talk to them and let them know what's on your mind.

> *I have walked many miles for breast cancer. I have golfed for breast cancer. I have even spoken about breast cancer advocacy to groups.*

LIPOMA
A lipoma is a benign tumor composed of adipose tissue. It is the most common form of soft tissue tumor. Lipomas are soft to the touch, usually movable, and are generally painless. Many lipomas are small (under one centimeter diameter) but can enlarge to sizes greater than six centimeters. Lipomas are commonly found in adults from 40 to 60 years of age, but can also be found in children. Some sources claim that malignant transformation can occur, while others say that this has yet to be convincingly documented.

I currently work for the State of California, Environmental Protection Agency, as a Senior Industrial Hygienist, but I will be retiring in mid-2012. I love to golf and read, and will be doing a lot of both when I retire. First I will have to perform some reorganization of the garage and a few rooms in the house, but look out golf courses—here I come! I also volunteer for a few local nonprofit organizations. I will be able to do more of that once I retire. I also plan on taking a bigger role in caring for my mother. My father died in May 2011, and my mother lives alone. She will be 82 in 2011 and has had her own health issues. My twin sister has spent a lot of time with mom, and now my older sister is living with her. I hope to play a bigger role in her life because I love her so very much. She has been very strong, and I admire her strength.

I will admit that I'm a little self-conscious of the scar on my left breast. If I wear a scoop-neck or v-neck top, or a swim suit, you can see the scar. I had a friend tell me, "You're a breast cancer survivor. Who cares if you have a scar?" My daughter has told me the same thing! So you know what? I don't shy away from a cute blouse or ball gown that doesn't hide the scar. If someone asks I just tell them how I earned it. I'm a breast cancer survivor.

As a Christian, when I think about cancer, I think about healing. The bible is full of verses about healing. One of my favorites is in Psalm 30:2, which reads, *"LORD my God, I called to you for help, and you healed me."*

If you have cancer, cry about it, pray about it, and talk about it. Otherwise no one will benefit from your experience and your knowledge.

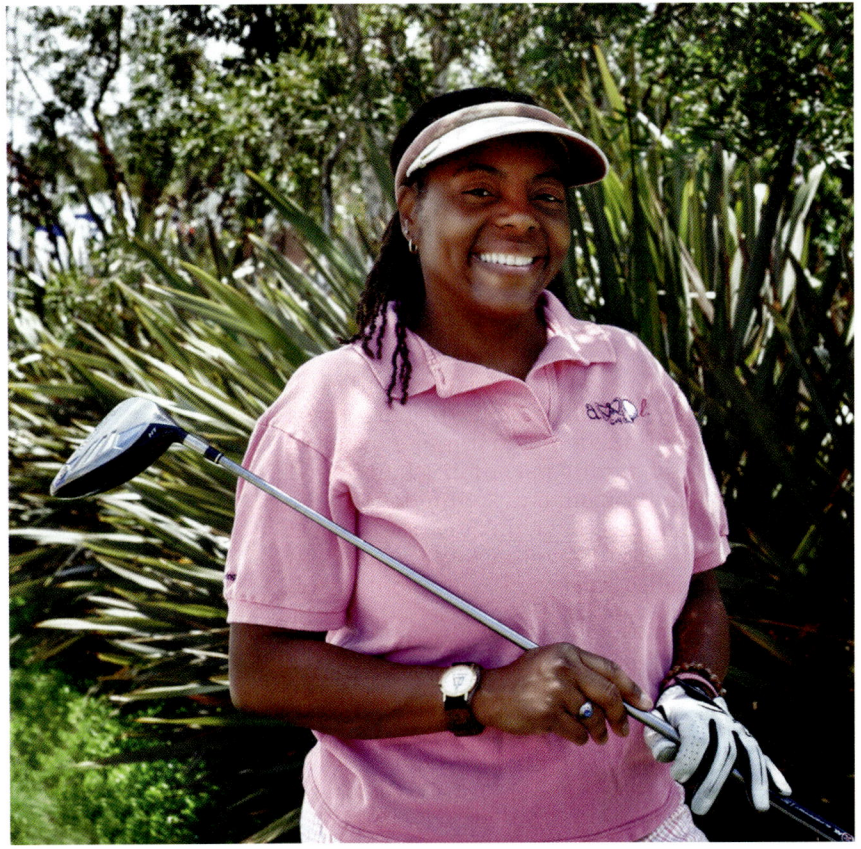

Photography by Joanna Herr

Laura

"My Severe Mercy"

Laura Farmer Sherman, 50. Diagnosed in 2003 at 42. Stage 3A.

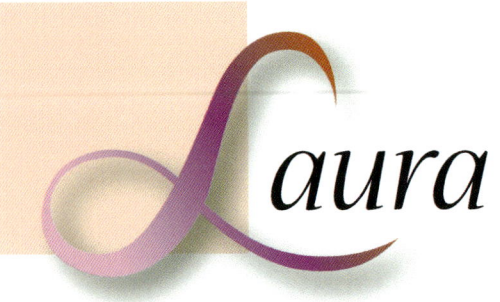

I honestly couldn't believe the diagnosis. I hadn't been sick a day in my life. And I struggled against the reality of what I considered a death sentence. I didn't know much about cancer—I honestly thought you had to have it in your family to get it. Not true. I found that out quickly along with a hundred other facts that made me a "likely candidate" to get breast cancer: My period started early in my life. I didn't have children. I led a very stressful life.

I was diagnosed on a Wednesday. On that Friday I was having a mastectomy. When I woke up, I learned that 15 lymph nodes were "taken" and that four had evidence of cancer. My path was now clear. Heal from the surgery. Start very aggressive chemotherapy followed by radiation.

I found as the days turned into weeks, I was having trouble "getting up" the will to fight. A grief counselor changed all that when she had me write my obituary as the person I was, and then a second obituary for the person I wanted to be. The "other person" became my reason for living. I wanted to live so that I could be a better friend, a better sister, a better Aunt, a more compassionate person. Notice I didn't say "a better worker." The old adage is true. No one on their death beds ever wishes they had spent more time at work. Why did it take a cancer diagnosis to wake me up to that reality? I'm not sure, but I'm grateful every day for the wake up call.

> *...she had me write my obituary as the person I was, and then a second obituary for the person I wanted to be. The "other person" became my reason for living.*

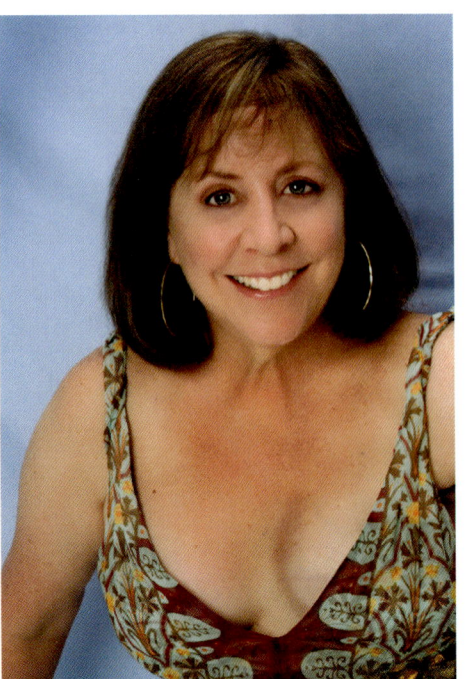

My friends and family—when they heard the news—were shocked and all reacted in different ways. The people I thought "would be there" weren't. Some of the people who "were there" were surprising to me. I learned that not all of us know what to say or do when faced with such a serious blow. Some people actually avoided me because they didn't know what to say. Total strangers came up to me to tell me their stories, and to encourage me.

One of the sweetest things that happened was that my dear friend's little girl—when she knew that I would lose my hair—shaved all of her Barbie's heads so that I "wouldn't feel alone." And I'll never forget her saying: Mommy says that Barbie's hair won't grow back—but yours will.

Breast cancer was the best thing that ever happened to me. For every "bad" thing that happens in our lives—look for the "yes." Every thing that happens has a gift. The trick is to be open to finding it. Breast Cancer allowed me to change my life completely. I quit my job. I found out what I really wanted to do. And now I'm doing it. When you face death—you can face anything. Nothing frightens me anymore. No one can ever hold me back. Cancer taught me that. And I am grateful.

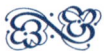

…my dear friend's little girl— when she knew that I would lose my hair — shaved all of her Barbie's heads so that I "wouldn't feel alone."

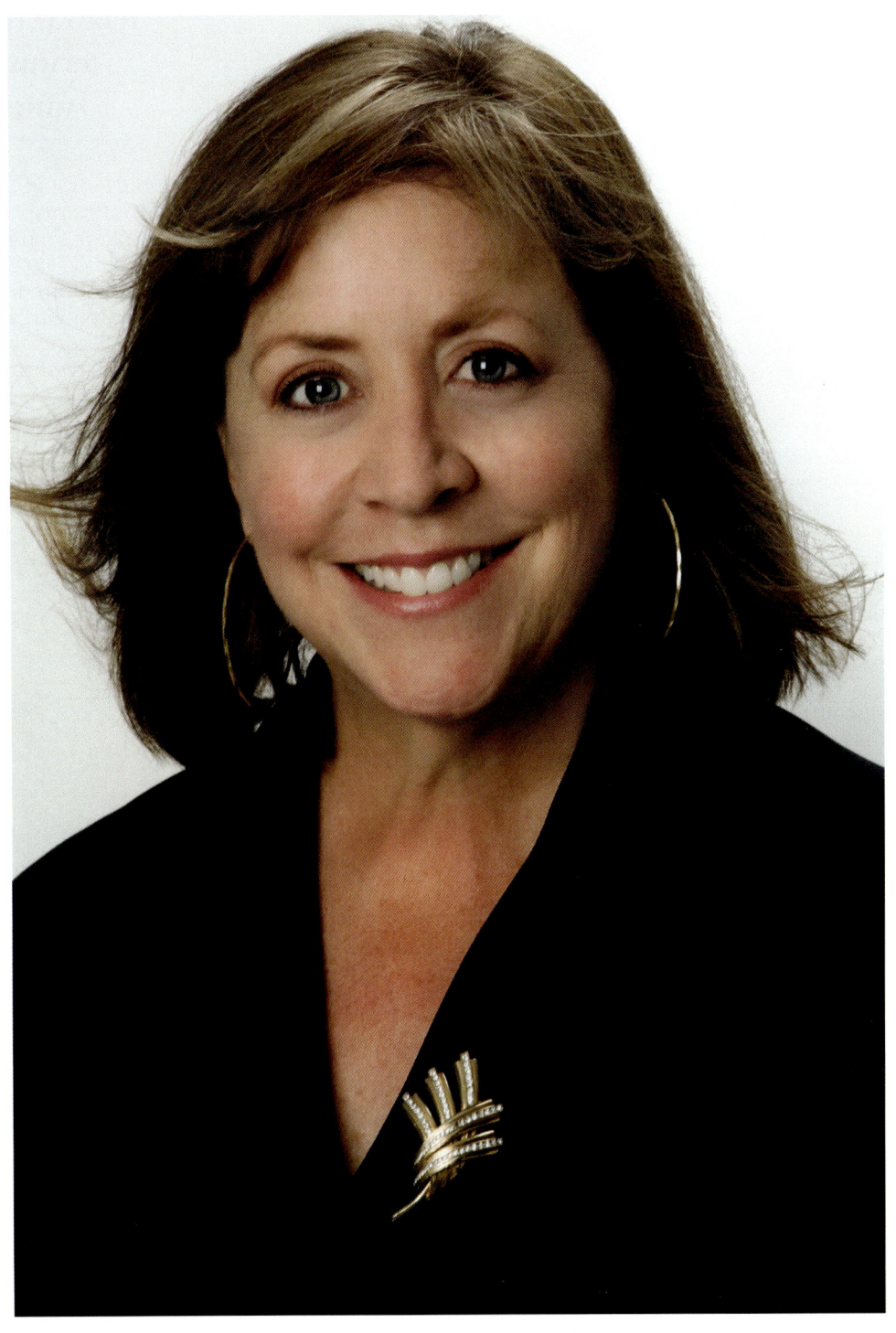

Dikla

"Nine years and Counting Many More..."
living, surviving, growing, thriving and loving.

My name is Dikla Benzeevi, currently 41 years old. I was diagnosed with breast cancer at age 32 in Los Angeles, California in August 2002.

8/2002 Diagnosis: Stage 3 infiltrating/invasive ductal carcinoma; Her2/neu positive, Estrogen Receptor (ER) positive, Progesterone Receptor (PR) positive, TOPO2 positive, BRCA1 negative, BRCA2 negative
— **Treatments:** *Lumpectomy + Lymph Node Dissection, chemotherapy (Carboplatin + Taxotere), Herceptin, Zoladex, Whole Breast Radiation, Tamoxifen*

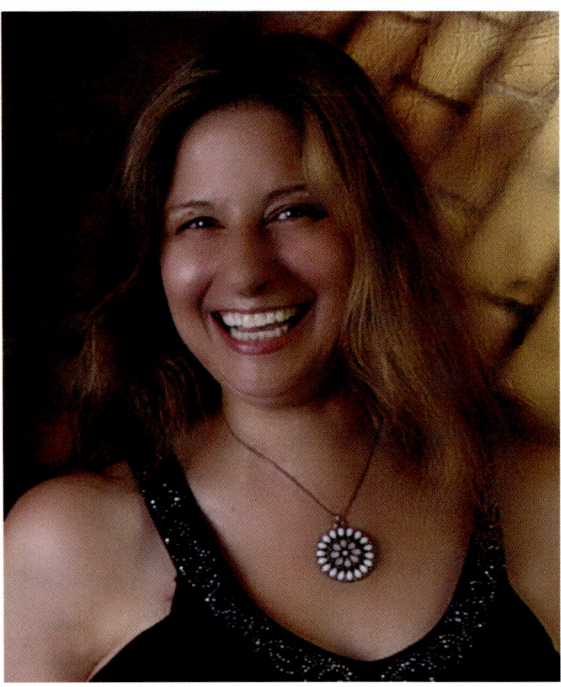

Photography by Joanna Herr

I was in shock. I received the diagnosis on 8/19/2002 in the radiologist's office at the Breast Center in Van Nuys, CA. This was after 2 weeks of firsts: first mammogram, first breast ultrasound, and 4 stereotactic biopsies. All this in response to my gynecologist feeling a lump during a routine annual breast exam, thinking it was just a cyst and sending me to get it investigated.

> *I was frustrated and upset that I was missing so much work to get all these procedures done and wanted to get them over with. I was completely clueless.*

I did not suspect at all that I may have something serious going on. I was frustrated and upset that I was missing so much work to get all these procedures done and wanted to get them over with. I was completely clueless. After I complained to my brother who is an ER doctor and lives with his family 3 hours away about all this disruption to my work, he calmly said he wanted to come with me to the final doctor appointment to discuss the biopsy results. I told him he can come but that it wasn't necessary since it is such a far drive for him. Even with his desire to come with me, I still did not understand the severity of my situation. I was clueless as ever. I didn't even understand that if the doctor wants to discuss the results with you in his office it means something serious, otherwise the office would just tell me over the phone that everything was fine. I only thought that this doctor visit was another inconvenience to me.

I am so happy my brother came with me to the doctor appointment. His wife waited for us at my apartment. I was in complete shock when the doctor told me I had cancer. Everything stopped for me. The sound died. The air stopped. I was in shock. I didn't know what to do with this information. It was a complete surprise. All I could say to the doctor was "c'est la vie" (such is life).

12/2004 Diagnosis: Stage 4 (aka Advanced aka Metastatic) breast cancer, metastasis to the bone: T7 vertebra in my spine
— **Treatments:** *Zometa, Faslodex, Zoladex, Herceptin, spine fusion surgery, spine radiation*

I felt the same way with my second diagnosis of advanced breast cancer that spread to my spine. Only this time I felt fear and pain, as well as shock. The cancer had eaten up my vertebrae, had caused it to collapse and posed a great risk to my spinal cord. This cancer which was causing great pain in my back could paralyze me. It hurt to walk. The pain felt like I had a 2x4 wooden board in my back under my skin juggling around every time I walked or moved. A sneeze or cough felt like an explosion in my chest. It was excruciating. I was panicked and

> *Over the past 9 years I've had to deal with new diagnoses, and each time it feels like the first time I was getting diagnosed.*

petrified that at any time and with any movement my spine could break and I would be paralyzed. I was immediately placed in a back brace and had to have spine fusion surgery to correct that risk. I was in a back brace for 6 months and physical therapy for 6 months before I fully recovered. What an ordeal! I never want to repeat it.

7/2007 Diagnosis: Stage 4 (aka Advanced aka Metastatic) breast cancer, metastasis to both my lungs
— **Treatments:** *Zometa, Faslodex, Zoladex, Herceptin, Tykerb, Chemotherapy (Navelbine), lung biopsy surgery (removed 10% of my left lung)*

My lung metastases diagnosis in 2007 also scared me, but at least I didn't run the risk of being paralyzed from it. I didn't know if lung metastases meant that it was the end of the line for me or not. I had a lung biopsy in 2008 that removed a few tumors and 10% of my left lung. This procedure left me anemic and suffering from constant migraines for 6 months until my red blood cell count increased to normal levels on their own.

Over the past 9 years I've had to deal with new diagnoses, and each time it feels like the first time I was getting diagnosed. Fear, uncertainty, having to educate myself quickly regarding each new type of diagnosis and what it means and learning to cope with the uncertainty and waiting period to see if each new treatment protocol I try is working and wondering if I should plan for the far future or not.

The Toughest Times.

The hardest part over these 9 years has been learning to cope with uncertainty and regaining a sense of normality and routine with each new treatment and its side-effects.

One of my brothers cried when I told him. My other 2 brothers kept a brave face on. One brother was working overseas at the time and he moved back to Los Angeles immediately and lived with me for nearly a year to help me out. My three brothers and sister-in-law were amazing. They put on a brave face and helped me move along with my scan appointments and doctor visits to find the best care for me. I know the diagnosis was hard on them. We had lost both our parents to cancer and our mom to breast cancer, and that pain still felt fresh. I know my family was scared and worried for me, and they kept a strong and optimistic face for me. I appreciate their help and support more than they will ever know.

I am from Israel and my family from Israel is very supportive. They also put on a brave face when I spoke to them on the phone and they talked to oncologists in Israel to assist me in confirming and finding the best therapies for me.

I had two most difficult times. My first one was dealing with my initial chemo treatment and working through treatment. The chemo made a mess of my stomach and I had awful GI issues. When I needed to go to the bathroom, the need was sudden and urgent, and finding a nearby bathroom at all times, and trying to avoid an accident in my pants was extremely stressful and embarrassing. Due to my chemo, I also lost my hair, gained 30 pounds and developed acne. I felt like I was going through a 2nd puberty. My body was changing without my consent and I didn't like it. The chemo and the steroids I

Photography by Joanna Herr

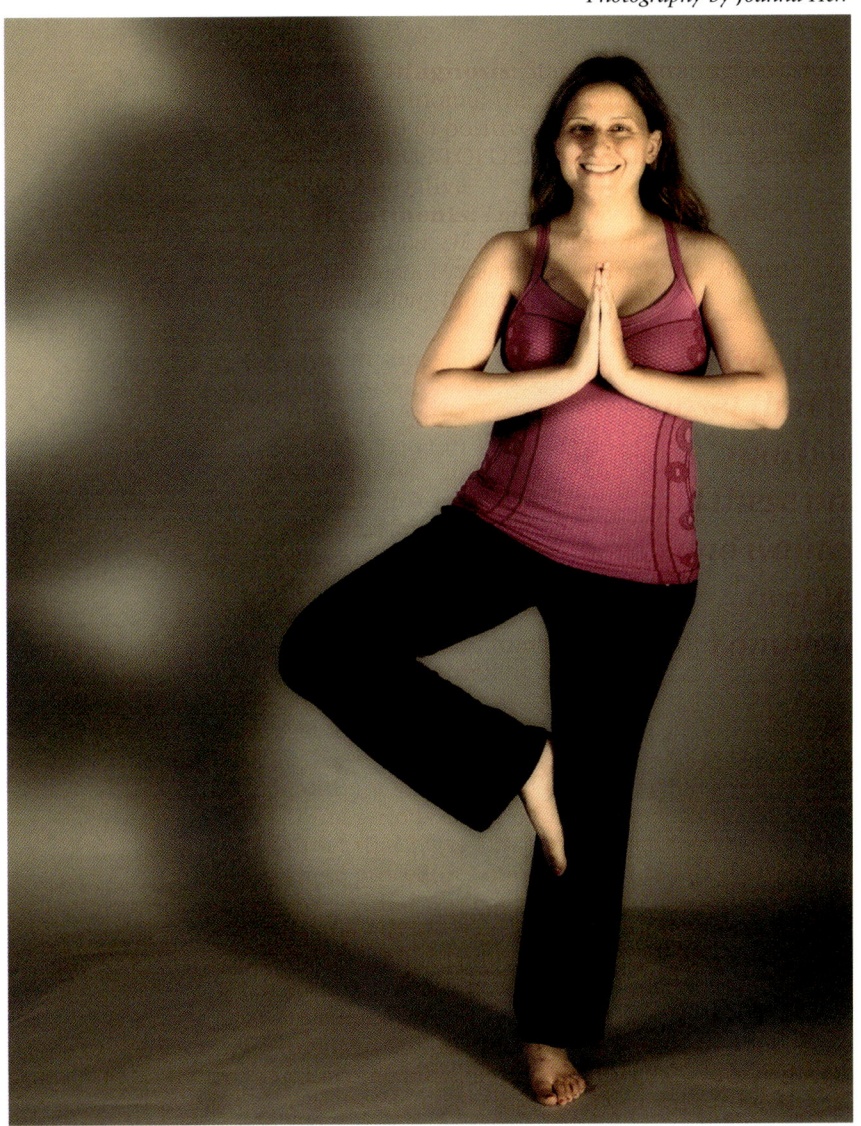

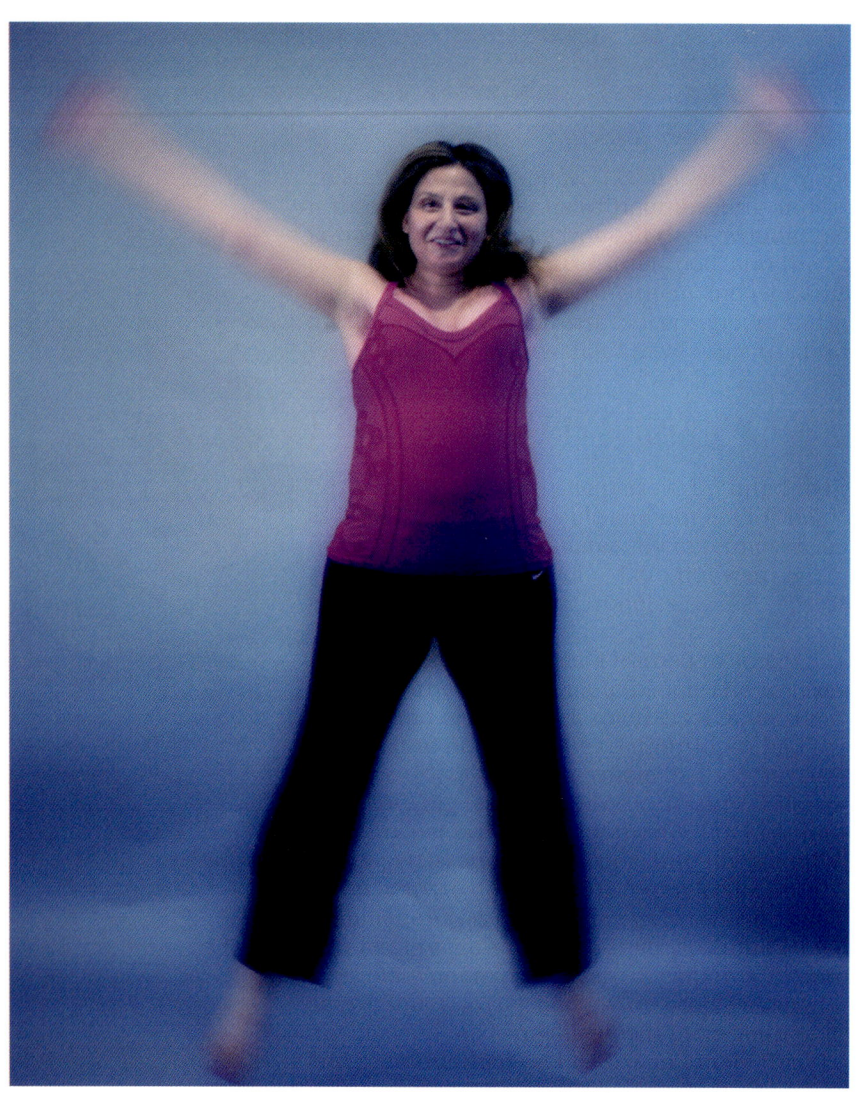

Photography by Joanna Herr

took to counteract the side-effects of the chemo also made me very moody and upset. All this together made for a very difficult 9 months. I worked 30 hours a week and this combined with my treatment and surgeries wore me out completely. I was thoroughly exhausted. I didn't want to admit it, but it was apparent to all who saw me.

My most difficult time after that was after my spine metastases diagnosis. I was petrified I would end up paralyzed because of the stupid cancer in my vertebra. In addition I had to wear a god-awful waist to chin back brace that I hated. At the time, I was a private person and did not want to advertise my cancer to the whole world. I dreaded hearing the words, "what happened to you" from people I met with my back brace on. I wanted to make up more interesting stories like "I had a hang gliding accident" or "it's from mountain climbing" or "skydiving accident" instead of trying to explain that my breast cancer spread to my spine and fractured my vertebra.

In addition, during this phase, I was not allowed to drive, bend over or lift anything above a gallon of water. Even that wasn't advised for me to do. I needed rides to all appointments, to all outdoor chores. I needed help with shopping, with placing items in bags, with loading and unloading items from the car and in my house. I needed help doing laundry since I wasn't allowed to bend over to put clothes in or out of the washer and dryer, or to carry laundry to the machines. I even had instructions from my doctor on how to get in and out of the shower carefully. I needed help trying on pants in a store since I wasn't allowed to bend over to put them on.

It was very tough. I was used to being a very independent woman, doing most everything myself. I was very proud of that. Now I had to ask for help with almost everything. During my first diagnosis and chemo, I was much more independent and still went to work. My brothers helped me, but I could still mostly take care of myself.

This time I couldn't work anymore. I was embarrassed to ask for help. I didn't want to burden already busy people with my needs. I felt like I had to eat humble pie and admit I was human, and needed help. I didn't feel like superwoman anymore. I don't know if I ever was one, but I had this image in my mind and tried to portray it.

My Best Supporters.

My family was of great support and helped me overcome the most difficult times. My three brothers and my sister in law were always there for me, supporting me in any way I needed— emotionally, intellectually, financially, and practically. They motivated me and encouraged me during very difficult and emotional times. My niece and nephew were very young at the time I was diagnosed. They're adorable and lovely and great and I love them very much. Wanting to see them grow up, finish school, and create their own independent lives inspired me to continue through these arduous times.

In addition, the wonderful women and counselors and staff at the 2 support groups, and cancer support centers I attended were and are a great support system. They listen, encourage, offer practical advice and inspire without judgment. They offered me rides to appointments, helped me with laundry and shopping, kept me company and made me laugh – all with the

> *I dreaded hearing the words, "what happened to you" from people I met with my back brace on. I wanted to make up more interesting stories…*

greatest love and support. I could not have made it through these 9 years without meeting and knowing and learning from all these wonderful peers in this breast cancer sisterhood, and the admirable people supporting them and working for the multitude of breast cancer support and research organizations that I have come to know.

How Cancer Has Changed Me.

I used to be a very private person. I wanted to be as independent as possible and not ask for help from anyone. I never shared my innermost fears and concerns with anyone. I did not want to burden anyone with my troubles.

During these past 9 years, I learned to accept help. I learned to open up to people and to take a chance and reveal myself to others. I understand now that to nourish close relationships I had to take the risk of being my whole true self, reveal and share my fears, my insecurities, my childishness, my pet peeves, all my thorns, not just the pretty petals, and allow people into my life fully. It was scary to do and the fear of rejection and humiliation was great. There were some people that left my life and that was very painful. However, many more open hearted, empowering, proactive, smart, loving and giving people entered my life, and made my life much more abundant and beautiful than ever before and more than I ever expected. I do not feel alone now.

My Advice to New Patients.

You are not alone. You have a wealth of support and resources out there to help make the journey as smooth and easy as possible. Please reach out and share and ask.

> **Many women before you and many going through breast cancer with you… have found and are finding loving and fulfilling relationships.**

Reach out to the people closest to you, who make you feel good and support you in a positive way. They want to help but probably don't know how. Be specific with them what your needs and desires are and you will be amazed how eager they will be to help.

If you feel there is no one in your life you can reach out to or trust, then reach out to your cancer support centers or national cancer support hotlines and talk to others who are going through similar situations. You will find a large family of supportive and encouraging and helpful breast cancer peers and professionals out there who want to help you, and want to help you find the resources you need.

Learn to accept help. You are also making others feel good if you accept their help – and especially if it is the type of help you truly need, and that you expressed to them specifically that you need.

Reach out to your breast cancer peers. They have a lot of useful information to share and reveal. You can do this by either calling a breast cancer center hotline or physically going to a support group at a cancer center in your area. If one support group doesn't fit your needs, try another. The right one will make you feel supported, encouraged, empowered and relieved.

It takes a community of loving, helpful, encouraging, empowering, resourceful and supportive people, in different fields and parts of life, to make the journey through breast cancer smoother and easier.

The help you need is out there. Even if you are not aware of it now, it is out there. Even if you think what you need is too far-fetched or does not exist, trust me it probably does exist. Ask around, ask your medical professionals, seek out cancer support centers, call the cancer toll-free numbers, request to talk to a social worker or have someone you trust do the checking for you. The services and support you seek is out there. Trust me, it is out there. You just have to seek it out.

**You are not "defective".
You are whole and lovely and good.**

There is dating and having loving relationships with new people during, through and after

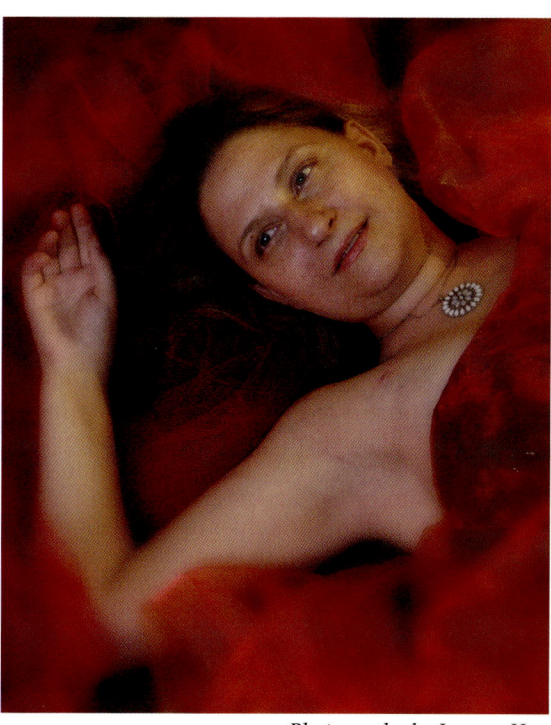

Photography by Joanna Herr

breast cancer, even with advanced stage 4 breast cancer, even if you lose your interest in sex or sex is painful or you believe you are unattractive because of multiple surgeries. Many women before you and many going through breast cancer with you, even with any physical and emotional hurdles, have found and are finding loving and fulfilling relationships. It exists, it can happen. Many good people are out there.

I am proudest of the informal email breast cancer Support network I created. I am proud of being a trained Peer match counselor. I am proud of being a Patient Navigator. I really enjoy helping others—it is extremely fulfilling. I am proud of all the wonderful people I've met through this journey that I would not have met otherwise. I am proud of my family and boyfriend for their constant support and love

My Inspiration.

The many amazing women that have gone through breast cancer before me and who have trail-blazed the way and continue to do so for better resources and services for breast cancer patients.

I am also inspired by the desire that no person go through breast cancer alone or without all the resources available to them. I want to make sure every patient feels provided for, cared for and guided through this difficult experience; with compassion, empathy, support, respect and expertise.

What do I do now? I used to work in the entertainment industry. Now I am a passionate breast cancer patient advocate / navigator. I love helping others diagnosed with breast cancer, and their loved ones and friends, navigate smoothly and as painlessly as possible through the breast cancer journey. I am a peer match counselor with multiple organizations. I founded and run a national informal email breast cancer support network. I was a charter member of the Komen Young Women National Advisory Council and am currently a board member of the Noreen Fraser Foundation.

For fun, I like to hang out with my family and my boyfriend and my friends, go on walks and easy hikes. I like to be pampered at spas and retreats. I like it when everyone around me is having a good time.

Take the Risk—Be Yourself!

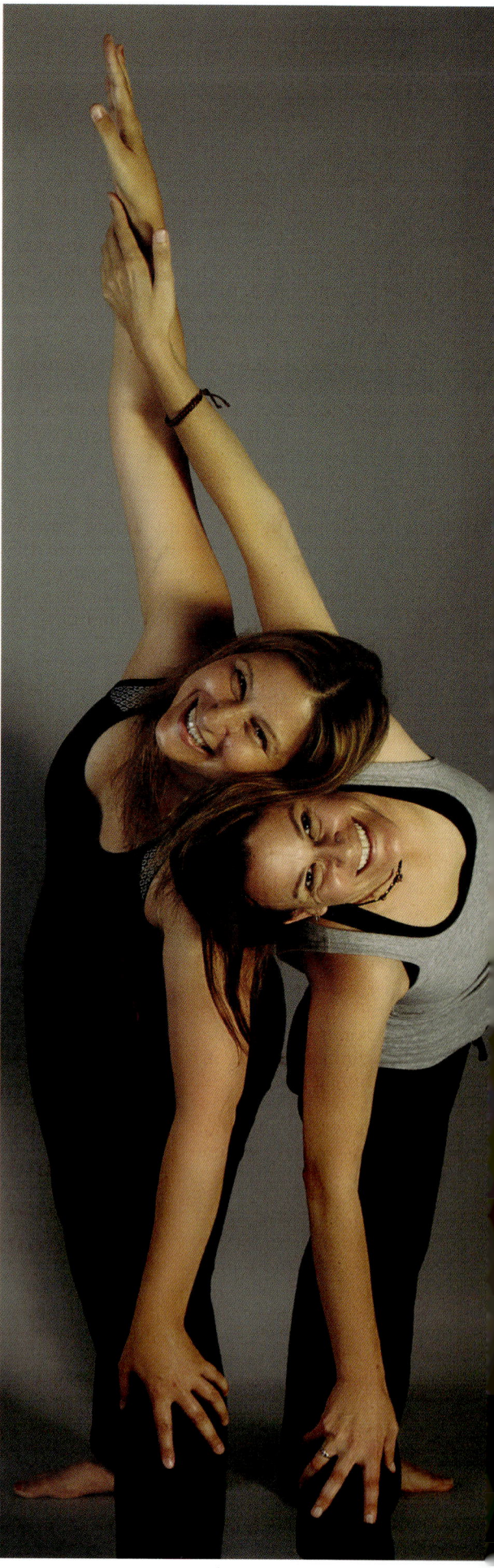

Dikla and Julie
Photography by Joanna Herr

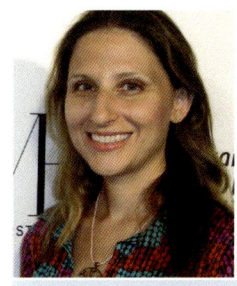

Humorous Tales…
by Dikla Benzeevi

"Through humor, you can soften some of the worst blows that life delivers. And once you find laughter, no matter how painful your situation might be, you can survive it."
~ Bill Cosby

THE DYE JOB ~

When I was first diagnosed with breast cancer and started chemotherapy prior to surgery, I did not tell many people at work. In fact, I only told my boss and 2 co-workers. I did not tell any of my other colleagues—dozens of them. Prior to losing my hair from chemo, I cut my very long hair short. It was still my natural hair, thank god. I became the new show & tell item at work and everyone would come by and stare at me from the entrance to my office. Some would ask questions which was fine, but others would just stand and stare. I thought it was so rude and it made me very uncomfortable. I thought to myself, how much worse I would feel with all this attention if I went directly from my naturally long hair to a short hair wig. At least the short haircut was my own hair. After several days of feeling like the main attraction at the zoo, I finally told the spectators to leave unless they had a work issue to discuss. So much for that.

Several weeks later my real hair fell out and I shaved my head and wore a short hair wig. The color and style were a little different than my real hair but the length was about the same.

The first day I wore my wig to work I was afraid of the same reaction from my colleagues. I was relieved when most everyone didn't care. The showcase to them was the major haircut not the change in color or style. Thank god I cut my own hair short first and didn't transition directly to a wig from long hair.

The funny incident was with one colleague who was trying to be friendly, but didn't know that her friendliness was making me uncomfortable. She didn't know I had a wig on. She just thought I got my hair colored and styled. She started asking me all kinds of questions regarding my hair—where did I get my hair colored, what brand of color I used, what number / name of color I used, and so on and so forth. I was flabbergasted. I was not prepared to answer those kind of questions. I almost wanted to pull of my wig and give it to her and say, "why don't you look it up?" God bless her, she didn't know I had a wig on. I somehow deflected her questions and said I was busy, if we could talk another time.

Later on she came by and said, "Just wait till your hair grows in, you'll have to go in and color your roots every 6-10 weeks". I thought to myself with a smile, "Yeah, I'll wait till my hair grows in—in about 6 months!"

She also asked how often I washed my hair since I had a dye job. I sort of flubbed the answer, but thought to myself "oh, about once a week in the sink, it's so easy. I just leave my hair in the sink and go". That made me smile. AT least I knew I had a great wig on—so great that no one even suspected I had a wig on. Everyone thought I got a dye job.

She eventually stopped asking questions about my supposed "dye" job and I eventually told everyone at work that I was going through chemotherapy and cancer treatment. Everyone was surprised! And everyone was very supportive!

SOMETHING'S MISSING ~

My normal routine included shower, dress up, makeup and out the door. Now I had to include wig time. However, some days I'd be rushing and I'd forget to put on my wig. I'd run out the door in my apartment complex to the elevator. Something would feel amiss and I couldn't figure it out. I finally realized as I waited for the elevator that I felt a breeze on my bald head and I had forgotten to put on my wig. So I'd run back to my apartment to put it on.

BLOWING IN THE WIND ~

I bought a convertible Lexus during this time and would drive it with the top down. Well, once I drove it with the top down and forgot that I had a wig on. I realized I had a wig on in the first quarter mile as I felt the wind tugging my wig off. So I ended up driving with one hand on the wheel and one hand on top of my head holding my wig down. I must have made an interesting sight to other motorists.

I WIN ~

I took an acting class at my cancer support center in my neighborhood. I was the only person in active treatment and bald in the class. I would attend wearing a cap. One exercise we had to do was to sit opposite another person and stare at each other. Each person took a turn trying to make the other one laugh or lose his composure during the staring session. I was pretty good at keeping a straight face. However, when it was my turn to make the other person react, all I needed to do was pull of my cap and surprise them with my bald head. End of story.

HOLDING HANDS ~

Because of my spine mets, I had to have spine fusion surgery. Big surgery—very scary. I even had a chest tube in me that drained all the excess fluid from my lung cavity into this huge container by my bed. Pretty disgusting, not to mention painful. So, on about Day 2 in the hospital, the thoracic surgeon comes by to remove the chest tube. I am very nervous, of course. The surgeon brings a resident or intern with him to watch the removal. The surgeon is on my left where the tube is and the resident is on my right watching. I am very nervous so I ask the resident if I can hold his hand while the surgeon removes the tube—basically by jerking it out really quickly and stitching up the little hole left over. The resident looks at me stunned. "She talks, and she is talking to me" "and she wants to hold my hand". The resident looked petrified and at a loss. He really wasn't prepared to interact with a patient. He only wanted to watch and basically ignore me. Poor guy. I didn't give up though. I was scared and wanted something to hold onto. So finally, the resident, with a panicked look on his face, gives me his pinky finger to hold. I laughed, but hey, I'll take what I can get and I grasped his pinky finger while the surgeon pulled out my chest tube. Thankfully it was quick. Painful, yes, but at least quick. However, for the state of the resident's pinky finger, I'm not sure of at all.

TOO SEXY ~

When I had to wear a back brace for 5 months, the brace was very uncomfortable and embarrassing for me. I did not like advertising my illness to all, and that is how I felt with the back brace on. However, I made the best of it and a friend of mine, Bonnie Grasse, was a huge help to me. She was a great buddy and we got along great. We made each other laugh and she helped me out tremendously with rides and assistance during this time with the brace. She even made me a jean jacket with the words "TOO SEXY FOR MY BRACE" embroidered on the back. I loved it. She also made me a T-shirt with a bulls-eye symbol in the middle, right where the opening in the front of my back brace was.

KEEP YOUR PANTS ON ~

Bonne Grasse was an amazing friend and help to me during my days in my back brace. My doctor's orders were very strict—I was not allowed to bend my back or carry anything over 5 pounds. At one point I needed to buy new clothes, and Bonnie went shopping with me. We would pick out pants and shirts to try out and then maneuver to the handicapped stall in the dressing room. We'd both get in there, and then the fun would start. Since I wasn't allowed to bend over, Bonnie had to help me off and on with any pants I tried on. The whole maneuver was hilarious. I'd stand spread-eagled against the wall of the stall, and Bonnie would help me off with my pants and on with any I had to try on. I felt like one of the Keystone Cops or in an episode of "I Love Lucy." I don't know what the people outside the dressing room thought about hearing two women giggling their heads of in the dressing room, discussing how best to take pants off and on for someone else.

*"If I have the belief that I can do it,
I shall surely acquire the capacity to do it
even if I may not have it at the beginning."*

~ Mahatma Gandhi

Cancer sucks…
Breast cancer sucks…
Advanced breast cancer
really sucks…
Metastatic stage four breast cancer
really really sucks…

Dealing with advanced
breast cancer for nine years:

UNBEARABLE.

Doing it alone:

IMPOSSIBLE.

Having the support, love, acceptance,
encouragement, assistance, empathy, and
compassion from family, friends, community:

PRICELESS.

My expectations for the future:

LIMITLESS.

Dikla

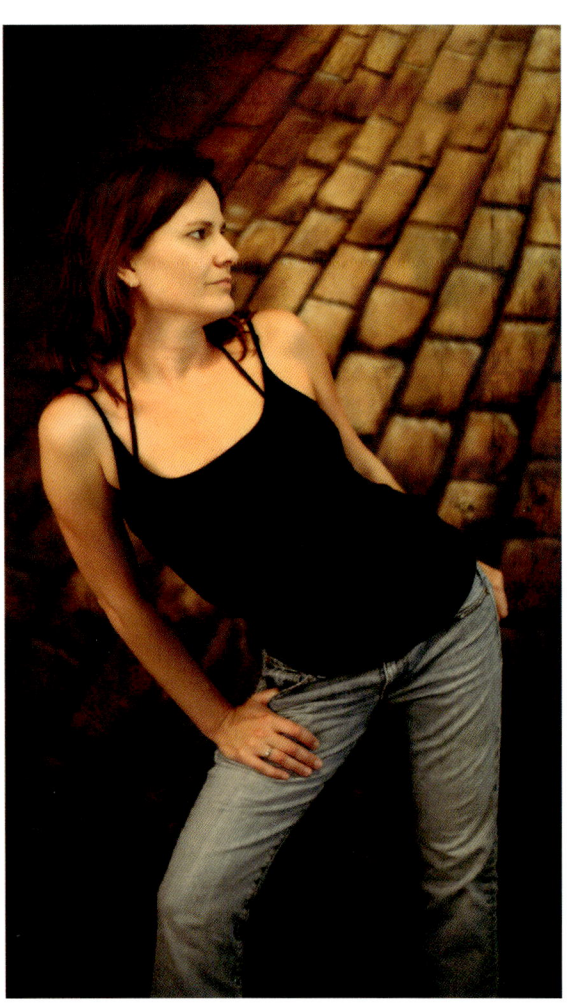

*Photography by Joanna Herr
Julie and Dikla*

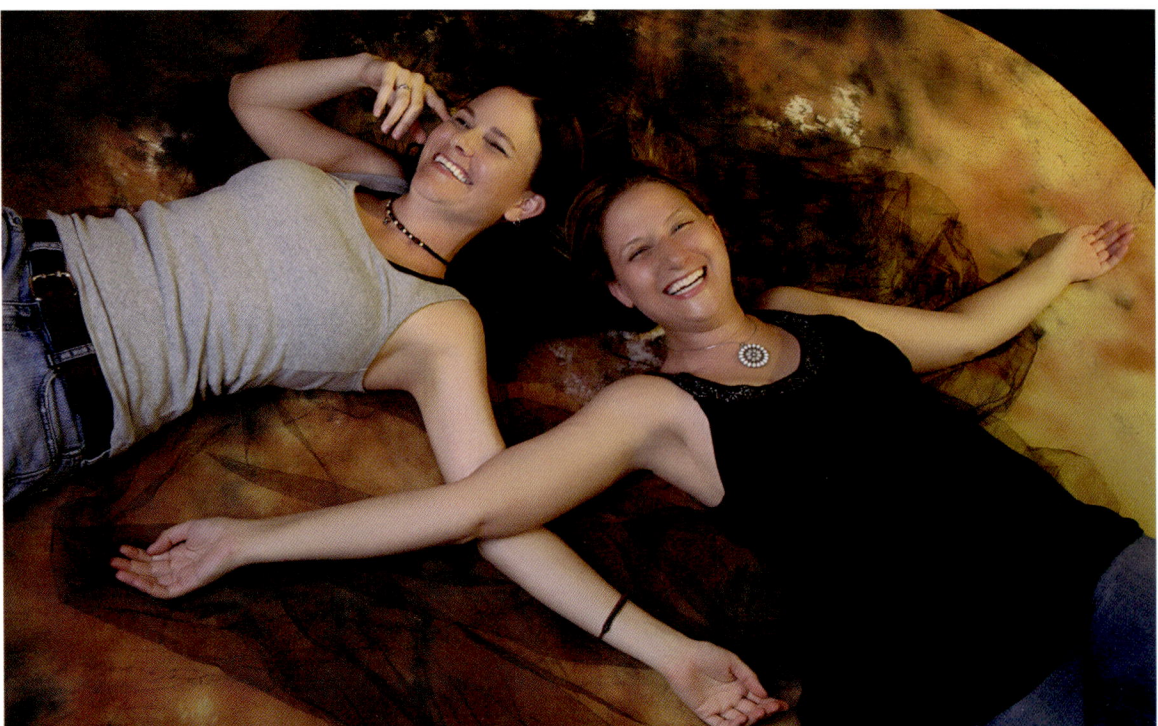

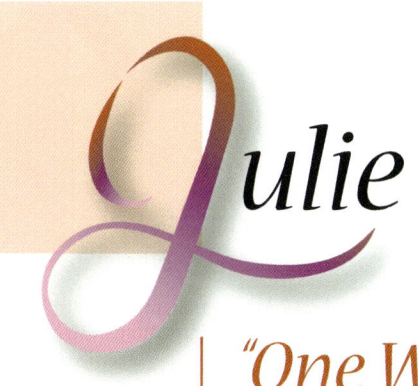

"One Way to Really Live…Beat Cancer Twice!!!"

My name is Julie Goiset. I am 36 years old. I was first diagnosed when I was 27 years old in November 2002. I had invasive ductal carcinoma er+/pr+, her2+, grade 3, stage 1, 0/6 nodes. I had a lumpectomy on my right breast with radiation and chemotherapy and Herceptin.

Of course when you hear you have cancer it is quite devastating. I questioned what I did wrong in my life. Why me? Then I realized I really had a choice. I could feel sorry for myself and wallow in all my misery, or I could take each step with power, knowing that I was going to be ok. I knew deep down that I was going to be a mother and that these harsh treatments were not going to stop that. There is always a risk in life, no matter which road you take. But I also new that something much bigger was needed to stop me and this was just a stepping stool.

> *Then I realized I really had a choice. I could feel sorry for myself and wallow in all my misery, or I could take each step with power, knowing that I was going to be ok.*

Cancer has taught me to be appreciative of all the people I have in my life. We don't live in this world alone. We don't accomplish things alone. Learning to work together has always been my working area. Cancer is a wake up call! Your time to live is now! Some people don't get that. Waking up is a process too. I stopped being afraid of dying. I took big challenges. I had 2 kids since and that journey has been so worth it. My kids have given me new meaning of community in so many ways.

I keep coming back to myself. Listening and nurturing my intuition. I recently have been diagnosed again with almost the same cancer. My gut told me to get another mammogram before I was due. Sure enough, a new primary. This time it is not hormone sensitive, but Her2+, which means it's fast growing. So I am doing chemotherapy again and this time having a double mastectomy with full reconstruction. None of this is easy by any means, but attitude makes a huge difference. It's going to take a lot more than this to stop me from living the life of my dreams!

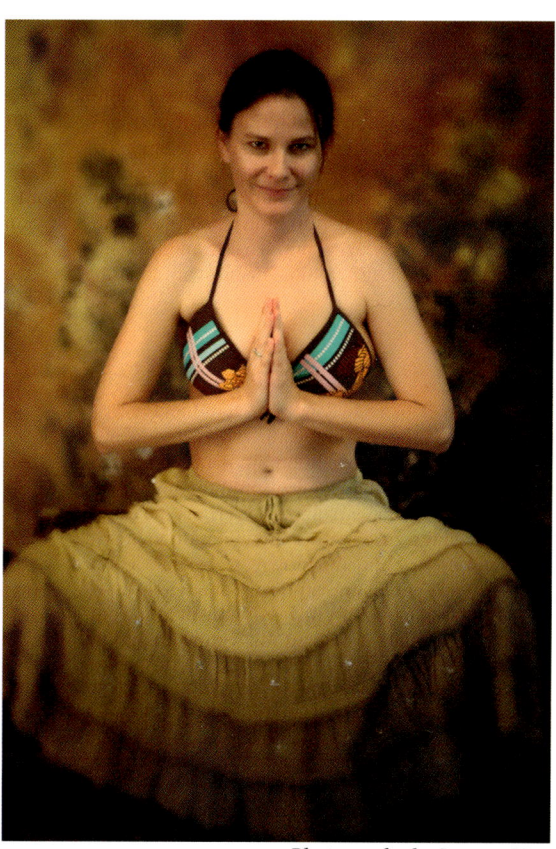

Photography by Joanna Herr

Sandy

"Getting to the Other Side of Breast Cancer"

I was diagnosed with Stage 3A breast cancer seven years ago at age 35. I had a left side mastectomy, 8 rounds of chemo, 48 rounds of radiation, and several reconstructive surgeries.

My feelings when diagnosed: shock, fear, and the overwhelming sense that I was in for the fight of my life.

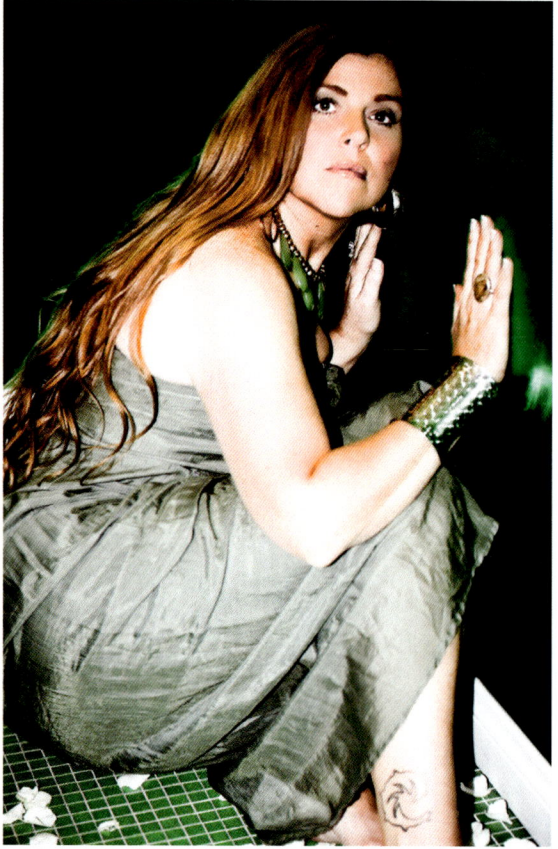

My family members were so supportive. My husband is the best co-survivor and caretaker in the world. There was a tremendous outpouring of love from everyone in my life and the people with whom I worked. I have the sense that you are never really alone when you go through a tragedy. Love and goodness prevail. It is comforting to walk through the rest of my days with that knowing.

The most difficult time that I recall was around the half way mark through the chemo treatments. I just felt so weak and defeated and like my body really couldn't take anymore. Being bald and having everything that made me feminine taken away was a difficult adjustment.

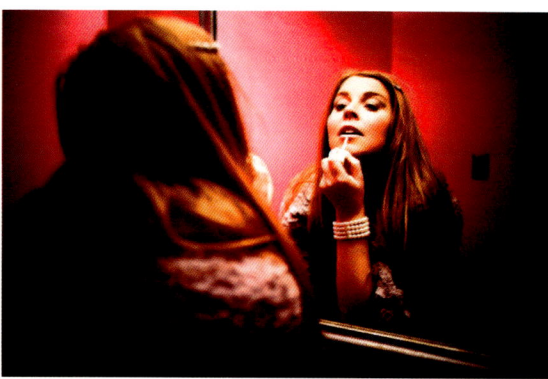

Going through breast cancer has changed me in so many ways for the better. I lead a very purpose driven life and my career path changed from being an executive in the publishing industry to being an activist for the nonprofit, Susan G. Komen for the Cure. I've emerged on the other side a more beautiful person internally because I have greater understanding of the depths of suffering.

> **When I was sick I had a wig of EVERY color. It was a social experiment to walk as a blonde, a brunette, and a redhead. I think blondes have more fun.**

My advice to patients is to reach out, you aren't alone. EVER.

I am FIRST and foremost proudest of my relationship with my husband and how much he stood by me through this. I'm also proud that I was able to channel my grief into something so positive. I am blessed in so many ways by the people I have met and the things I get to do with Susan G. Komen for the Cure.

What has inspired me? The many survivors I meet along the way and the many young women I have met who come to volunteer at Susan G. Komen… a great number of these young women in their early twenties have lost their mothers to breast cancer. They are brave and amazing young women that I get to mentor. I do not have children of my own, so in many ways they are my children, and I'm thankful that I can nurture them for their moms who have passed on.

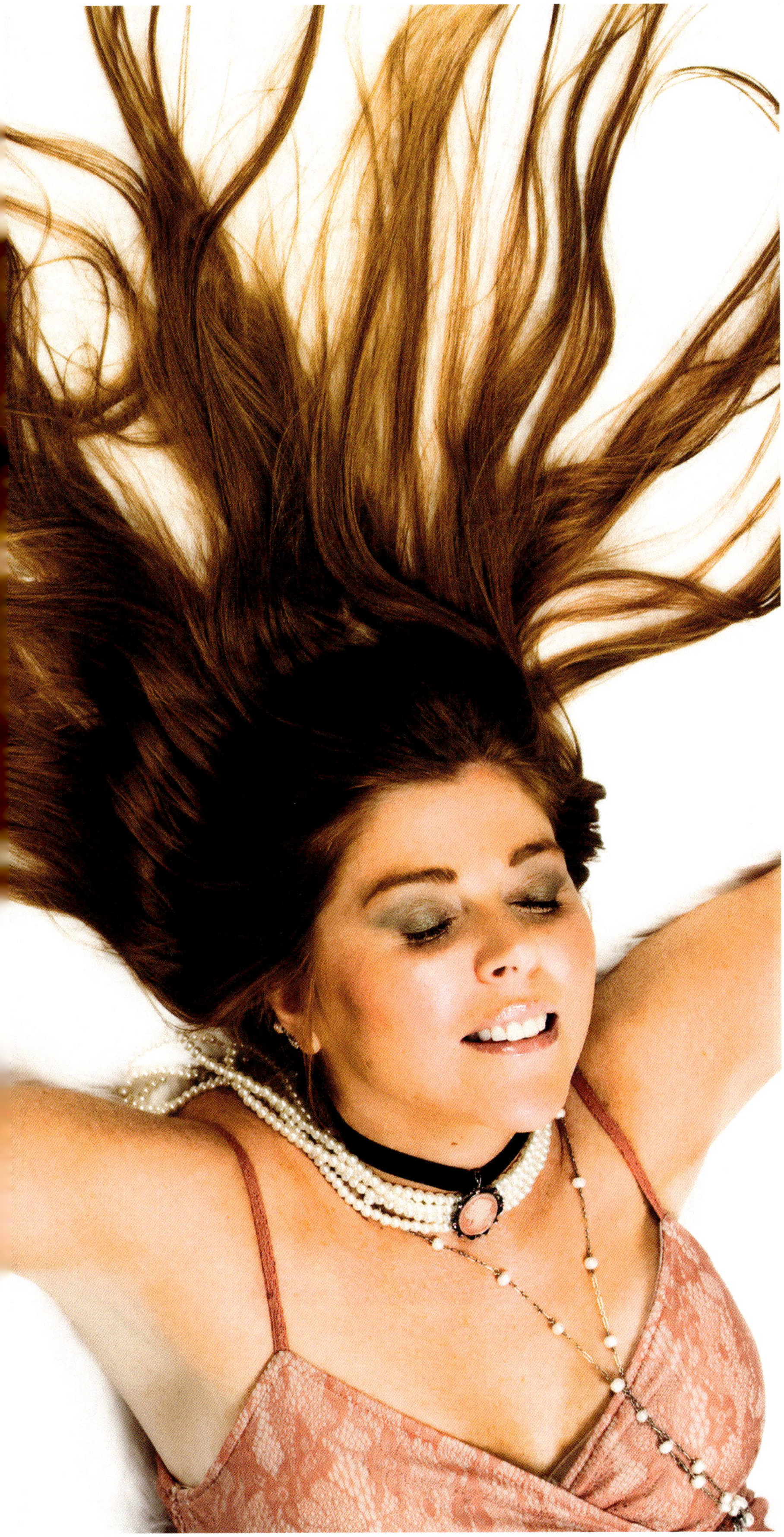

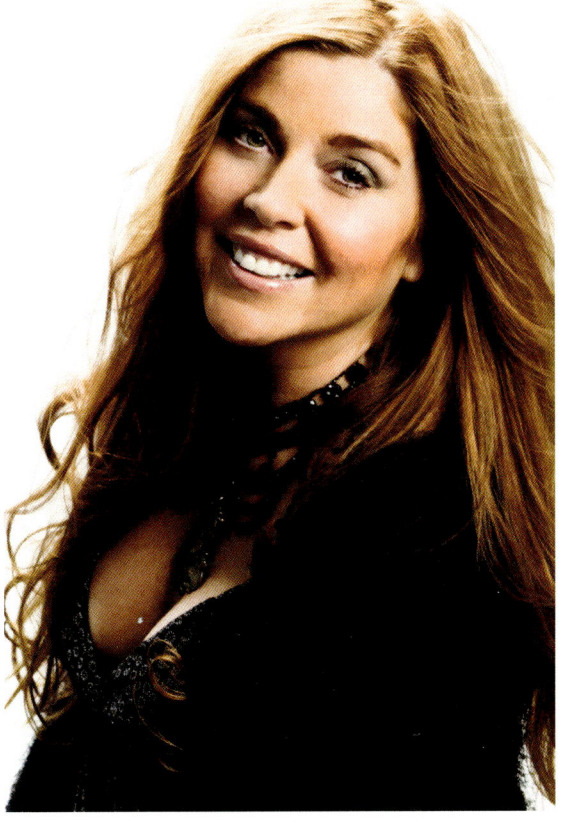

*Channel Your Grief.
It is not what happens to you
that defines your life.
It is the way in which you handle
what happens to you that
defines your life.*

Director of Development
and Marketing Communications for
Susan G. Komen for the Cure

Rosalie

"You Talkin' to Me?"

My name is Rosalie. I am a Breast Cancer Survivor. I was 48 years old when I was diagnosed. I think I'm 49 years old now—I dunno—Chemo Brain. I've been married to Dale for almost 19 years. My daughter Kayla is now 13.

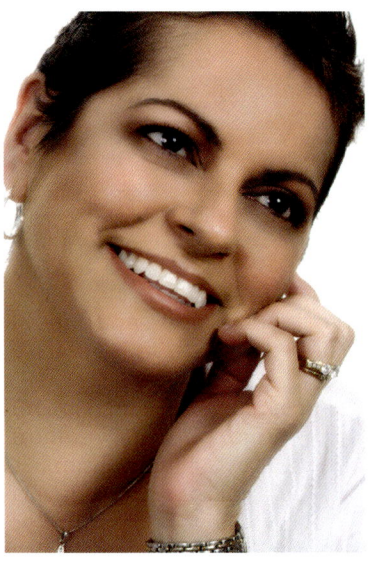

My diagnosis was Stage 2 Breast Cancer 3.5 mm Triple negative. I had 2 biopsies, 2 lumpectomies, 4 chemo treatments and 36 radiation treatments. I did not have a lump. I did not have pain. My cancer was found in a mammogram. It was a mass inside me, growing and spreading. I skipped a year, I don't know why. I thought I went. Why didn't I go? Thank God I finally went.

My Doctor called me on Friday August 6th, 2010, 4:10 p.m. I think I was drunk by 4:30 p.m. (Patron shots).

Dale arrived home right as I hung up the phone with my doctor. I cried when I told him. I was scared and felt guilty. I didn't want to put my family through this. What did I do wrong to make us go through this? Will I be here for my daughter? Will I be at her graduation, at her wedding? Will my husband remarry? How will my parents react? After the tears I decided to be strong, brave, and positive to get past this.

Dale went into "Let's fix this" mode. My parents cried. I didn't want to tell my best friend, Mary, right away since she had other things going on in her life. But she knew something was wrong. Of course she did, we've known each other since the 2nd grade. She kept on calling me and I kept on hanging up on her. Finally she got it out of me. She cried with me. My parents cried.

My daughter, Kayla, was confused. Didn't know what Cancer does. She was scared of the unknown. My parents cried.

My aunt Nancy listened and said, "you will be ok". She said she will tell my parents not to cry. But…My parents cried.

After the initial blow, my husband started calling family, friends and neighbors. I called one of my neighbors, Robin. I wanted her to hear the news straight from me. I asked her to tell her husband, Mike, for me. I couldn't tell him 'cause I didn't want him to see me cry. Mike came over later with about 6 get well cards. He didn't know which one to get me so he bought all of them. That's when I realized I have people on my team. I decided I will be ok.

Chemo treatment was tough. Not the treatment itself, but the few days after. Everything hurt. It hurt to stand, sit, lie down, walk, breath, blink. Everything hurt all the time. Then there was the lack of taste. Everything tasted like dirty metal. Water – yuk. Ice cream – blah. French Fries – no thank you. Once my taste came back I had a new appreciation for the flavor of a banana.

I did struggle with my appearance. I lost my hair about 2 weeks after my first chemo. That wasn't fun at all. I had hoped that if I saw Kenny Chesney he would autograph my bald head. The worst was losing my eye lashes. You see—I'm all about my eyelashes. Fake eyelashes wouldn't be the same. I wanted MY eyelashes. Is there patron saint of eyelashes? I dunno.

> *I lost my hair about 2 weeks after my first chemo. That wasn't fun at all. I had hoped that if I saw Kenny Chesney he would autograph my bald head.*

My daughter turned 13 after my 2nd chemo. I felt I cheated her out of a milestone birthday. But a neighbor saved the day and entertained her for the evening. Thanks Robin.

I'm not sure how I overcame the hard times. My husband helped a lot, kept me laughing. He made lots of mashed potatoes since that was the one thing that didn't taste bad. I love his mashed potatoes.

I allowed myself to cry 5 minutes a day. The remaining 23 hours and 55 minutes…no crying.

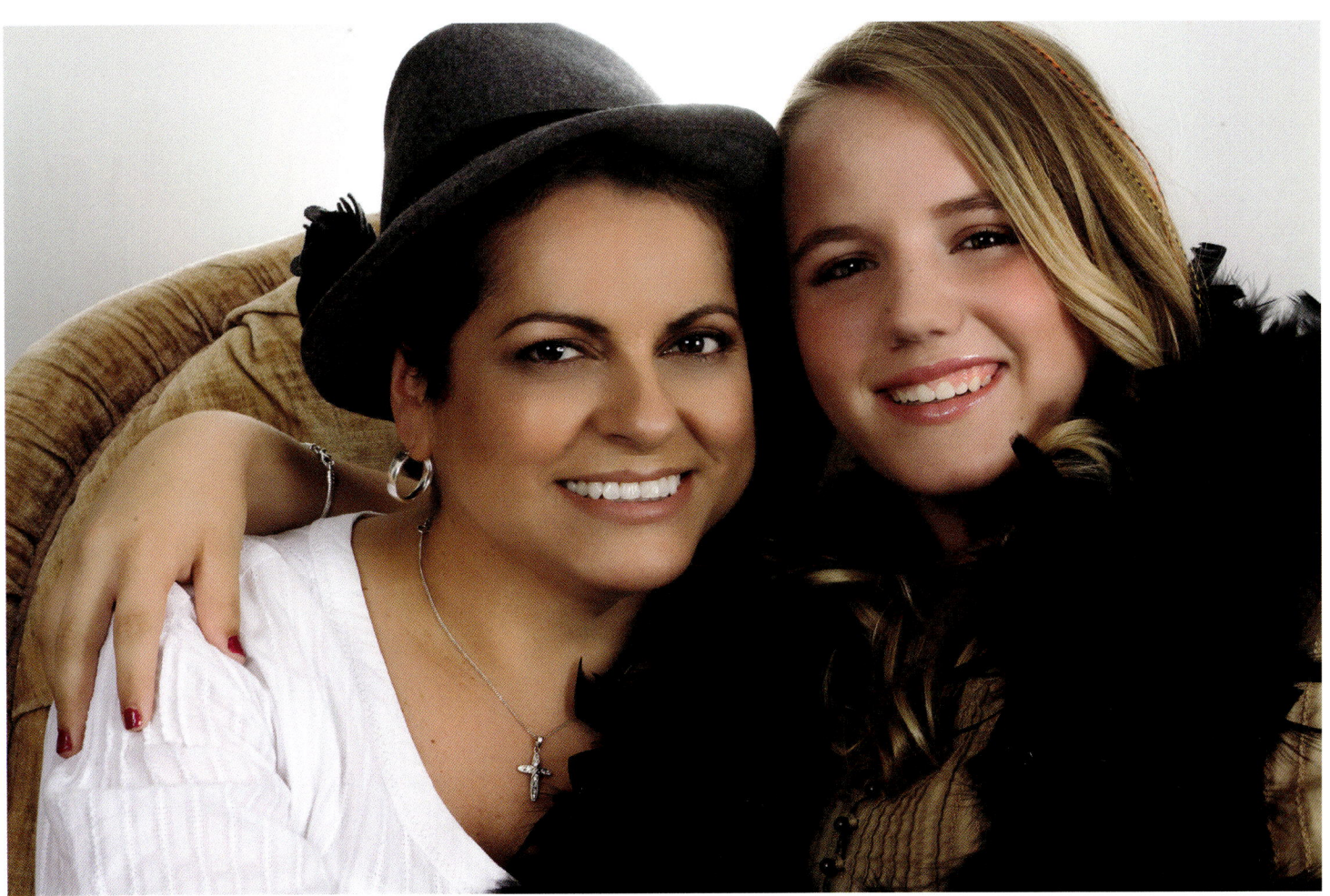

I found ways to laugh. Crying made me lose my eyelashes faster anyway. I talked to GOD a lot!!!

Breast Cancer did change me. I have new friends from my support group. Thanks Bunny! I love all the gals there. Friends for life. So much love there. My hair came back darker and curly. I gained 18 pounds –UGH. I'm eating healthier…haven't had a Big Mac in months. No more Hershey bars. I don't buy Ruffle chips anymore. I "goofie-dance" a lot more. I sing a lot more too—but I forget the lyrics now—chemo brain.

My neighbors and friends helped with meals during my chemo treatment, delicious meals. Now my husband expects me to follow those recipes and cook. (yeah, right). I do have aches and pains still from surgery and chemo. I noticed that being in crowds bother me now. Weird. But overall I feel that I am a better and stronger person since my diagnoses.

I have no "advice" for new patients. I'm not a breast cancer pro (I don't want to be). I will say that you will feel the sunshine again. You will laugh. Treatment will end. Love your medical team. They will become your good friend while you go through this journey, and after. It's ok to cry in front of them. My surgeon wiped my tears.

Tell your husband to go out with the guys. They need to de-stress from the issues at home. They need to be one of the guys, not just the husband of a BC patient. They need a break too.

> …there is a photographer who wanted to do a photo shoot at one of my radiation treatments. I guess he didn't realize that I would be topless.

I'm proud of my husband. He quickly educated himself so much on Breast Cancer. He has answered all my questions. He went to all my appointments. He made my treatment easier. He was and still is my Team Captain. There should be some type of award for husbands of BC patients. He deserves the best.

My daughter tried using my cancer as an excuse for messing up in school. Ha! I nipped that one right away. Good try though.

And you know what…I'm kinda proud of myself. I gotta give myself a little credit for getting through it. I decided that I was gonna make it.

I was inspired by many people during my challenge. My surgeon is so freaking smart. I'm glad she paid attention in school. The women in my Breast Cancer Support Group inspire me each time we meet. They are incredibly strong women.

I continued working through my treatment. I didn't want to sit home just thinking about BC. I wanted to keep busy. Plus I got tons of support and love from my friends at work.
Once I got my doctors ok, I went back to the gym. I got my daughter a membership. We go about 5 times a week. Gotta keep strong.

God sends angels to us every day. I left work early one day, I had no energy and everything hurt. I had to get gas in the car or I wouldn't make it home. I pulled into the local AM/PM. I had no strength. I struggled with the gas hose. Out of nowhere a gentleman appeared to help. I think he said his name was Ken. He said he had family with Cancer and recognized that I had it too. He helped fill my car and just talked to me. He made me smile. Thanks Ken.

My daughter asked me one day if I was going to die of Breast Cancer. I thought that no child should need to ask their mom that question. I told her "No, not of Breast Cancer". I told her that I might die when I open her closet doors and everything falls on top of me. She shook her head and walked away.

A funny thing…there is a photographer who wanted to do a photo shoot at one of my radiation treatments. I guess he didn't realize that I would be topless. And he wasn't gonna pay me for it….not even dinner. Who is this guy?

Breast Cancer was definitely the hardest thing that I've gone through. I made it! Onto the next journey…My parents are not crying anymore.

"You Talkin' to My Momma?"

My name is Kayla. I was 12 years old when my mom was diagnosed with breast cancer. I turned 13 after my mom's 2nd chemo.

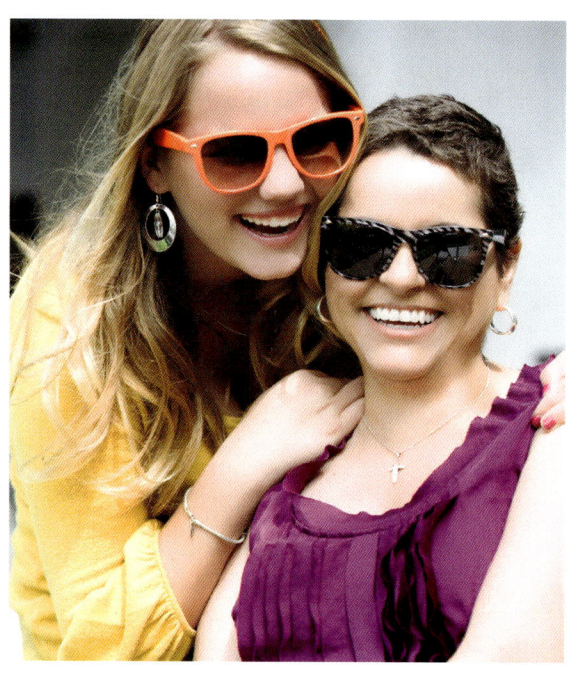

When I found out I didn't understand. I asked myself "why my mom, why?"

One day I decided that I wanted to meet her doctors. The day I had gone to meet them, Susan Heath, told my mom that they got all the cancer. My mom would be OK.

I had a late start at my school one day. My mom took me to her radiation. I got to do her radiation. It was cool learning how to work the machines. I got to do it two different times. I feel like I helped my mom get better.

I know my mom cried, but I remember my dad, mom and I laughing a lot too.

Jennifer

"Not Too Young"

I was diagnosed at 28. I am now 31 and mother and student. I love the beach, any sport, volunteering, my dogs, anything with the kids, and photography.

I first heard I had cancer after my biopsy. I found a lump and went to a doctor. He told me not to worry because I was too young to get cancer. I wanted that to be true but was still worried. It was a small lump and could only be felt at certain angles. I read an article in a magazine about women of all ages who had breast cancer and that stuck in the back of my mind.

> "I found a lump and went to a doctor. He told me not to worry because I was too young to get cancer."

I moved to a different city and mentioned the lump to my new doctor. The doctor felt the lump and immediately scheduled me for surgery. I was a newly single mom of two children under the age of five. I was in shock that this could actually happen when my previous doctor told me nothing was wrong with me.

My children didn't really know what was going on. My oldest daughter just knows mom was sick a lot. I didn't want her to worry about me knowing I wasn't going to be alive anymore. She will know her history but isn't old enough to understand what cancer really is. I always tell everyone to do checks and trust yourself. A doctor isn't a god and if you really feel something is wrong get a second and third opinion.

I'm proud of making it through this. The hardest thing to overcome is the fear. Every year after the mammogram I wait for the letter saying they didn't find anything new. I used to be embarrassed of the scars but now I feel like they are a badge that I've earned from getting through this.

I feel a new understanding for my Nana who died of breast cancer. I feel like I learned from her. She didn't want to go to the doctor and have them touch her chest. She was of a different generation. The difference between her experience and mine was early detection. In some way she taught me even though she wasn't here anymore.

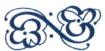

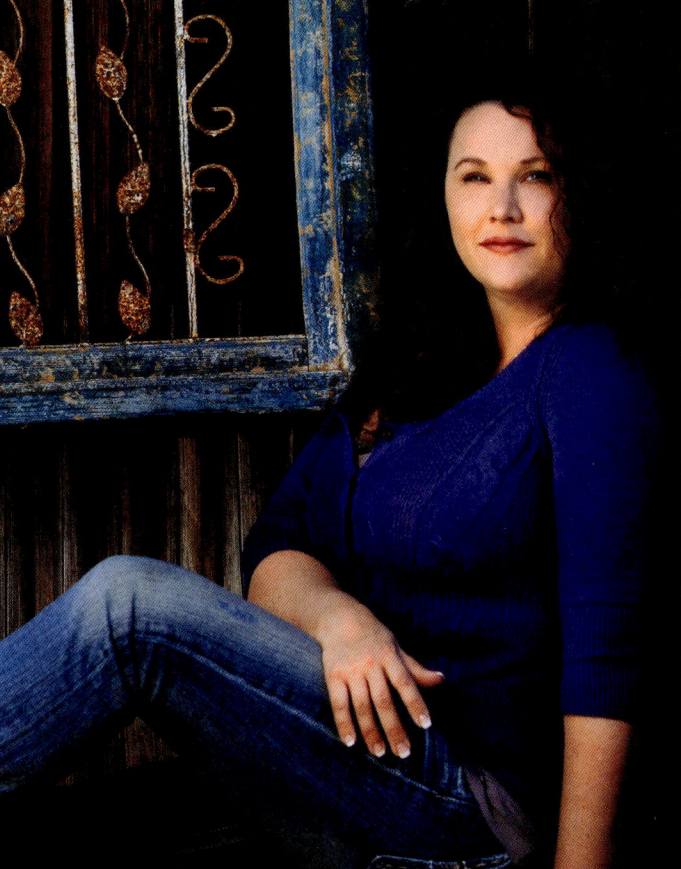

SOME LIKE IT SHOT PHOTOGRAPHY
~ Photo by Alisha McGraw ~

*Alisha is the principal photographer at **Some Like It Shot Photography**, located in San Diego, CA. Together with husband Holland, they are contributing photographers for local, regional, and international publications. Their forte is photographing people with their pets, as well as pinup artwork.*

Email: info@somelikeitshotphotography.com
Web: www.somelikeitshotphotography.com/
Join Our Facebook Page.

Love… No Matter What

by Petra Van Baar

Q: What is **Love…No Matter What**?

A: *What started out as an inspirational card business has blossomed into a full service outreach program. I like to think of it as a resource to express oneself and a place to find hope and inspiration. Giving and receiving is what we provide, an outlet or community for people to share their experience, courage and hope through extremely difficult times; a sounding board and also a resource for spiritual and emotional tools. We provide a place where people can sign up at a "blog" to share their journey. We also offer a hotline for survivors for whatever their needs may be. Cards, calendars and other inspirational media are available.*

Mission Statement

A blossoming place where people are invited to come and share their experience, or find inspiration, courage, strength and hope, through:

Love…No Matter What.

The set up is like a forum; open for people to cross communicate about their struggles in life and how they overcome them.

When we find ourselves living with a situation that seems frightening and painful, we have to remind ourselves that our immediate experience, our now, is what really matters. It is the shift from walking through our lives, to walking *IN* our lives. Gratitude for what *IS* can shine light into our darkness.

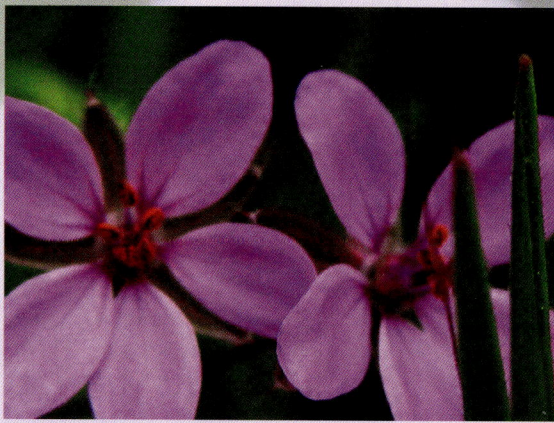

Photography: "LoveNoMatterWhat.com" by Petra

We are grateful for the people we touch, and that touch us, during times of pain and suffering, and they remind us of the blessings that are sometimes hard to see. Remember then that everything we do matters. Every time we are truly grateful it creates a ripple of positive energy that travels infinitely, touching countless hearts and lives along the way. We can change the world…not only our perception of it, but truly change it. What a gift to be thankful for! We need only to ask and the answers, love and support we need will be granted to us, if we are open to receive it. I can think of no better gift than to experience relief of my own suffering by, in some way, relieving the suffering of another. Our gratitude and service are what matters on this journey… it is what we are here to do. By truly living our lives, leading by example, we have purpose and joy.

"It is during our darkest moments that we must focus to see the light."

~ Aristotle Onassis

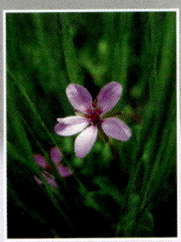
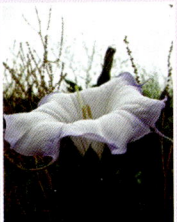
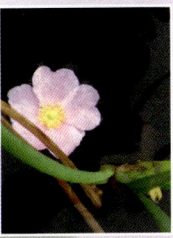
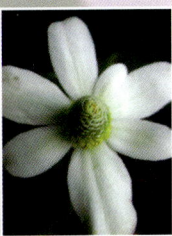
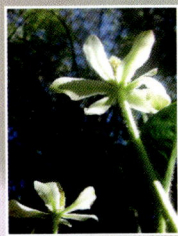
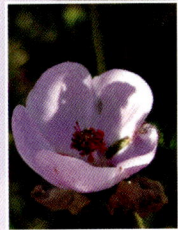
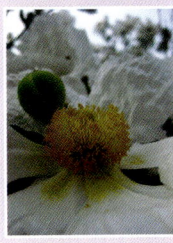

Examples of
***Love…No Matter What* Cards:**

I love you… no matter what
no matter what…you are safe
I am here for you…no matter what
I will stand beside you…no matter what
always know, you can lean on me…
no matter what

No matter what…
believe in the power of love
no matter what… you are never alone
let love guide you…no matter what
we will get through this together…
no matter what

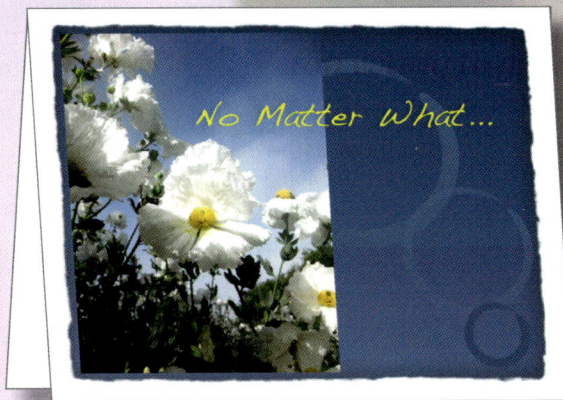

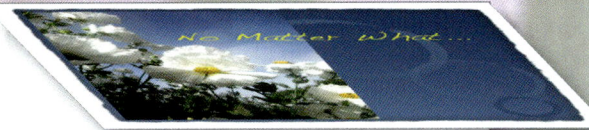

You are safe.

Contact Info:

Petra Van Baar
www.lovenomatterwhat.com • petra@lovenomatterwhat.com

cards ~ encouragement ~ inspiration

Sonia

"I'll Never Win the 'OWIE' Game."

My name is Sonia Encinias. I'm a 41 year old woman who was diagnosed with Stage II B breast cancer at age 40. I was misdiagnosed at 37.

When I first learned that I had breast cancer, I was confused because my family did not have a history of breast cancer (41 females in my family). It was heartbreaking once it became a reality. I felt like my life was over.

How did my family react when I told them? My daughter took it very hard, but kept all her feelings in. My long time boyfriend closed down and soon after my surgery decided he needed to be single. My mom cried so much it killed me to tell her. And my granddaughter did not understand what was going on.

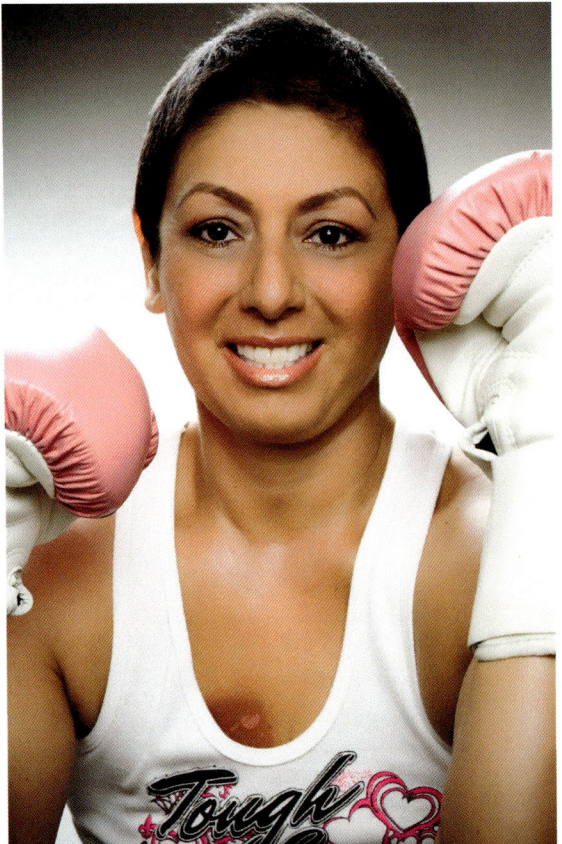

My most difficult time was losing my hair, my eyelashes, and my eyebrows. I felt like ALL my feminine qualities were stripped away. I really struggled with being bald. I was mistaken for a man numerous times…losing my hair sucked the life out of me.

I never overcame the baldness…it took over. I hid behind black beanies and hoodies…I hated it! I bought wigs but could not wear them, I did not feel like myself and I felt like everyone was looking at me.

> **ALL my feminine qualities were stripped away. I really struggled with being bald. I was mistaken for a man numerous times…**

At first I became withdrawn and stayed in my house as much as possible. Now that I have completed my treatments and am cancer free… I have a new breath of life. I live by myself for the first time ever, I am trying new things… I am finding myself.

My advice to new patients is to talk about your feelings. Your cancer is your cancer and only you can decide to fight. No matter how hard it gets, let your family and friends help you.

I am proudest of my daughter Sydney…she is a single mother and graduated from Kaplan College with her Medical Assistant Certificate while I was undergoing chemotherapy. She is so strong and totally amazing!

My family and friends have inspired me through my entire journey. But I have to say that volunteering at Susan G. Komen has truly inspired me. Laura, Sandy, and Mary Beth opened my eyes to life as a woman and as a survivor. They are truly angels, they taught me it was okay to cry or be upset because after all that, we can laugh and smile.

I now enjoy riding my beach cruiser daily, and walking on the beach as much as possible. I am seeing the beauty in life again so my camera is always with me. I am spending more time with friends, and volunteer weekly at Susan G. Komen (best job ever). I will return to my full time job soon.

Through this journey my then two year old granddaughter and I have had this "game" of comparing our "owies"… hers from preschool and mine from chemotherapy. The day finally

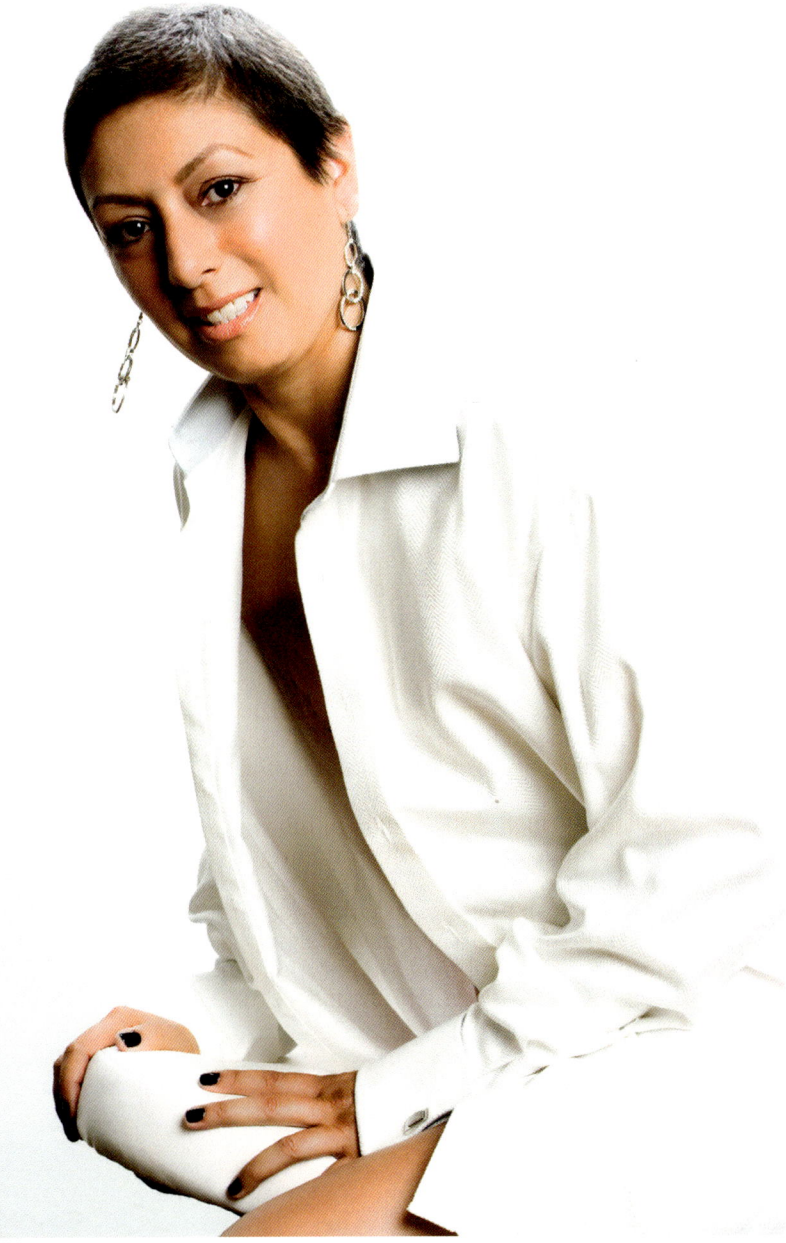

All wounds heal, scars are the beauty left behind.

came when I was scheduled for my bi-lateral mastectomy; I told her that morning that when I got home I would have something to show her. I was so excited I was finally going to win the competition on who had the best owie! When she got home that evening I called her to my room and of course she had a new owie to share. I then told her that I had the best owie ever…I lifted my shirt and showed her my scars and tubes and all she said was "that's it? Where is it?" I pointed to the scars and said "right here" and she replied "I see that, but where is your owie?" So I guess I will never win at the owie game.

All wounds heal, scars are the beauty left behind.

OMG! I have never and I mean never seen myself like this before…these pictures brought tears to my eyes. I now see that it was not my hair…not my brows or eyelashes…not my boobs that made me beautiful…it was just me.

"Nunca Ganaré en el Juego de el Moretón."

Mi nombre es Sonia Encinias. Soy una mujer de 41 años que fue diagnosticada con etapa II B cáncer de mama a la edad de 40 años. Fui mal diagnosticada a los 37.

En un principio cuando comprendí que tenia cáncerde mama, estuve confundida porque en mi familia no hay un historial de cáncer de mama (41 mujeres en mi familia). Se me rompió el corazón una vez que me di cuenta que era una realidad. Sentí como si mi vida había terminado.

¿Cómo reacciono mi familia cuando les dije? Fue muy duro para mi hija, pero mantuvo todos sus sentimientos ocultos. Mi ex-novio también mantuvo sus sentimientos ocultos…el nunca mostró ninguna emoción. Mi mama lloró tanto, que me mató decirle. Y mi nieta no comprendía lo que pasaba.

Mi tiempo más difícil fué cuando perdí el pelo, las pestañas, y las cejas. S entí como que fui despojada de TODAS mis cualidades femeninas. Me fue muy difícil quedarme calva. Me confundieron por un hombre en varias ocasionés… haber perdido el pelo me quitó la vida.

¡Nunca vencí la calvicie… me venció a mí! ¡Me oculté detrás de gorros y sudaderas negras…lo odiaba! Compré pelucas pero no pude usarlas, no me sentía como yo misma y sentía como si todos me veian.

En un principio me aparté y permanecí en mi casa lo más posible. Ahora que he terminado mis tratamientos y estoy liberada de cáncer… tengo un nuevo aliento de la vida. Vivo por mí misma por primera vez en la vida, estoy intentando cosas nuevas… me he encontrado a mí misma.

Mi consejo para nuevos pacientes es que hablen de sus sentimientos. Tu cáncer es tu cáncer y solo tú puedes decidir luchar. Por muy duro que se ponga, permite que tu familia y tus amigos te ayuden.

Estoy muy orgullosa de mi hija Sydney…ella es una madre soltera y graduada del colegio de

Kaplan con un certificado de asistente médico mientras que yo experimentaba la quimioterapia. ¡Ella es muy fuerte y totalmente asombrosa!

Mi familia y amigos me han inspirado por toda mi travesía. Pero tengo que decir que ser voluntaria en Susan G.Komen realmente me ha inspirado. Laura, Sandy y Mary Beth me abrieron los ojos a la vida como una mujer y como una sobreviviente. Ellas son verdaderos ángeles, y me enseñaron que esta bien llorar o estar molesta porque después de todo eso, nosotros podemos reírnos y sonreír.

Ahora disfruto de andar en bicicleta a diario, y caminar por la playa lo más posible. Veo la belleza nuevamente en la vida y mi cámara esta siempre conmigo. Estoy más tiempo con amigos, y soy voluntaria semanal en Susan G. Komen (es el mejor trabajo que he tenido). Pronto regresaré a mi trabajo de tiempo completo.

Durante esta travesía, mi nieta entonces de dos años de edad y yo hemos tenido este "juego" de comparar nuestros moretones… los suyos del jardín de niños y los míos de quimioterapia. ¡Llegó por fin el día en que fui citada para mi mastectomía bilateral; y le dije en la mañana que cuando llegara a casa yo tendría algo que mostrarle! Yo estava muy emocionada porque por fin iba a ganar la competencia de quien tenia el mejor moretón! Cuando ella llegó a casa esa noche yo la llamé a mi cuarto y por supuesto ella tuvo un nuevo moretón que compartir. Entonces le dije que yo tenia el mejor moretón… Levante mi camisa y le mostré mis cicatrices y tubos, y ella solo dijo "eso es todo? ¿dónde esta?" ¡Le señale las cicatrices y le dije "aquí mismo" y contesto, "yo veo eso, pero donde esta tu moretón?" Ahora creo que nunca ganaré en el juego de los moretones.

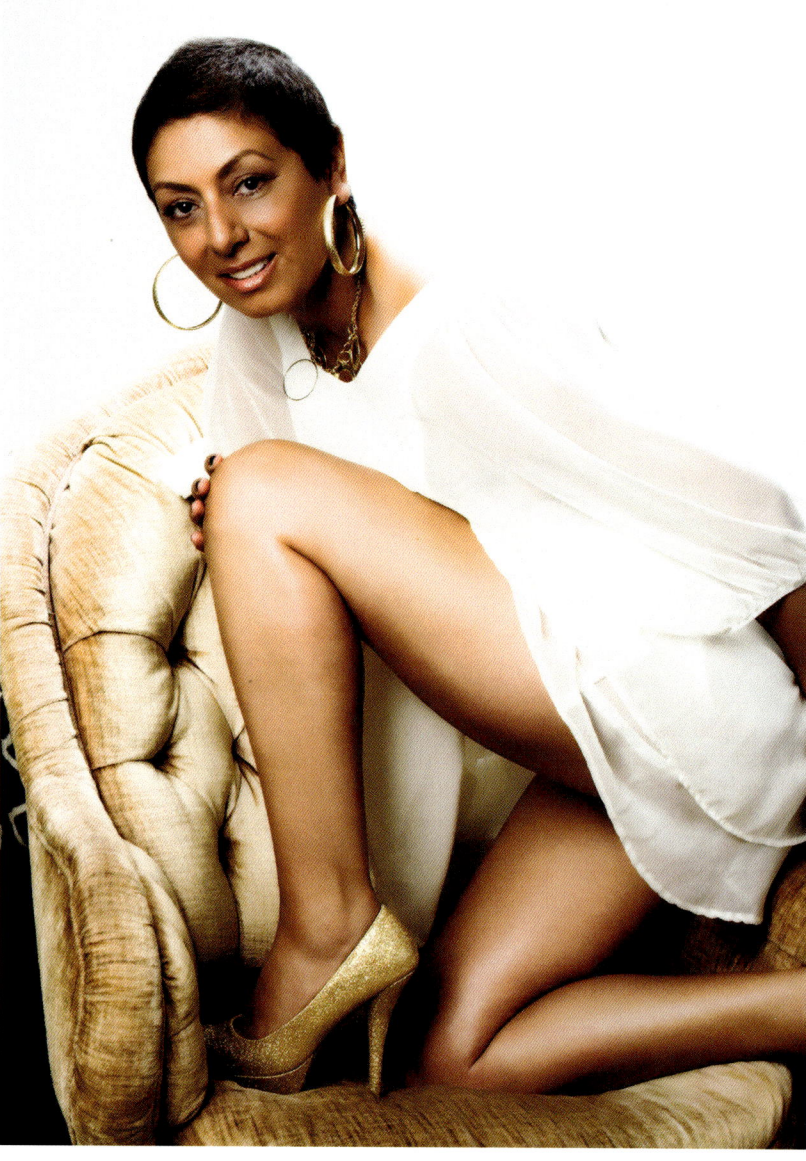

> *Ahora veo que no es el pelo… ni mis cejas o pestañas… ni mis pechos lo que me hacen hermosa… solo era yo.*

Todas las heridas sanan, las cicatrices son la belleza que queda atras.

Dios mio! Anteriormente nunca, y digo nunca, me he visto así… estas fotos trajeron lagrimas a mis ojos. Ahora veo que no es el pelo… ni mis cejas o pestañas… ni mis pechos lo que me hacen hermosa… solo era yo.

Sherry

"Tradin' Chevys for Ferraris"

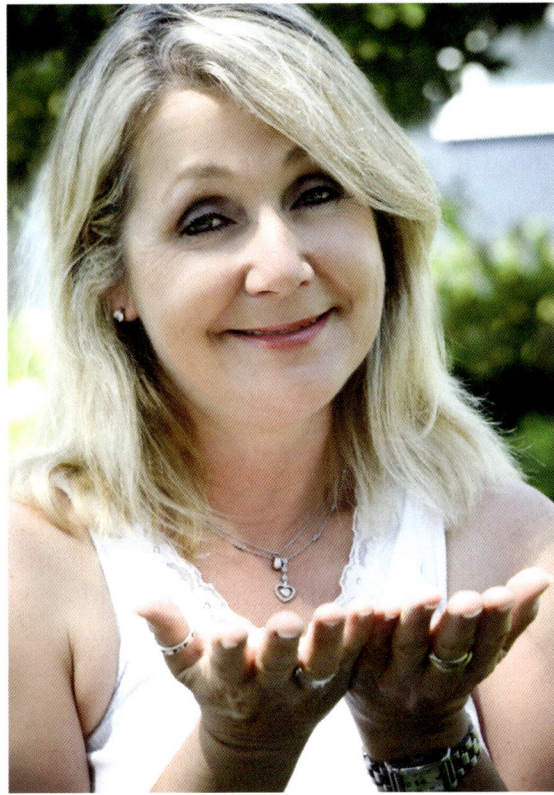

At the age of 41, I was diagnosed with breast cancer. I had a lumpectomy, chemo, and radiation. I continued to maintain a healthy lifestyle of eating right and regular exercise. Then 14 years later I was diagnosed again. So I traded in my 1956 Chevys for a pair of 2011 Ferraris.

> **Now as before I do not let breast cancer slow me down. Nor do I allow it to change my positive attitude.**

Because of regular mammograms it was caught early. Now as before I do not let breast cancer slow me down. Nor do I allow it to change my positive attitude. Our bodies get diseases. There is no getting around that. I'm very fortunate that I surround myself with wonderful friends and I try to stay up-to-date with new breast cancer treatments.

I am a fashion designer and I try to use my work to help others. I participate in fundraisers and fashion shows that help breast cancer organizations. Remember, in today's world, breast cancer is not always life threatening. Like anything else in life, it is what you make it.

Also, every day there are some things that I try to do. I try to say hi to 3 new people, give a stranger a compliment, say thank you, do one good deed, meditate, go for a walk, hug a friend, hug my dog, hug my Ferraris…life is good :)

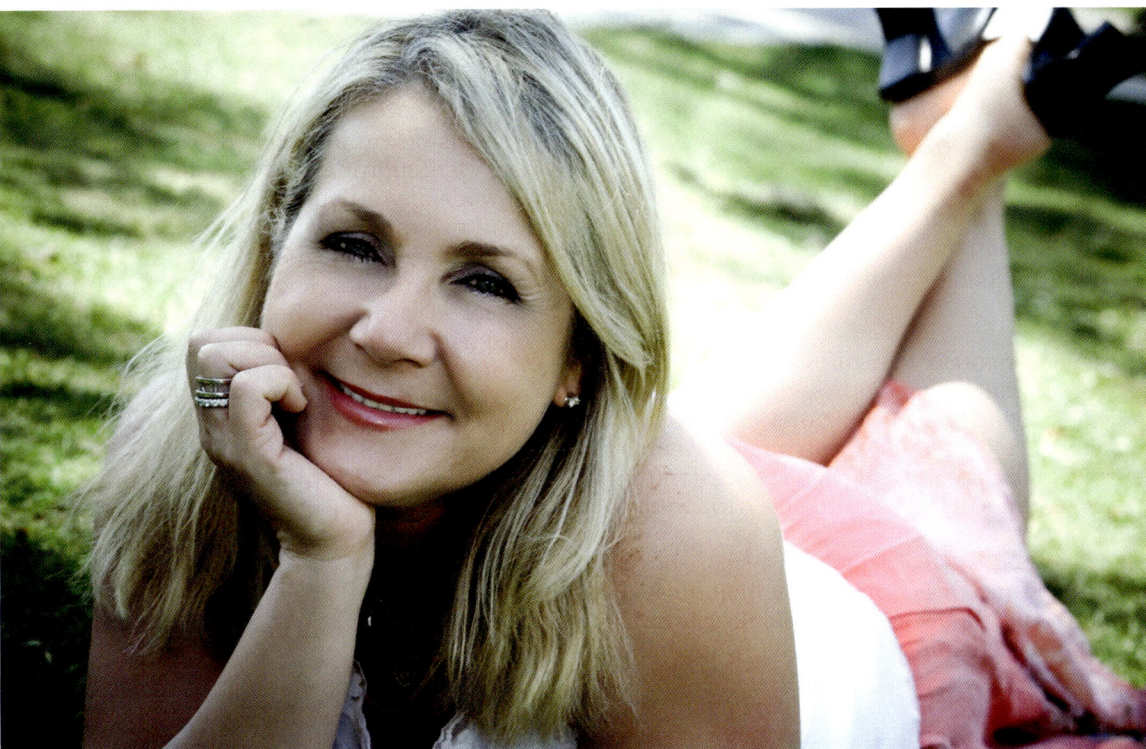

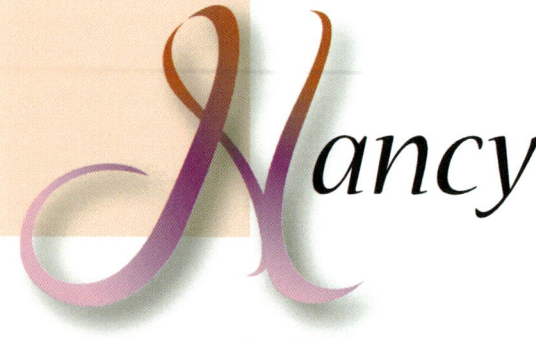

Nancy

"A Breast Is Just That…a Breast."

My name is Nancy Barnes. I am 44 years old and I am a 12-year cancer survivor! I was first diagnosed with breast cancer at the beginning of 1999. At the time, I was nursing my 8 month old daughter, Emma, when I felt a lump. I thought it was a fibroid tumor since I'd had one removed about 10 years prior. So, I told my ob/gyn I wanted to have it removed. Thank goodness I did! (I'm also thankful he didn't tell me it was just a clogged milk duct.)

Anyway, I had a lumpectomy and it was at that point we discovered that the tumor was malignant and there were also two more lumps. When the surgeon told my husband, Eric, that I had cancer, we both just sat there in shock. He tried to tell us how important it was for Eric to be supportive, but in the process of him telling us a story of a man who was not supportive of his wife, and therefore his wife died, all we heard was that I had cancer and I was going to die (like the lady in his story).

At the time I was diagnosed, I exercised regularly, was nursing my daughter, and had been a vegetarian for 10 years. Plus, cancer did not run in my family. How could this be happening to me?! When we came home from visiting the surgeon, Eric had to call our families and friends and inform them that I had a lumpectomy and I have cancer. The entire time he was making phone calls, Emma lied there, not making a sound while I sat on the bed, crying, wondering if I was going to live to see her grow up. This was the second time I had seen Eric cry. (The first time was when Emma was born.)

When I was diagnosed, I was told I wouldn't be able to have anymore kids. I couldn't harvest any eggs, because of the type of cancer I had. (Ductal Carcinoma in Situ, estrogen receptor positive and progesterone receptor positive. As well as, HER-2/neu positive.) It was so difficult to think that I was just going to have one child. (I was happy I had Emma, but I didn't like being told I couldn't have more kids, if we wanted to.) Well, I finished all of my treatment in December 1999. On January 22, 2001, I gave birth to a healthy baby girl, Elleanna. She is my miracle baby and just as I couldn't imagine life without Emma, I can't imagine not having Elleanna around either.

Now, back to 1999. On February 22, 1999, I had a mastectomy, with reconstructive surgery, followed by 4 rounds of chemotherapy (Adriamycin and Taxotere) and 31 rounds of radiation. Before the surgery, I had to wrap my chest in bandages so I would stop producing milk. It was so painful! I had an allergic reaction to the chemotherapy, so I had to have Benadryl (through IV) before each chemo session and they had to drip it very slowly. So, each chemo session took approximately 6 hours. During this time, Eric and I sat in a private room and watched movies.

I didn't know anyone else who had ever had breast cancer. I thought only old people got cancer. I was only 32 years old. I never considered going to a support group because I had a lot of family and friends close by and everyone was so supportive. We scheduled family and friends to come over every day for the week after I had finished chemotherapy, to help take care of Emma. The hardest part, besides the nausea, was that no one

> **When I was diagnosed, I was told I wouldn't be able to have anymore kids. I couldn't harvest any eggs, because of the type of cancer I had.**

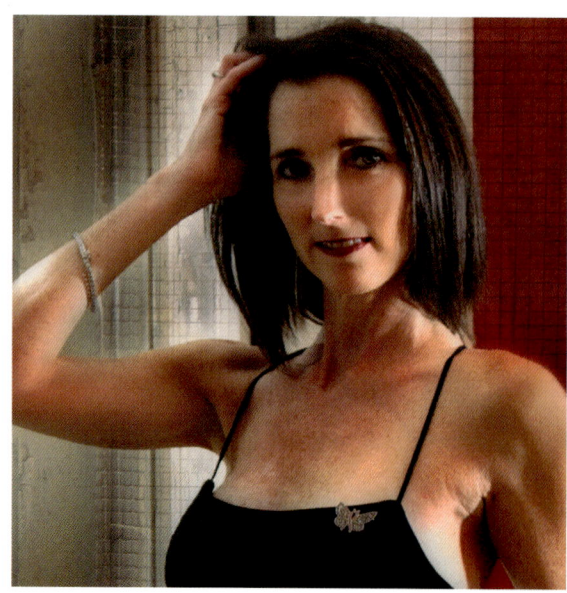

Photography by Joanna Herr

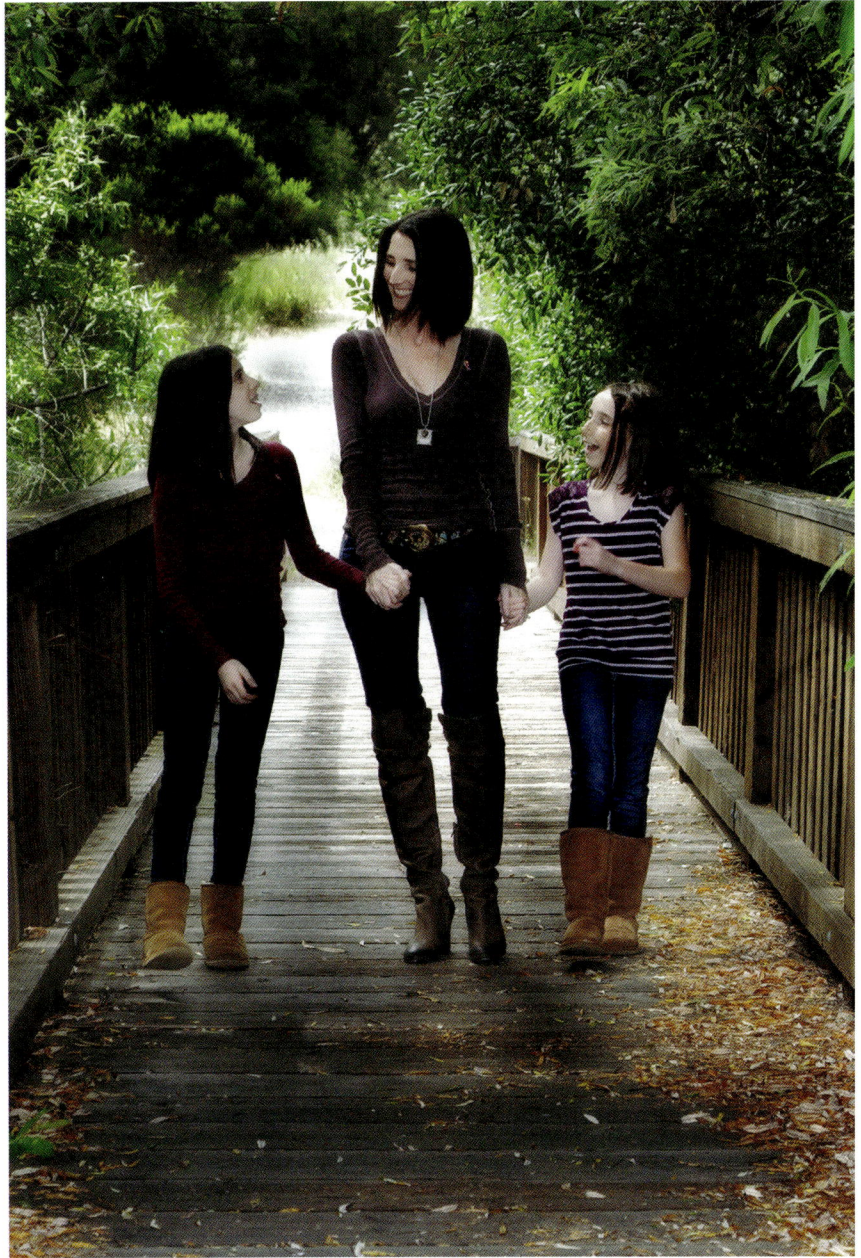

Photography by Joanna Herr

really understood what I was going through. Everyone was very positive, which was great. However, I got very tired of hearing "You'll be fine," and "We'll get through this, just do what the doctors tell you to do." Sometimes, I just wanted to be allowed to feel sorry for myself. That's one thing I would definitely tell new patients…It's okay to be angry. It's okay to think "Why is this happening to me?" My sister-in-law, Evangeline, bought me a journal and suggested that everyday I write down 5 things that I'm grateful for. That was one of the best gifts someone could've given me. Some days, it was so difficult to come up with 5 things to be grateful for. I still have the journal, and look back on it now and again. It taught me to

> *My sister-in-law… bought me a journal and suggested that everyday I write down 5 things that I'm grateful for. That was one of the best gifts someone could've given me.*

appreciate the little things. (i.e. "I'm alive!, I don't have cancer in my left breast., I didn't feel as nauseated today as I did yesterday.", "Emma smiled at me.", etc…). Another thing I would tell new patients is: shave your head before your hair starts to fall out. It is so difficult to see hair come out in long clumps. When it's short, it's still traumatic, but it's definitely not as bad. Plus, it's a lot more difficult for a baby to pull out hair that is very short. I shaved my head and wore a wig. I think if I had to do it over again, I wouldn't bother with the wig. It would be easier if people knew what I was going through. Perhaps, I would've met others going through the same thing.

For me, having the reconstructive surgery at the same time as the mastectomy made the entire experience of cancer a little easier. I never left the hospital flat on one side. So, it definitely helped me emotionally. I highly recommend having reconstructive surgery at the same time, if possible.

Cancer has changed my life in so many ways. It taught me to appreciate what I have, especially friends and family. I only surround myself with good, positive people. I don't waste time with people who are negative or who like to have a lot of drama in their life. At the time I was diagnosed with breast cancer, my aunt had just been diagnosed with lung cancer. She lost her battle with cancer, and she was an amazing person. It was hard for me to accept the fact that she passed away, and I was still here. I used to have a hard time getting older. Around my 41st birthday, for some reason I was having a really difficult time. I was at our store, "Jump 'n Jammin," in Arcadia, and it was the month of October. So, we had a big pink ribbon up, for breast cancer awareness month. I was speaking with a lady, having a private party at our store, and we were discussing birthdays, cancer, etc…She told me she used to have a hard time having a birthday until her niece died of cancer. She realized that the alternative to having a birthday is to not have a birthday. Wow! Did that statement hit me hard! I then realized how silly I had been. I'm a cancer survivor and I am so happy to be getting older.

When I was diagnosed with cancer, my sister-in-law, Francine, had just finished walking the Avon (at the time) 3-day walk (60 miles). Her feet were swollen and she didn't want to do the walk again. I went to the closing ceremonies and told her I wanted to do the walk with her. So, at the end of October 2000, Francine, my dad, Eddie, and I walked 60 miles for breast cancer. My brother Michael worked the crew. I was just starting my last trimester pregnant, but no one could tell because it was pouring rain. So, everyone had a poncho on over their fanny pack. Everyone looked pregnant. It was one of the most amazing experiences! I did the 3-day walk for a second time in April 2002 with my husband Eric, and for a third time in November 2008, with my best friend Anna. I don't know if I would've ever done even one 60 mile walk had I not gone through cancer treatment. We all had an incredible adventure and raised a lot of money for breast cancer research.

I've also done the Susan G. Komen Race for the Cure, almost every year with Emma. It's been our thing and she even sits with me in the survivor area. I love that even if others join us in the future, we've had this, just the two of us, for a couple of years.

Before having cancer, I never had my hair shorter than my shoulders. After being bald, I realized hair grows back. So, now, not only have I donated my hair three times, but Emma (my 13 year old) has donated her hair 4 times and Elleanna (who is now 10 years old) has donated her hair 3 times, all for "Pantene Beautiful Lengths," to help women undergoing cancer treatment (only 8 inches is needed).

My entire family also volunteers every year at the Orange County St. Baldrick's Event to raise money for pediatric cancer research. This is our fourth year being involved with that organization.

Plus, my sister-in-law Francine started From Chrysalis to Wings, and the A.W.O.L. Retreat (A Way of Life after diagnosis) for breast cancer survivors (partly because I was a survivor). When she first mentioned the retreat to me, I told her I didn't want to go, because I didn't want to sit around with a bunch of old people feeling sorry for themselves. (I still felt that's who had cancer.) Anyway, she informed me that this retreat was not about that. It was about massages, nature hikes, yoga, etc. So, in June 2003, I went to the first retreat and had the most incredible experience! I met other women, like me, who had had breast cancer. There were all ages there, from 28 years old to 84 years old. It was so incredible to not only be pampered, but to actually speak with others who knew what I had been through, because they had been through the same thing. I now go every year, not as a guest, but as a volunteer.

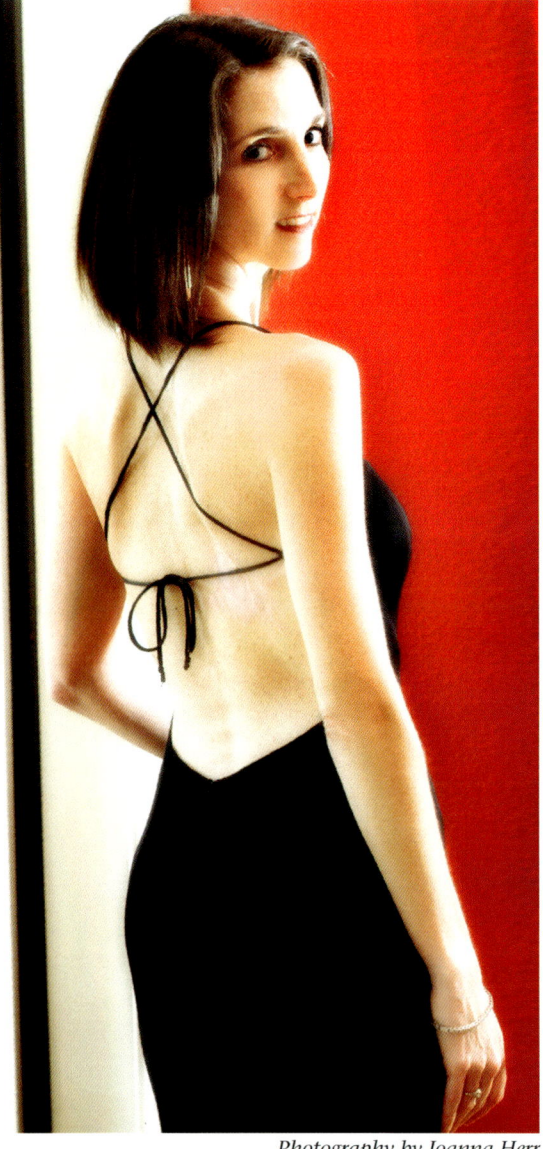

Photography by Joanna Herr

> ...so the implant had to be removed. This was the first time I had seen myself flat on one side. For me, this was one of the most difficult things I've ever had to deal with.

In July 2009, I got an infection around my implant. Apparently, since I had the mastectomy ten years earlier, that was the weakest part of my body. Even though it wasn't cancer again, it had just as much of an effect on me as the cancer. I was put on IV antibiotics for 2 weeks, to make the infection go away. After the 2 weeks, the infection was still there, so the implant had to be removed. This was the first time I had seen myself flat on one side. For me, this was one of the most difficult things I've ever had to deal with. I sat in front of the mirror, staring at myself, and just cried. (Remember, I never had to deal with this after my mastectomy.) I think having two girls (11 years and 8 years old at the time) helped me realize what was really important. They wanted to see what I looked like, without a breast and at first, I didn't want them to see me flat on one side.

Then, I realized, I didn't want my girls thinking that how they look is so important. So, I showed them what I looked like. Emma looked at me and didn't say much. She was processing everything. Elleanna (my 8 year old) looked at me and said, "Mommy, you should be in the Guiness Book of Records." I told her I couldn't because unfortunately, I'm not the only woman who looks like this. I didn't know if she thought I looked freaky or if she just thought it was so rare to be missing a breast. After the girls saw what I looked like, they were fine. I let them know how upset I was, not having a breast, but also told them how happy I was to be alive and be with them. I told them that this was all temporary, and a breast is just that…a breast. After the infection was gone, the implant could not be put back in, since my skin had been radiated, scarred, and stretched 10 years earlier. I had to go through 5 surgeries in 7 months. (No chemo or radiation though.) I had lat flap surgery, expanders, my back opened up. It wasn't fun, but I believe the whole experience helped me be a stronger person, and my girls too. I have a huge scar on my back now and for the past year, I didn't want anyone to really see it. Now, I'm at the point that I don't really mind if anyone sees it. It's part of who I am. Doing the photos for this book, and putting on my black backless dress that I hadn't put on since my infection, helped me to feel pretty again, with my scars. I think me being okay with my many scars has shown my girls that it's okay to not be perfect. Plus, I have an amazing husband who loves me just the way I am (with all of my scars).

Living through cancer has helped me become a stronger, more confident person. It has helped me to realize what is important in life and who is important in my life. I don't believe I'd be the person I am today, had I not had cancer. I am so thankful for all of my friends, my family, and for just being healthy.

> **Living through cancer has helped me become a stronger, more confident person. It has helped me to realize what is important in life and who is important in my life.**

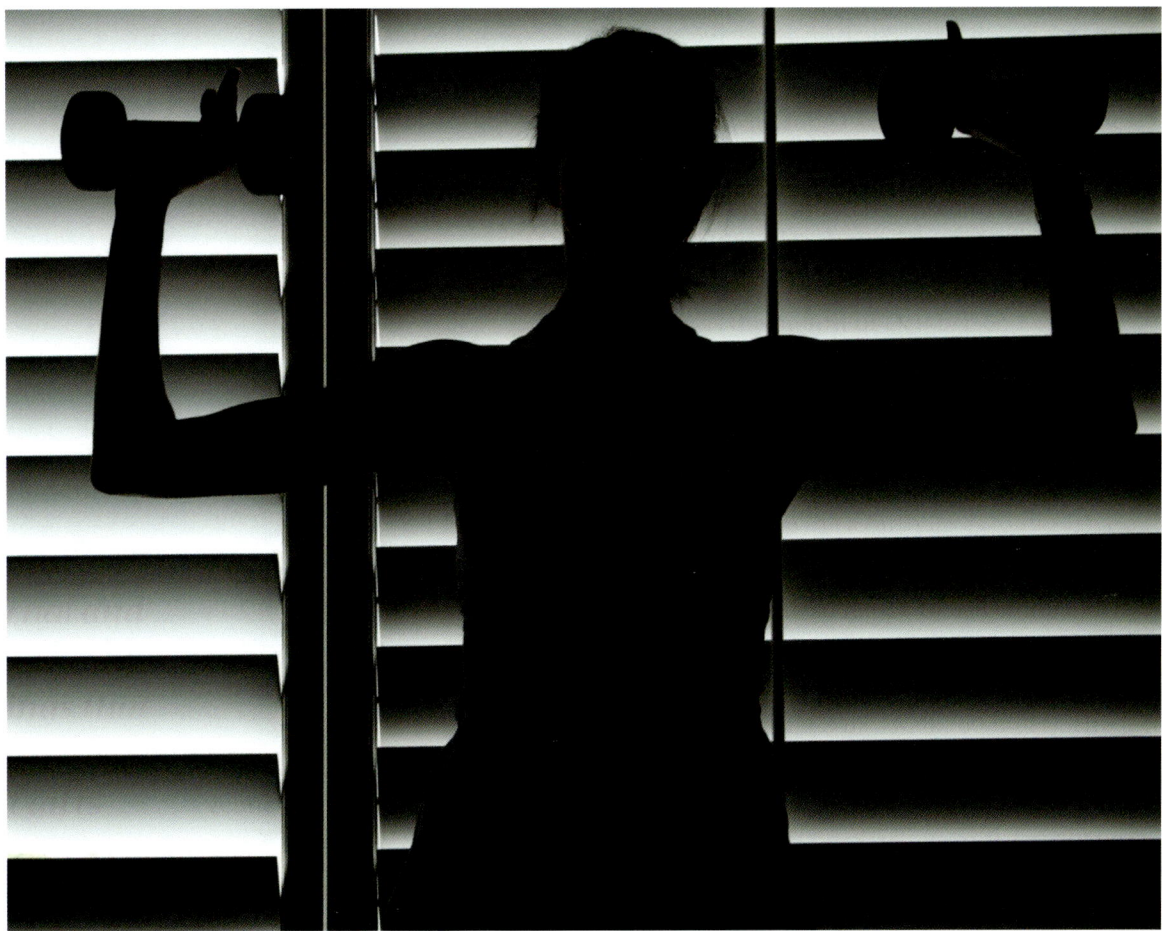

Photography by Joanna Herr

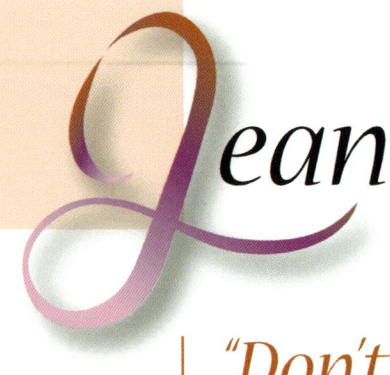

Jean

"Don't Sweat the Small Stuff"

My name is Jean Stringer. I am 71 years old and was age 59 when diagnosed with Stage I Ductal Carcinoma.

Because I had fibrocystic breast disease I was very diligent about having my annual mammogram and seeing the breast surgeon for an exam and to aspirate any lumps that needed it. I always felt great relief after the visit was over and that I had survived another year without hearing the dreaded "C" word.

In early July 1999, I had started a new job with the State of California, Employment Development Department. I was very excited to be working in an office with wonderful managers and colleagues who were positive and supportive.

I had gone for a stereo tactic biopsy because there were changes in the calcifications on the mammogram from the previous year. The good thing was that every year I went to the same radiology group for my mammograms so they had every one that had ever been done.

On the day that I received the call from the radiologist, I was preparing to attend a meeting outside of the office. He calls me and the minute he began with the words, "I'm sorry", etc., my heart skipped a beat. I asked him if he could just tell my Dr. and he said no, he had to tell me. I can't even remember everything that he said, but when I hung up, I immediately called my Dr.'s office and asked to speak to him. He was busy at the time so I left a message for him. When he called me back at work, everybody was gone except my boss and he told her to have me call him at his home that evening.

> *He calls me and the minute he began with the words, "I'm sorry," etc., my heart skipped a beat.*

He was so wonderful and reassured me that I wasn't going to die, which was my greatest fear. He had me immediately come in to see him, gave me a book to read and asked me if I wanted a second opinion, which I didn't as I trusted him completely. What also helped prepare me for the surgery was one of my best friends' mother was a survivor and she met with me and we were able to talk. By the time of my surgery which was a couple of weeks away, I felt much, much better and less fearful.

All of my family lives in Florida, so I told my close friends and boyfriend before my family. When I did finally tell my family, they were at first scared, but I was able to reassure them that it was caught early and I would be fine. It seemed that my boyfriend had a more difficult time with the news than I did.

As I said previously, the most difficult time was waiting for the results of the biopsy and the many hours before finally talking to my surgeon who reassured me everything was going to be OK. What I struggled with the most was the fear of reoccurrence.

I overcame the difficult times by reading all that I could. I also got involved with the Wellness Community where I joined a support group and met other cancer survivors. That was one of the best things I did. I then participated in the San Diego Komen Walk for the cure where I found out about Healing Odyssey, a retreat for women

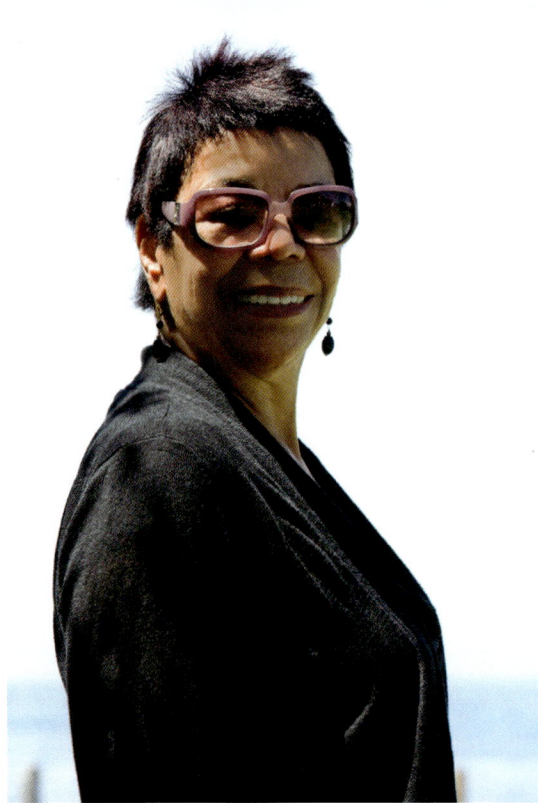

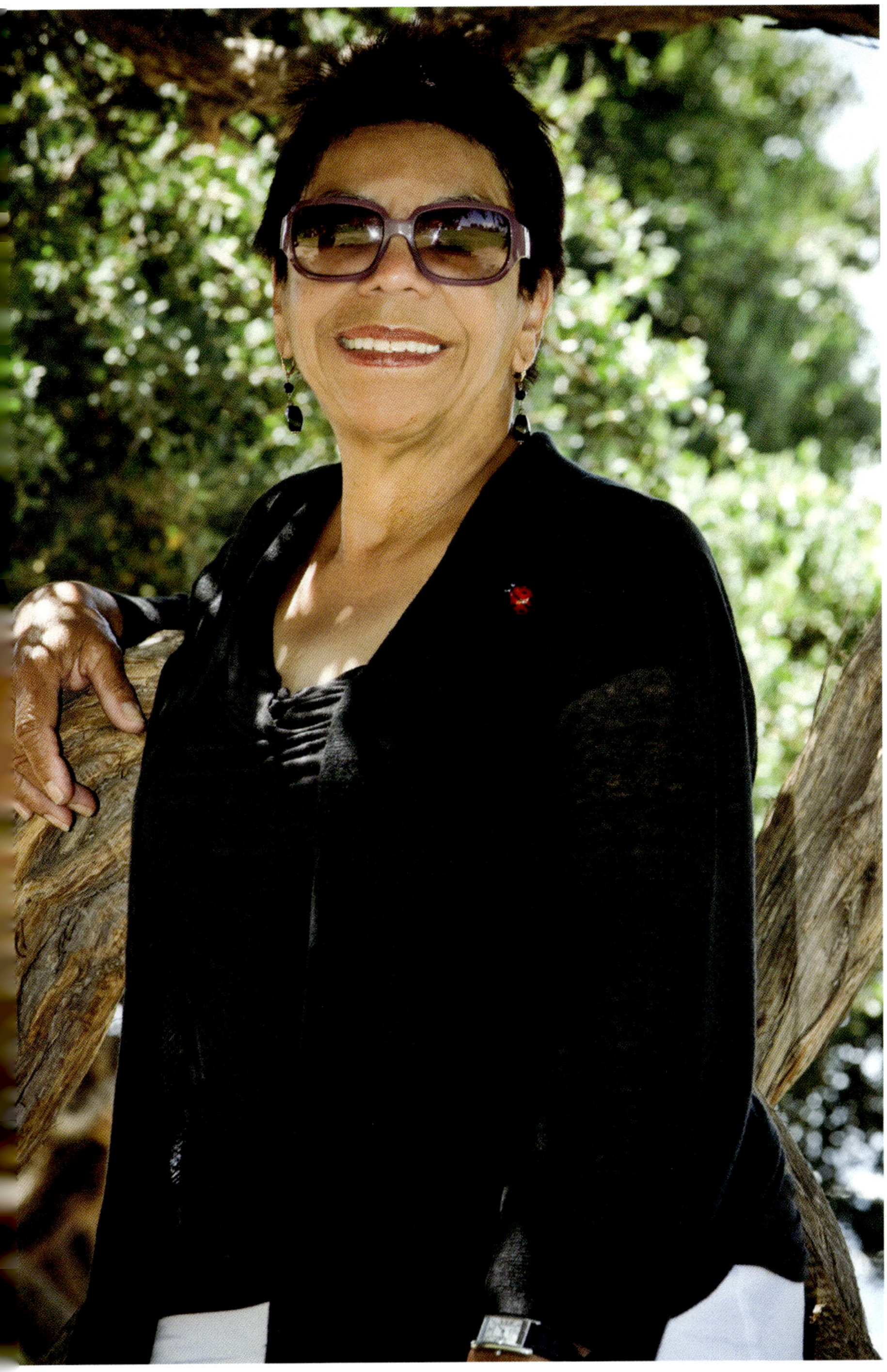

I wouldn't ask to have Breast cancer, but since I was diagnosed, it has changed my life for the better. In becoming involved and giving back, I've met so many wonderful people and have made many new close friends and colleagues. It has also taught me not to sweat the small stuff, and to always reach out and help others whenever I can.

For me, early detection is the key. My advice is to get yearly mammograms and if possible with the same radiology or breast care center, so that there is consistency and they have a copy of all of your records. Also, do breast self-exams. You have to trust your own intuition. If you think something is not right and the Dr. says let's wait and see, get a second opinion.

I am proudest of using my survivorship to become involved in helping others to not only survive, but to thrive as well.

I feel very fortunate to have had great medical care and supportive friends and family. This has inspired me to help others who may not be as fortunate as I have been. That is why I spend a lot of time volunteering for Breast Cancer.

I am a psychotherapist, and also still work for EDD. In addition to giving workshops, I help both employees find work and employers find candidates. I don't have any hobbies per se, but during the summer, I like to go to the races at Del Mar. My most relaxing time is getting together with friends and having a glass of wine. I do like to go wine tasting as well.

I am proud to say that after 12 years of living with an expander, I recently had the Tram Flap reconstruction surgery. It was one of the best things I finally did for myself.

"That fear of something is actually greater than what one is afraid of."

cancer survivors. I attended the next retreat which was in about four months. There I saw that other survivors were also struggling with some of the same issues as I was and that they had workshops to give us tools to help cope. At the same time, the Scripps Polster Breast Care Center was starting a new program of volunteers called the Breast Buddy Program, which would pair up newly diagnosed women with a buddy who would be there for them. I immediately signed up to become a volunteer because I remembered how valuable it was having my friend's mother to talk to.

> **I am proudest of using my survivorship to become involved in helping others to not only survive, but to thrive as well.**

Sara

"Get a 2nd, 3rd or 4th Opinion"

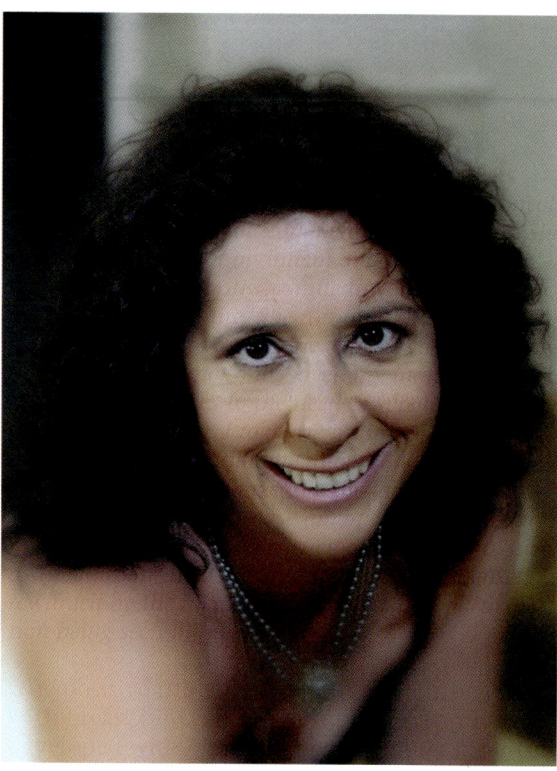

Photography by Joanna Herr

November of 2005 was a time that contradicted the festivities that were meant to revolve around Thanksgiving. I had been experiencing pain in my left breast for approximately 7 months. I had regular mammograms, and results were always clear, yet the pain continued. In November, my OB/GYN requested that I come in to examine this pain. I told him my internal medicine doctor said it was just a nerve causing the pain. That day, the OB/GYN found a lump in my breast along the chest wall. How could this be?

Nothing was detected on my mammogram and there was no family history. I took the next step in seeing a radiologist. The lump in my left breast was diagnosed as an early stage of breast cancer. Disillusioned, my world stopped in that moment. The word "cancer" screamed fright into my mind. Was I to live?

My husband and I spoke with the recommended surgeon and agreed the best option of treatment was a mastectomy of the left breast. But what about the right side? The surgeon insisted the right side was fine. My husband questioned this certainty; the surgeon's response was merely, "because it is statistically unlikely."

Following my diagnosis, I received a call from a friend, who just went though breast cancer and insisted that I see her surgeon, Dr. Lisa Curcio. At first, I didn't feel it was necessary since the surgeon we met with was a highly respected surgeon, whose wife also had breast cancer. However, seeing no harm in getting a second opinion, my husband and I met with Dr. Curcio—it was a completely different experience.

She said I had dense breast tissue and needed an MRI and PET scan of both breasts in order to get a proper diagnosis of this disease that was invading my body. What the other surgeon never mentioned was that having dense breast tissue, imaging through mammograms would not be sufficient. We were convinced that Dr. Curcio was far more thorough and needed to proceed.

> *She said I had dense breast tissue and needed an MRI and PET scan of both breasts in order to get a proper diagnosis of this disease…*

Given that she, herself, was a breast cancer survivor, we had full confidence that the tests she recommended would provide us with the answers we need to pursue the best route of treatment. With the testing Dr. Curcio had prescribed, results showed I had bilateral breast cancer. Again, how could this be? I never felt either of the lumps. All my mammograms were clear every year since my 30's, and I had no family history of any type of cancer. The culprit hiding the cancer was my dense breast tissue. I was never told that I was at higher risk or that dense breast tissue could have cancer hiding out. Now, whenever I share my experience of breast cancer with other women, I always ask if they have dense breast tissue. They usually don't know the specifics about their tissue formation, so I encourage them to find out and demand baseline MRI's and ultrasounds if they have dense breast tissue.

I am most proud of my daughter who was in high school during my treatment. My cancer experience has shaped her life. She wrote a touching essay for her English class that depicted her reaction and how having a mother with breast cancer influenced her life. I would like to share a segment of her words with you:

"I was raised in a fairly typical suburban Southern California environment. I am the only child of two working parents, heavily involved in sports and academics. Everything was proceeding according to plan. Aside from the typical, yet sometimes volatile changes that occur in high school, life was fairly predictable. The night of December 1, 2005—a day that will never be erased from my memory, everything that I thought I knew about life would abruptly change. My mother was diagnosed with breast cancer.

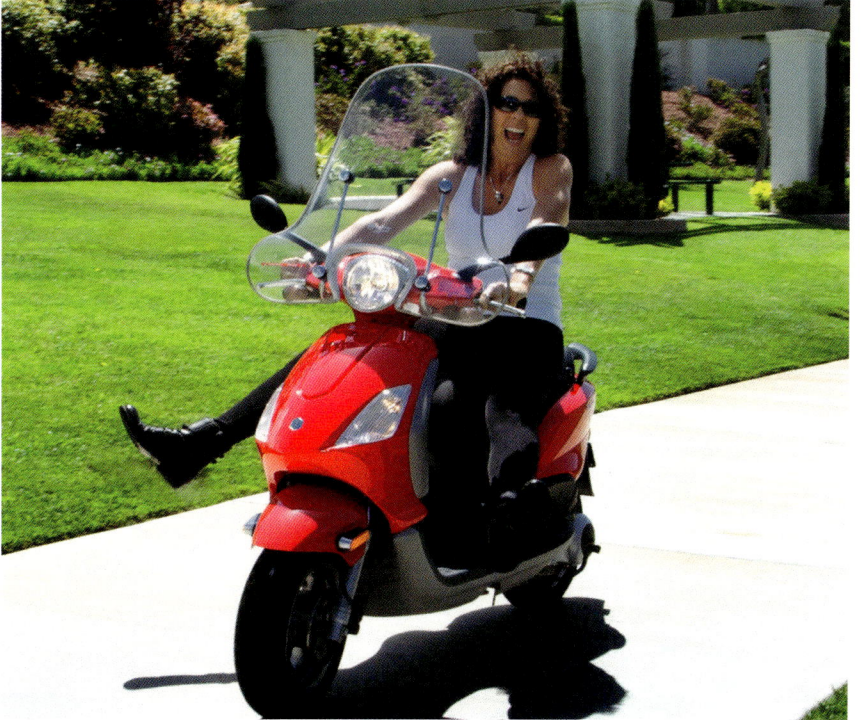

Photography by Joanna Herr

Confusion followed. The life-altering announcement simultaneously impacted me on so many different levels it is nearly impossible to describe. Would she die? How long did she have to live? Would she see me graduate from high school? How could we survive without her? All of these questions and more raced through my head. The only answer I had was "we don't know." In an instant, everything I thought I knew was thrown into chaos.

> **I have been inspired by so many strong women… She is a "chemo queen" who continues to live each day without a single complaint.**

When she was first diagnosed, we quickly discovered how much we didn't know. Treatment began. Her curly brown hair that I used to play with as a child fell lifeless to the ground. Her face grew pale. Her body lay motionless in bed for days. However, her spirit and love for us stayed strong. Her vision to be cured was never out of sight. She set her mind firmly upon her goal – life.

Over the course of the next twelve long months, my mother slowly and steadily regained her health, remission in sight. It was at this time that I was introduced to Dr. Curcio, my mother's surgical oncologist, whom herself had conquered breast cancer. She was a woman full of optimism and charisma, one who could always bring a smile to your face. She saved my mother's life. She ran tests that other physicians wouldn't to assure the cancer was completely in remission. She not only saved my mother, but also opened my eyes to the need to spread awareness about breast cancer. I took the initiative to found and direct the Pink Ribbon Club at San Clemente High School. I was amazed by the lack of knowledge about this merciless disease among the students at my school. I encouraged participation in events such as the Race for the Cure and have been immensely rewarded by the increased awareness and participation being seen in my community."

One positive thing throughout my journey with breast cancer was the support network that developed with other women with breast cancer. I joined a yoga group for breast cancer patients and survivors when I was first diagnosed and continue going to it currently. Getting connected and involved with other women who are, or have, experienced what you are going through, I feel is imperative in defeating cancer. Having that support as my backbone helped me to persevere. I have been inspired by so many strong women. One in particular is my friend Helen who has metastatic cancer. She is a "chemo queen" who continues to live each day without a single complaint. Her motivation to survive is amazing.

One special life changing experience that I was privileged to attend several months after treatment ended was the AWOL…A Way of Life After Breast Cancer retreat. My hair was not back yet, but I was able to do a Glamour Shot, something I always dreamed of. I put on a cute wig and posed away. I keep this special picture in my living room as a display of living hope. The retreat was a weekend of joy and peace being with a group of special surviving women. The retreat was meticulously thought out to every detail. I was speechless and amazed by the love of all the women. I will be forever touched by this experience.

Since my treatment, my life has changed. My heart reaches out and I have a yearning compassion for those battling cancer. I talk to women about the hidden dangers of dense breast tissue and the need for additional preventative studies. I also advise of multiple medical opinions after my experience of one bad opinion after another. My hope is to save lives by prompting women to catch breast cancer early. The best protection is early detection. This is my story - this is my hope.

Nataly

"Honor Your Intuition"

Nataly Pluta, age 53 and diagnosed at age 45 with Stage II Invasive ductal and DCIS of L breast.

At first, I received my diagnosis while driving in my car. When the surgeon suggested that I pull over, I knew it was cancer right then and there! I was in shock, took a few deep breaths, and then pulled

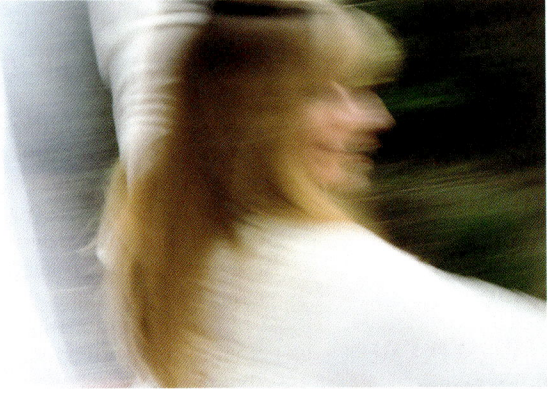

right back on the road, which in retrospect and metaphorically, is how I handled the whole treatment too.

I just considered the cancer as a need to take pause, get off the road of a hectic life, deal with the surgeries and treatments, and then get back onto the road of life... But not that same road, I took another road or path. One that includes time for myself by working a bit less and playing a lot more. One that enhances my femininity through belly dancing, massages and facials. One that certainly does not "sweat the small stuff." One that is full of GRACE and GRATITUDE as I say a prayer in the shower each morning and one as I start my evening meal.

The biggest lesson I learned through this process is to honor my intuition and I would advise all women to tap into this wonderful gift we all have. When spiraling through the labyrinth of medical appointments, tests and procedures you can get caught up in the "Western Medical Model's" philosophy of treating just the disease and excising all of the tumor. My intuition taught me to look at the whole picture of my body as one system, not just as a diseased breast... I chose to make my medical decisions based upon my quality of life at the moment and in the future. I chose not to get chemo since my lymph nodes were negative and I wanted to keep my entire immune system functioning optimally post-op and not knock it down with Chemo drugs. I was comfortable with my decision then, now, and will be in the future even if the cancer comes back. I just had to find an oncologist that was also comfortable with my decision and I did!

> *I just considered the cancer as a need to take pause, get off the road of a hectic life...*

I think the most difficult time was unveiling my chest to my boyfriend for the first time post-op. I had an expander inserted during the mastectomy surgery but the scars and inequity of size and disfigurement was difficult to visualize. Luckily he accommodated to the less than normal visuals of my chest and eventually became my biggest confidant and fan...

But later when we broke up, I was confronted with when do you tell a potential date/mate about breast cancer. Before, upon, or after a

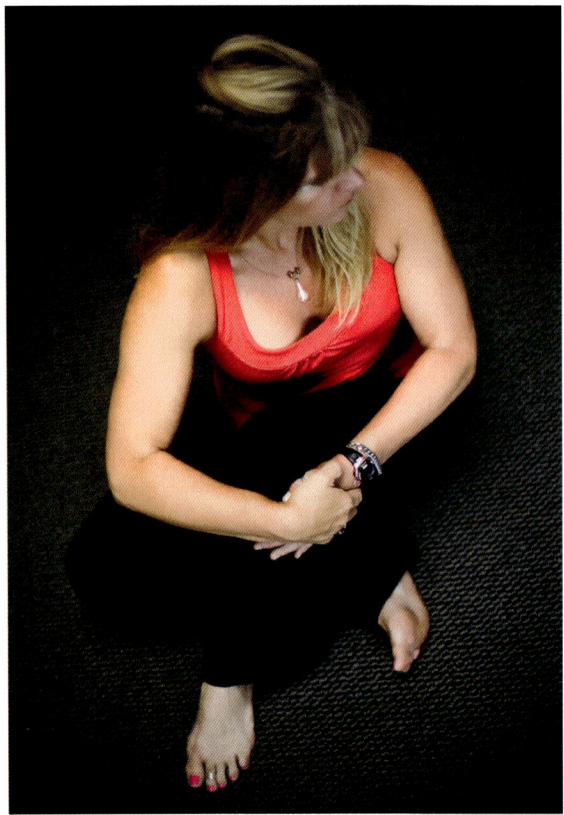

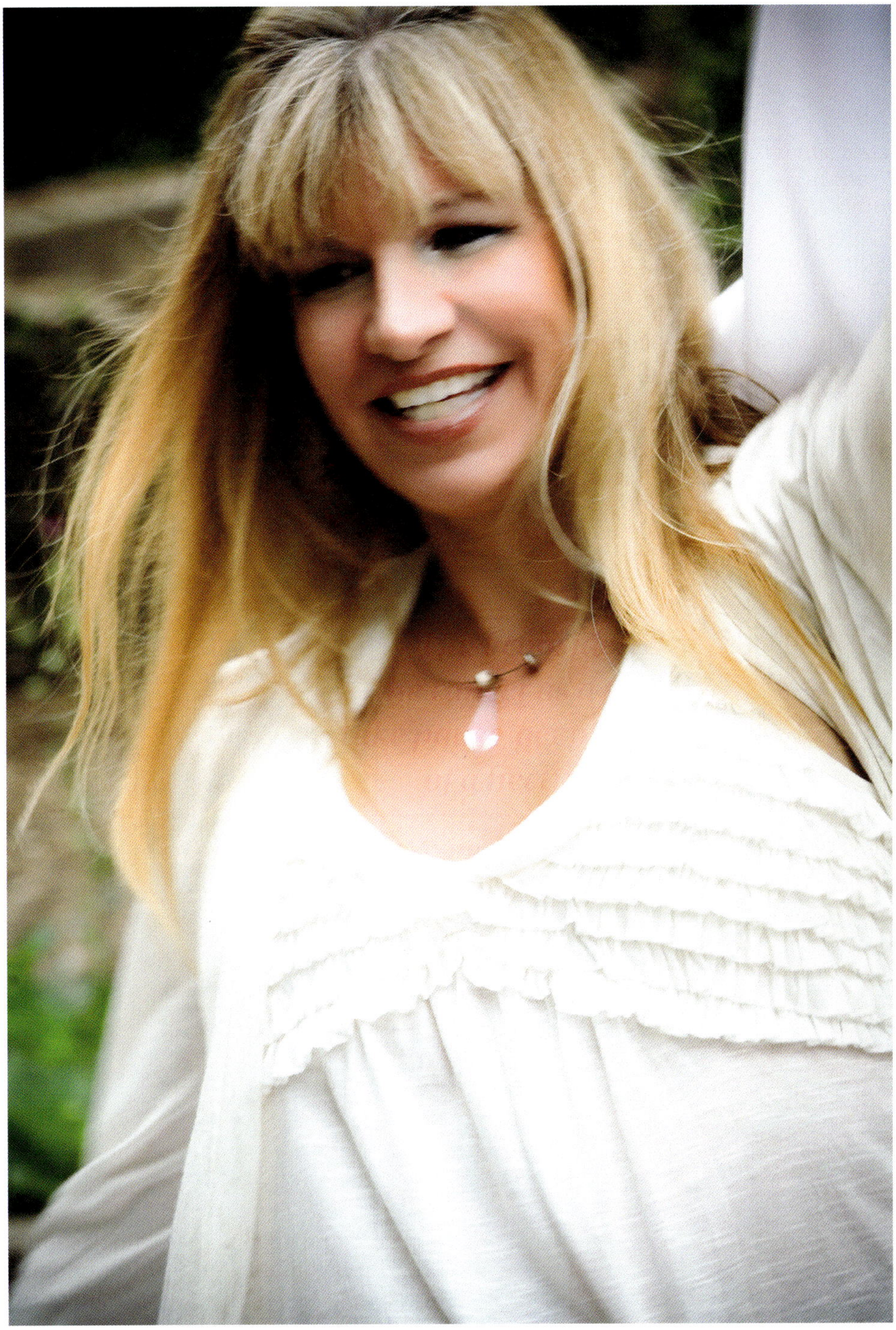

> *I think the most difficult time was unveiling my chest to my boyfriend for the first time…*

romantic intimate encounter, upon your first internet date, after the first kiss. When is it the right time? I suppose this dilemma is not different than other diseases, but since men are so visual… and maybe even "breast men." When do you mention it???

Oh… and did your breast surgeon tell you that when you go above 2000 feet altitude, your breast implant will squeak when you raise your arm??? Oops, they forgot… Warning… Warning!!!

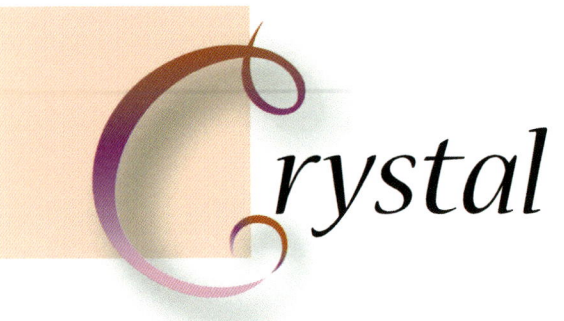

Crystal

"Cancer Taught Me How to Live"

Crystal Crawford—54 years old as of June 17th, Breast Cancer at 32½, and Breast Cancer again at 45—unrelated to the first.

Diagnosis: Lumpectomy and radiation in both instances. Early detection and prompt treatment were keys. Chemotherapy was an option but not required in both instances. I declined chemo and adjuvant treatment.

My family was very supportive. Unfortunately, they are no stranger to cancer. I had an aunt die from breast cancer when I was pretty young. I had a first cousin who had a brain tumor in the late 60's and suffered terribly with what now seem like primitive radiation and chemo therapies. My mother has had cancer 4 times—twice before I had breast cancer. I've had lots of first cousins with cancer and some have died.

I'm from Louisiana where the cancer rates are very high. So it's a common disease in my family and in Louisiana. You get it, you get treated, and you hope you don't get it again.

I was very young the first time I had cancer and not much was known about treating younger women at that time. So, the biggest challenge was getting access to information and figuring out my options. The internet was talked about in 1990, so I was reading articles in medical journals trying to figure out my options. Because I was so young, my team of doctors wanted to be very aggressive in treating me. It was a struggle for me to get the information about my tumor, my prognosis, and my options in order to make treatment decisions that I would live with for the rest of my life.

> *I faced my fears, I learned to trust my gut in order to decide what was right for me, and I was able to grow and learn from the experience.*

I asked a lot of questions. I insisted on second opinions and on changing doctors when I didn't have good communication with a doctor. I talked to other women who were breast cancer survivors and listened to their stories. I spent time with myself meditating and listening to my inner voice and acknowledging my fears and anxieties. I leaned on my friends and I made new friends among other cancer patients who I saw at my daily

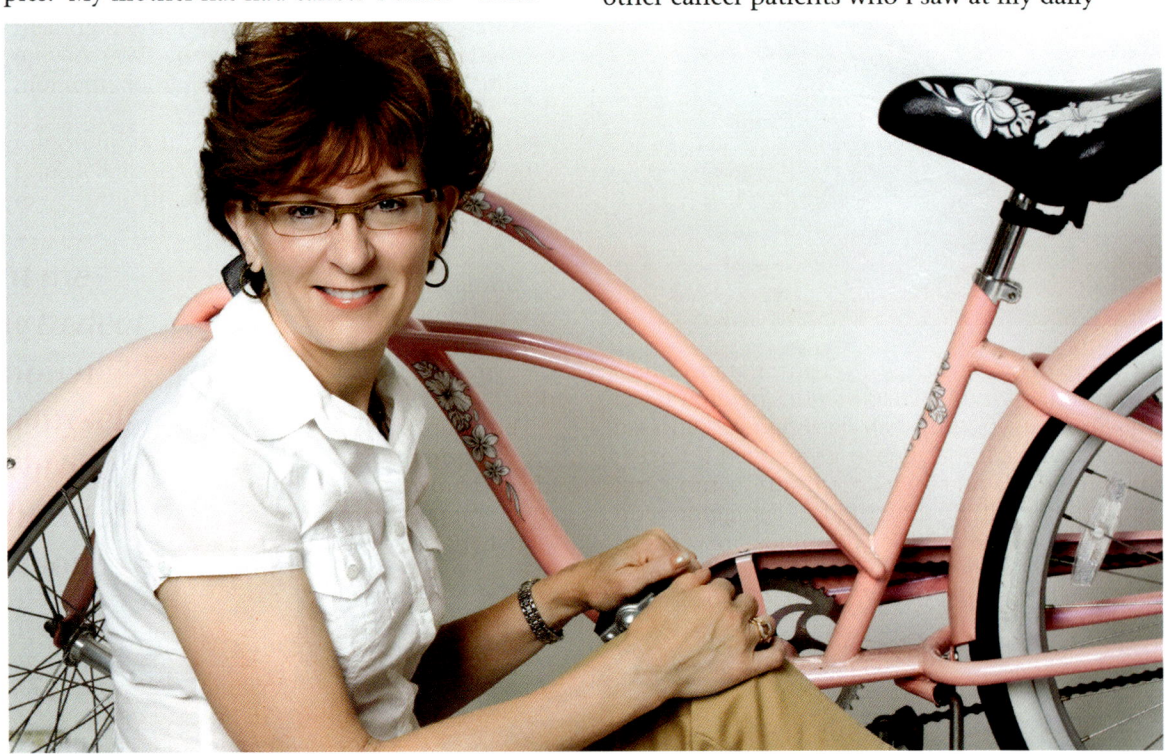

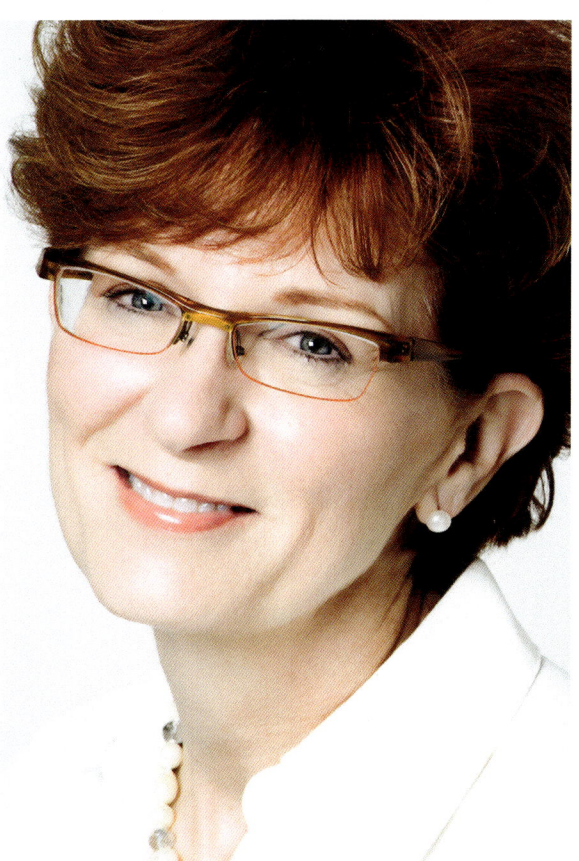

radiation sessions. I faced my fears, I learned to trust my gut in order to decide what was right for me, and I was able to grow and learn from the experience.

I'm a better person for it. I count my blessings, of course, and know how lucky I was to have had things work out so favorably for me. When I find myself in a funk, I snap out of it pretty quickly. All I have to do is remember to smell the roses and enjoy the day.

For new patients, take the time to feel your feelings: to cry, to be afraid, to be vulnerable, to be human. And then to figure out what you (the patient) need, and to ask for it.

I remember returning to my office after a harrowing appointment with a new doctor on my team. It was awful. I saw a co-worker as I walked in and went straight into her arms and burst into tears. She took the time to listen to me that afternoon and that very day I ended up calling and changing doctors. I ended up with a wonderful person treating me, and what started off terribly, ended up very positive. But I needed support at that moment, and I got it from a wonderful friend.

I'm proud of myself for finding the courage that I needed at 32 to make difficult decisions about my treatment and to have lived to know that I made the right choices!

> *Cancer taught me how to live—how to deal with the unknown, how to believe in myself, how to breathe through each day, and how to be a better person.*

Knowing that I'm not alone in my experiences and that so many others have lived through enormous challenges—far greater than I have faced—with grace and courage and good humor has been so inspirational for me. Knowing that the human experience equips us to rise up and meet the challenge and be better for it.

Presently, I'm in house counsel for a biotech software company. I recently retired after 12 years in elected office, but continue to be involved in my community and in politics and will be campaigning for another office soon.

In my free time, I garden and hike and paddle for a dragon boat team. I absolutely love dragon boat paddling for many reasons: the wonderful people I've met, the challenge of learning a new sport and how to work together, the pride at seeing our team improve over the three years that we've now been paddling together, the thrill of competing and winning!!! And, the pleasure of being on the water with friends…

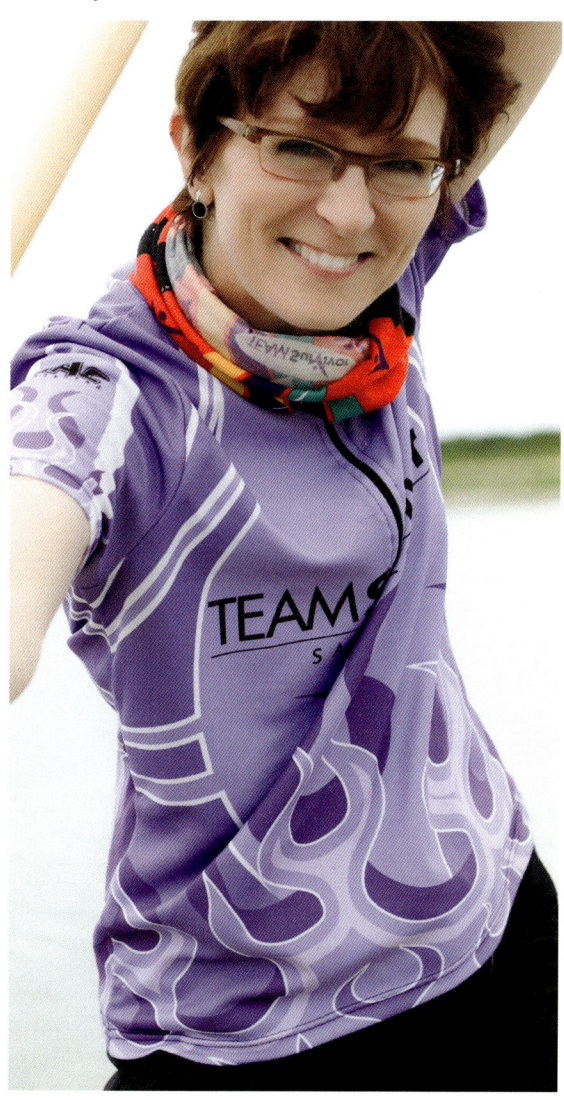

Cancer taught me how to live—how to deal with the unknown, how to believe in myself, how to breathe through each day, and how to be a better person. I have never been bashful about saying I'm a cancer survivor. There's no shame in it, it's not contagious, it's just a fact of life that people get sick and some get sick with cancer. I'm lucky —I don't have heart disease, diabetes, thyroid disease, or any host of other ailments!

TEAM Survivor SAN DIEGO

by Angie Bagnas

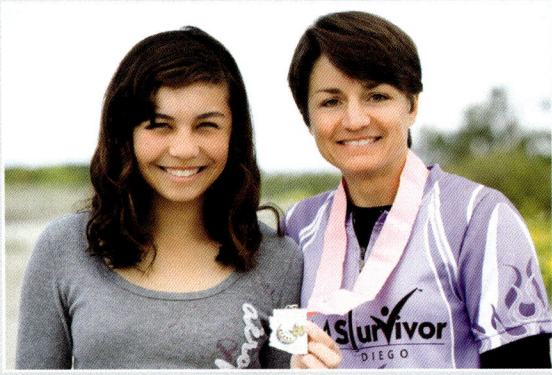

I started the SD chapter of TEAM Survivor eight years ago in May of 2003. TEAM Survivor's mission is to provide free fitness and supportive programs to women survivors of all ages and fitness levels. We welcome female survivors of all cancer types and in all stages of treatment and recovery.

As a 27-year survivor of neurofibrosarcoma and amputee (due to cancer—I was 13), I found that continuing to exercise and stay active while I was dealing with the challenges of cancer, helped tremendously during treatment and in my recovery, by counteracting many of the physical and emotional effects of such a disease. At the time, I was a competitive ice skater. Jumping, spinning, gliding across the ice took cancer far away and made me feel so good, even if it was for a brief moment. I remember how exercise made me feel back then, and what an important role it has played in my entire life, and I wanted to share those experiences with other women survivors in San Diego.

We currently offer 3 SD programs:

1. Gentle Yoga
2. Dragon Boating
3. A Walking Group

During the summer, a small group of members will usually start training for a sprint triathlon—my sport of choice—held this year in Palm Springs, CA.

Mission Statement

Our mission is to help improve the health and well-being of women cancer survivors in San Diego County, through FREE group exercise and support programs. Our programs combine fun fitness activities with emotional support and are an important part of the ongoing healing process for women living with cancer.

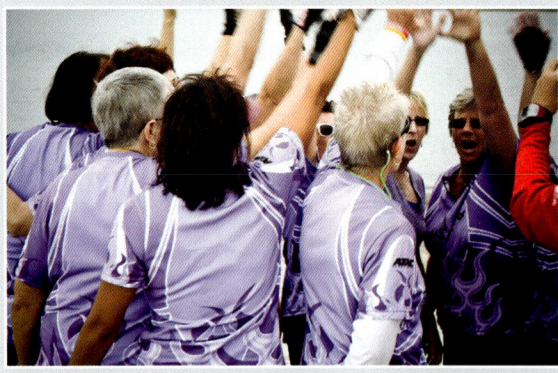

Contact Info:

TEAM SURVIVOR SAN DIEGO
Phone: (858) 578-5731
Email: teamsurvivorsd@yahoo.com
www.teamsurvivorsd.org

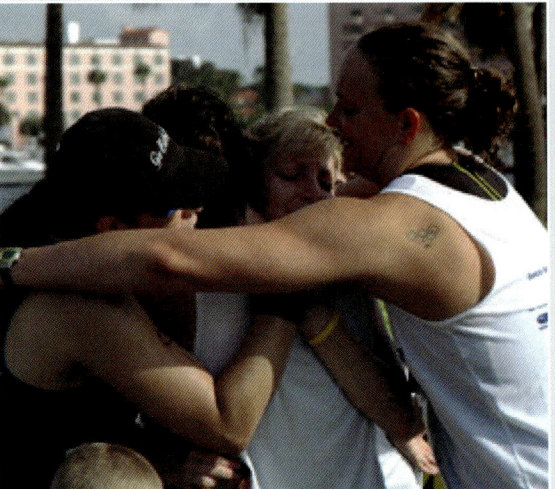

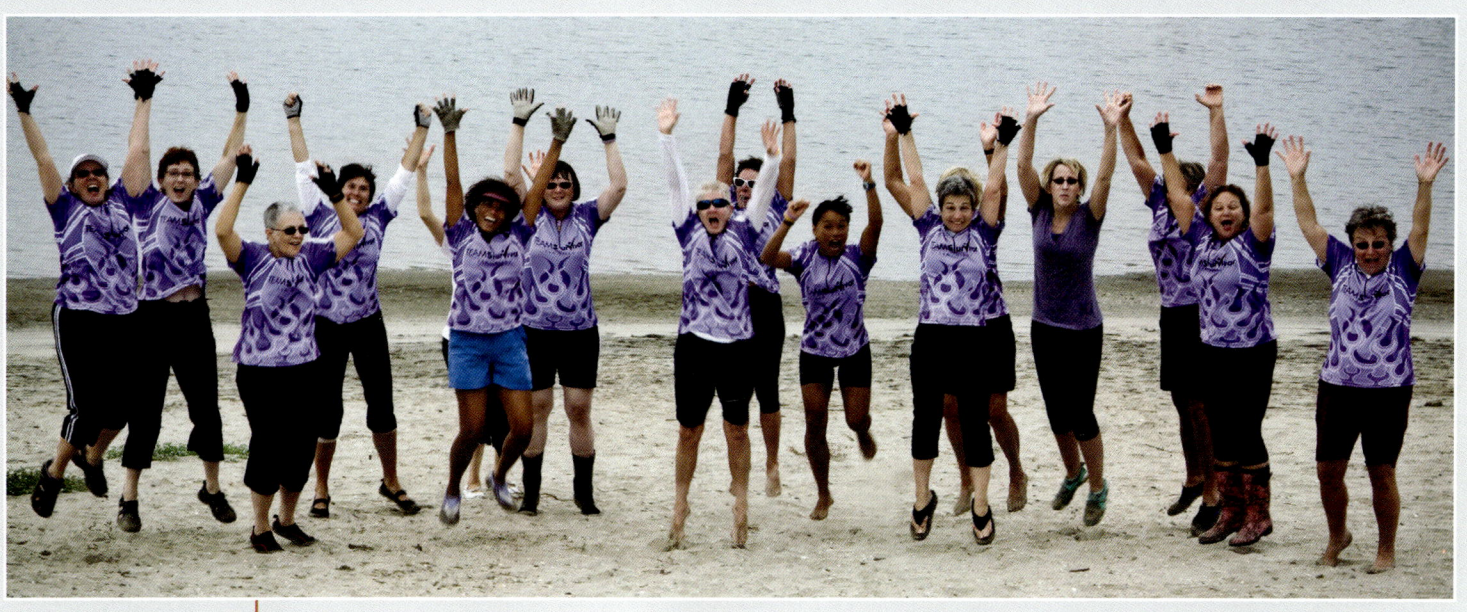

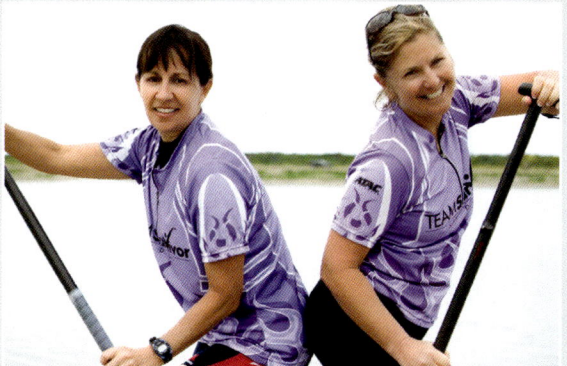

Raylene   *Andi*

Raylene

I've been paddling outrigger for 11 years and dragon boat for about 6 years. I'm sure being active has helped my recovery. My doctor knew I was an athlete and when asked prior to scheduling surgery why I was so upset, that my type of breast cancer had a great recovery rate, my friend answered, "She's afraid she is going to miss the first race." Well my doctor assured me I would not miss it. I was in the gym the morning of my surgery and two days after doing light lifting and cardio work. Three weeks later I was back on the water, first time doing a time trial for the national dragon boat team and made the crew. Also practicing 12 miles in the open ocean for out iron outrigger races. I didn't miss a single race.

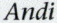

Jean

Jean

"I love Team Survivor Dragon Boat racing! I get to meet lots of women from a wide variety of backgrounds while we each work to conquer cancer with fitness and camaraderie. Outdoors, friends, exercise, on the water—what could be better!"

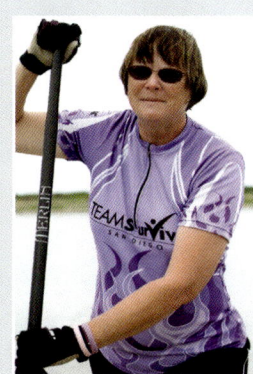

Mary

Mary

Team Survivor has kept me active in a fun way. I always feel better after a session on the water!

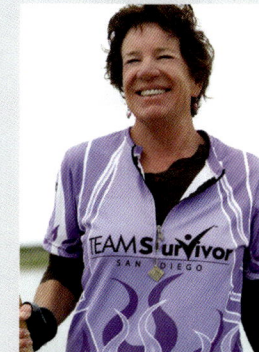

Kim

Kim

It is not about fighting dying, something we will all do. It's about living every day. Thank you SDTS for helping me live every day. I am honored and blessed to be apart of such a special and rocking hard team of ladies.

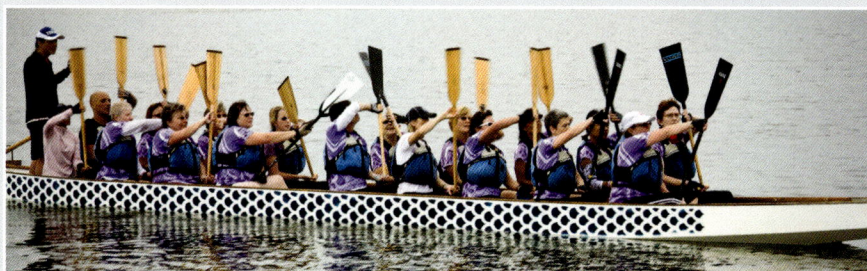

page 53

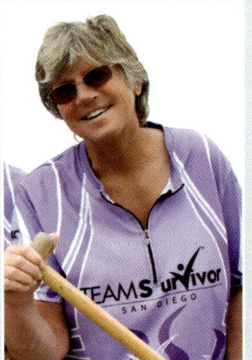
Ann

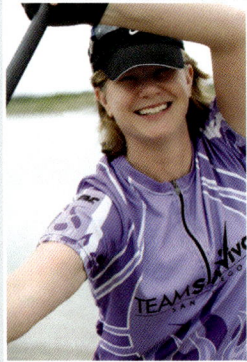
Trisha

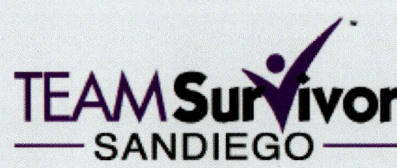

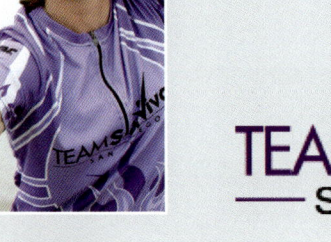
Donna

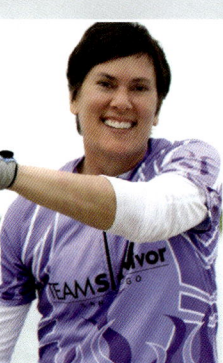
Susan

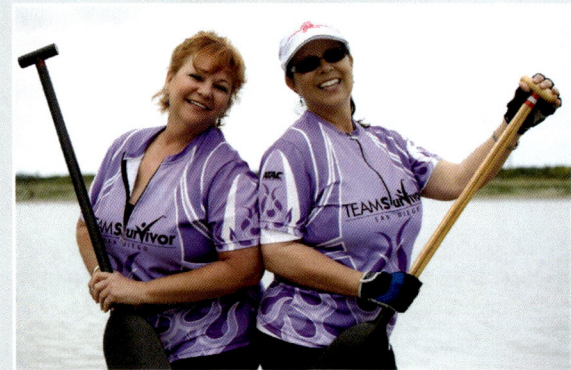
Lucy   *Penny*

Cheance... the coach

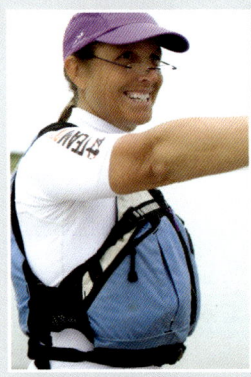

They did great—we had a our typical battle with the Central Coast (Team) SurvivOars. We actually surged past them in the semi—finished ahead of them by a dragon's nostril. Then the second heat we battled it out again, and this time they edged us out. They got the gold in the Survivor race and we got the silver, then we raced in the Women's C final, and fought to the finish- every stroke mattered- it was another photo finish- no one could call it—we waited for the posting on the results board—a GOLD in that race.

They are FANTASTIC! And have improved leaps and bounds in race execution—they are focused and determined. They held onto their start and powered thru the middle of the race, and came back strong and in concert at the finish! It was a great opportunity to race with them.

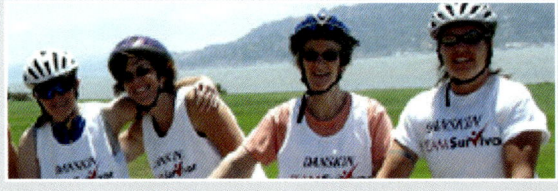

Penny

I will be celebrating my 10 year anniversary as a cancer survivor this September. I was one of the lucky ones whose cancer was caught early and therefore only had a lumpectomy with a little radiation thrown in! I could not have done it without the wonderful support of my family and friends. That's the number one piece of advice I would give to anyone who receives a cancer diagnosis—don't try to do the journey alone! Even if you have to seek out a buddy at a cancer support group, at bunko or online—do it! Because there will be those days when you just can't get up without assistance.

Although I had been a survivor for several years before I joined Team Survivor, being part of such a dynamic group of women can only improve your life. Most have had a more difficult journey than I did but if nothing else it makes them even that much more inspiring. The physical aspect of dragon boating has brought me the confidence to pursue other sports which is not what I expected to be doing at the age of 56!

Cancer will only beat you if you let it. The journey is like any journey we travel—up & down, twisting & turning, never fast enough or too fast. And even when you hear the word "cured" the journey will continue, just along another avenue with fellow survivors who become lifelong friends. Who would have thought there could be an upside to cancer?

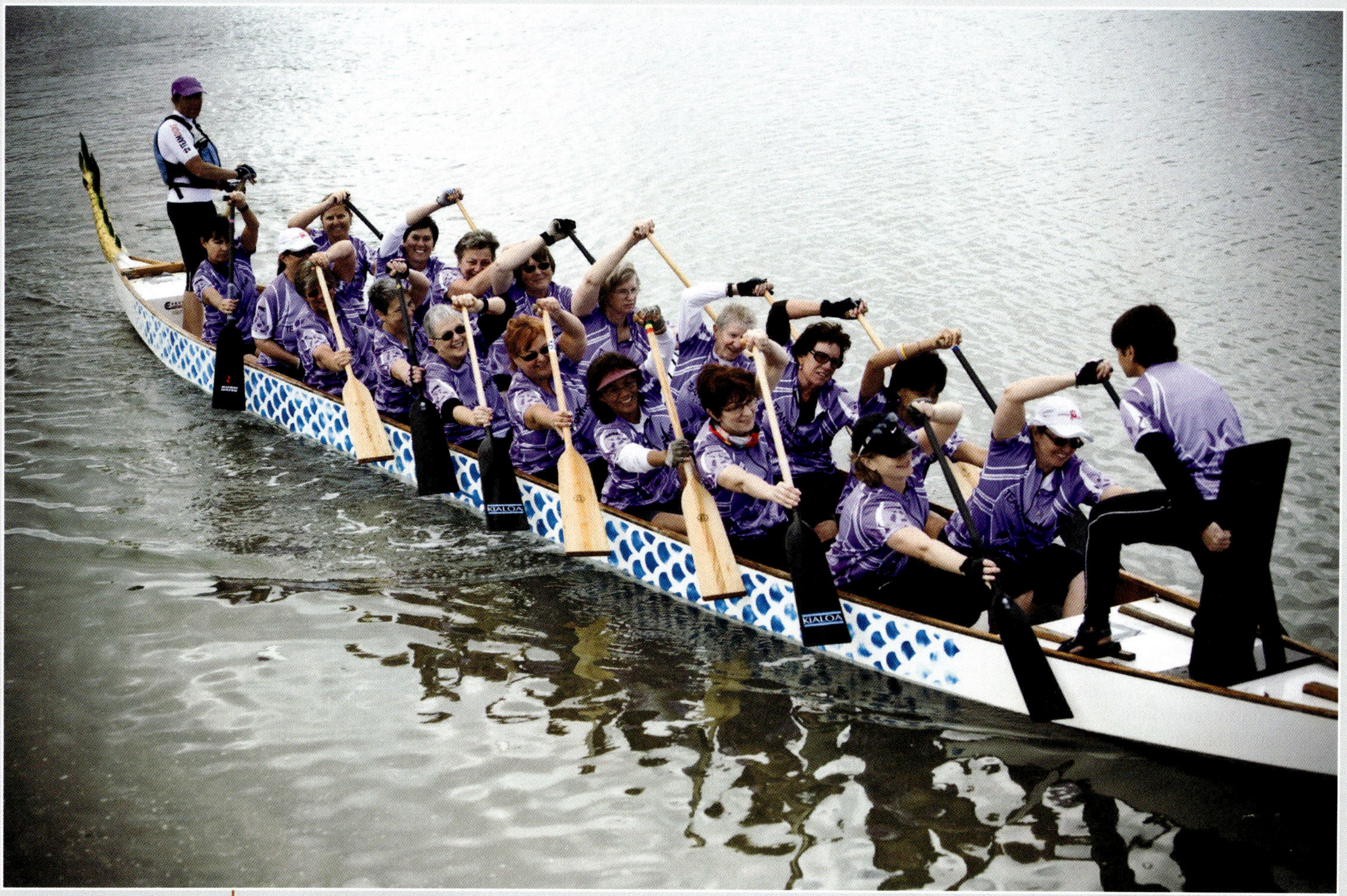

Ronni

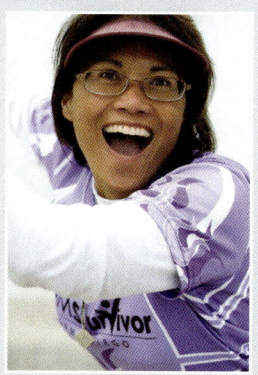
Ronni

When I was diagnosed at the age of 38, I was running 4-5 miles a day and eating healthy. My physician wanted me to wait until 40 for a mammogram since my risk factors were so low. Thank goodness for self exams; it saved my life.

Team Survivor has saved my spirit and has given me another outlet to bond with women who have similar experiences. I love being around women who love the outdoors and don't mind getting their hair wet!! (Now that we all have hair again!)

BTW—Bob Marley tunes helped me get through chemo…

"Don't worry 'bout a thing, cause every little thing is gonna be alright."
~ Peace ~

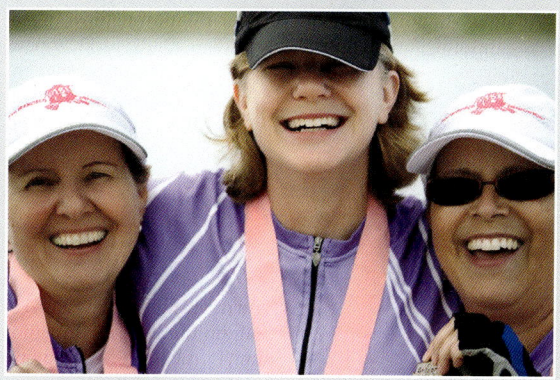

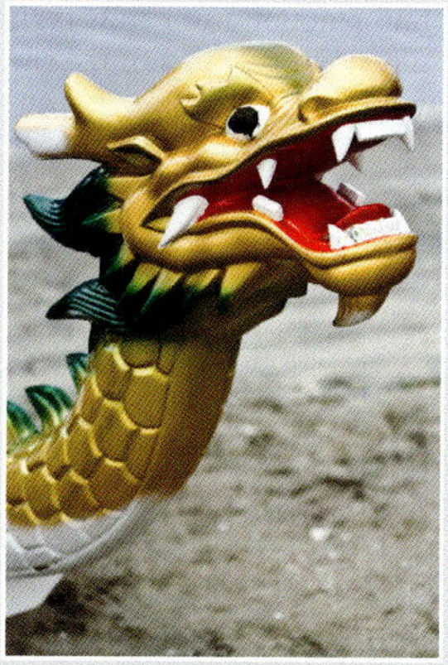

Join Us!

Eleanor

"Just a Bump in the Road"

I was diagnosed with breast cancer four years ago when I was 66.

I was a little numb when I first got the news, but my immediate reaction was that I was very thankful that I had just retired and did not have to deal with it while I was still working or had children to care for.

All in all I was extremely fortunate. My cancer was caught early (everyone should do self-exams and have mammograms). I just had to have a lumpectomy. My lymph nodes were not involved and I had to have radiation but did not have to have chemo. I don't think I really had a difficult time.

Having breast cancer has reminded me that life is finite. I am trying to live a healthier lifestyle, better diet, and more exercise. And I am trying to practice the philosophy to, "do it while you can".

My advice to new patients is to get a physician team that you feel good about. Follow their advice. Practice positive thinking and avoid negative people. Don't let cancer and cancer treatment be your whole life. Find something else that you are passionate about and do it.

> **My advice to new patients is to get a physician team that you feel good about. Follow their advice. Practice positive thinking and avoid negative people.**

After I finished my cancer treatment, I joined San Diego Team Survivors and started dragon boating. For the first time in my life I am participating in a competitive team sport.

My Team Survivor team members have really inspired me. Most of these women have had a much harder time of it than I did - and at a much younger age, yet they are active and positive and are leading fulfilling lives.

Presently, I read, play bridge, go to the theater (and usher), travel, and of course dragon boat.

Be sure to do self-exams and have routine mammograms. When you catch it early, it is much more likely to just be a small bump in the road.

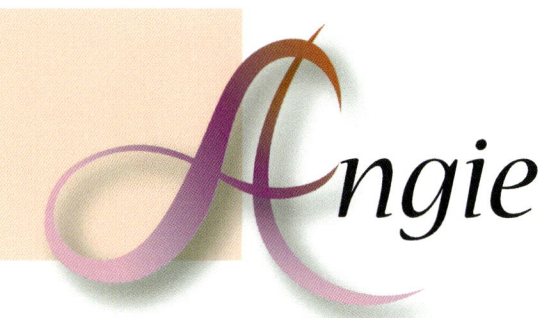
Angie

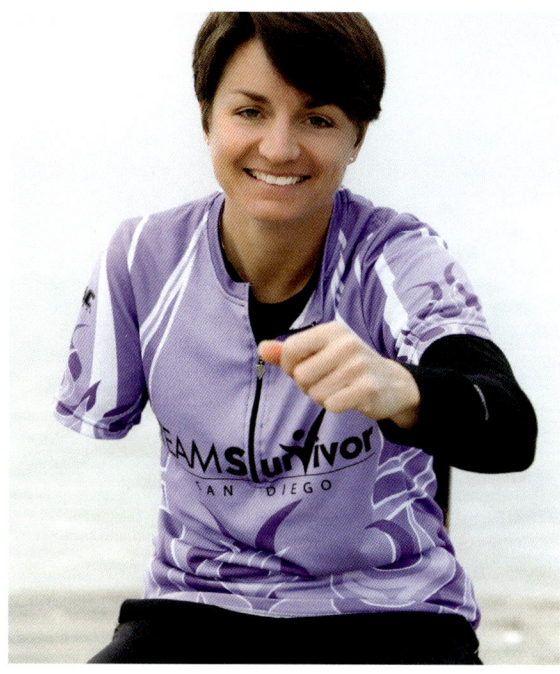

"Twenty-Seven Extra Years"

At the age of 13, I was diagnosed with neurofibrosarcoma in my right elbow—a malignant peripheral nerve sheath tumor. It is a form of cancer of the connective tissue surrounding nerves. It lead to amputation just above the right elbow.

When I understood that it is a form of cancer, I was very afraid. I was scared to die so young. Not ever having had the chance to experience anything in my life—never having a boyfriend, getting married, having a family, going to high school or college, never having the chance to experience life on my own.

My parents, were of course, with me when the doctors gave the diagnosis. They took it very hard; they didn't want to lose their only daughter at such a young age. They just put their full trust in God, in my doctors and staff at Children's Hospital, and confided in and leaned on good friends.

Amputation was very difficult—extremely painful physically and emotionally at age 13. Not only were my parents just divorced, but I was diagnosed with a life threatening disease. It still can be difficult to deal with at times. I still struggle with the stares and ignorance of others, and their sometimes very hurtful reactions to my disability. It is always out there, every day, for everyone to see.

My mother was always there for me, even though she was falling apart inside, she still was able to hold things together, and be there for me. My faith kept me strong. I pray to God and know that no matter what, I am loved. And I know that, after I get through it, I will be stronger.

It has made me fully appreciate what I have been blessed with in this life—I have received 27 extra years on this Earth. I have been given so many wonderful blessings, opportunities and life experiences.

> **Amputation was very difficult—extremely painful physically and emotionally at age 13.**

Even though what you are going through can seem like hell at the present time, it will get better. Seek out those who have been in your shoes, for encouragement and support—lean on others. We have made it through, and so can you.

I am proud of my wonderful family—my husband, Manny who supports me in all endeavors, including my leadership of TEAM Survivor San Diego, my beautiful daughter Alanna (13), and handsome son Ethan (10), who are so smart, and have really filled my life with joy. I am so thankful that I had the chance to grow up and be a woman, mother, wife, athlete, daughter. I had the chance to become ME!

I am inspired by other physically challenged people, not just cancer survivors, but other athletes, who have come up against difficult challenges in life and have prevailed. They chose to meet the challenges head-on and not to get discouraged. Every day, they just keep moving forward. They choose to take life as it comes and deal with it, with a positive attitude.

I am a stay-at-home Mom. I am the Founder and CEO of the San Diego affiliate of TEAM Survivor—a nonprofit organization that provides free fitness and supportive programs to all woman cancer survivors. I founded this group in San Diego in May of 2003. I am a triathlete. I love scrapbooking, spending time with my family, training and cycling with my husband.

If I had to provide one quote with regards to my experience, it would be "if I can do it, you can too."

Pam

"Quench My Spirit –No Way"

In January, 2001, a small lump was found in my left breast with mammography. A biopsy showed it was cancerous so I had it removed. The surgeon was confident that it wouldn't be in my lymph nodes because the tumor was small and nothing had been there the year before when I had a mammogram.

However, it was in one of the lymph nodes that they removed, so I started on a clinical trial of chemotherapy followed by radiation. The whole process took about a year.

Like most people, I was shocked when I got the call after my mammogram…the Dr. wanted to see me…I couldn't believe he was talking to me!

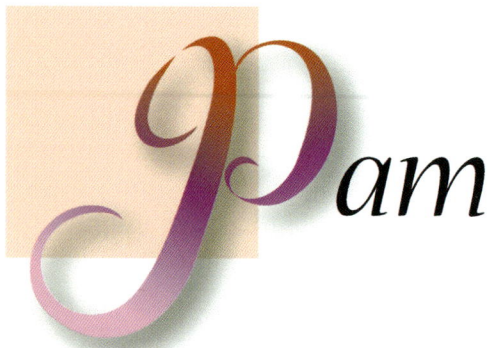

I had no BC history in my family (though now a number of cousins and my sister have had it).

Naturally, my family was upset. One son was just about to move 3,000 miles away and thought he shouldn't go. I insisted that he go. The younger son balked at my request for him to shave my head even after I showed him the toilet full of hair. I think he was in denial somewhat.

It was difficult telling my mother. She had Alzheimer's. I tried to keep it from her because I knew it wouldn't be easy. One day I was driving her to visit some friends. It was extremely hot and humid and I was wearing a wig. She kept saying that my hair looked funny. I finally got so exasperated that I pulled off the wig and yelled, "I've got BREAST CANCER."

Later, at the dinner table, still wigless, she didn't recognize me and asked where I was when I was sitting right across from her. For the rest of the weekend I wore turbans (luckily we were not living in the same city—this actually was the last time I saw her—she died Sept. 18th). She would say: You're not going out like that, are you?!? (She had never been an easy woman to live with!)

> **I finally got so exasperated that I pulled off the wig and yelled, "I've got BREAST CANCER."**

Luckily I am blessed with a very good sense of humor and actually managed to see the humor in it all.

Having breast cancer has certainly affected my life. I am more relaxed about a lot of things, though I do get a little impatient when people complain about petty things to me.

My advice to new patients is loud and clear, YOU CAN DO IT!! IT'S NOT SO BAD!!

I never thought that I could give myself injections in my abdomen. But I did. I was able to maintain a good attitude through it all. I was very lucky though. I stayed quite well throughout except a few times when my white blood cells would get too low, and I did end up in the hospital once.

It's great to have friends to help you along. My friends were fabulous—someone accompanied me to chemo each time. I protested at first but it was a great idea.

I just retired from teaching (hardly took any time off during treatment) a year ago and I am loving it. I am trying to prevent a recurrence by exercising, water aerobics, strength training, and dragon boat paddling. Unfortunately, I love cooking and eating way too much. I also enjoy traveling, reading, movies, music, wine…

This is kind of personal…I first discovered that I was losing my hair when I was going to the bathroom! I hadn't thought about this happening! I became like a young girl again!

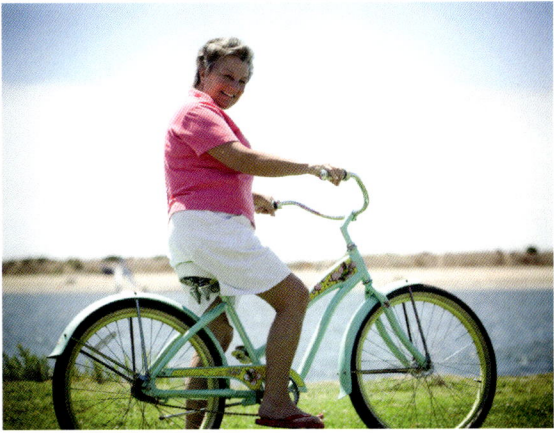

I always liked the poem about what cancer can't do:

What Cancer Cannot Do

Cancer is so limited.
It cannot cripple love.
It cannot shatter hope.
It cannot corrode faith.
It cannot eat away peace.
It cannot destroy confidence.
It cannot kill friendship.
It cannot shut out memories.
It cannot silence courage.
It cannot reduce eternal life.
It cannot quench the Spirit.

~ Author Unknown

My advice to new patients is loud and clear, YOU CAN DO IT!! IT'S NOT SO BAD!!

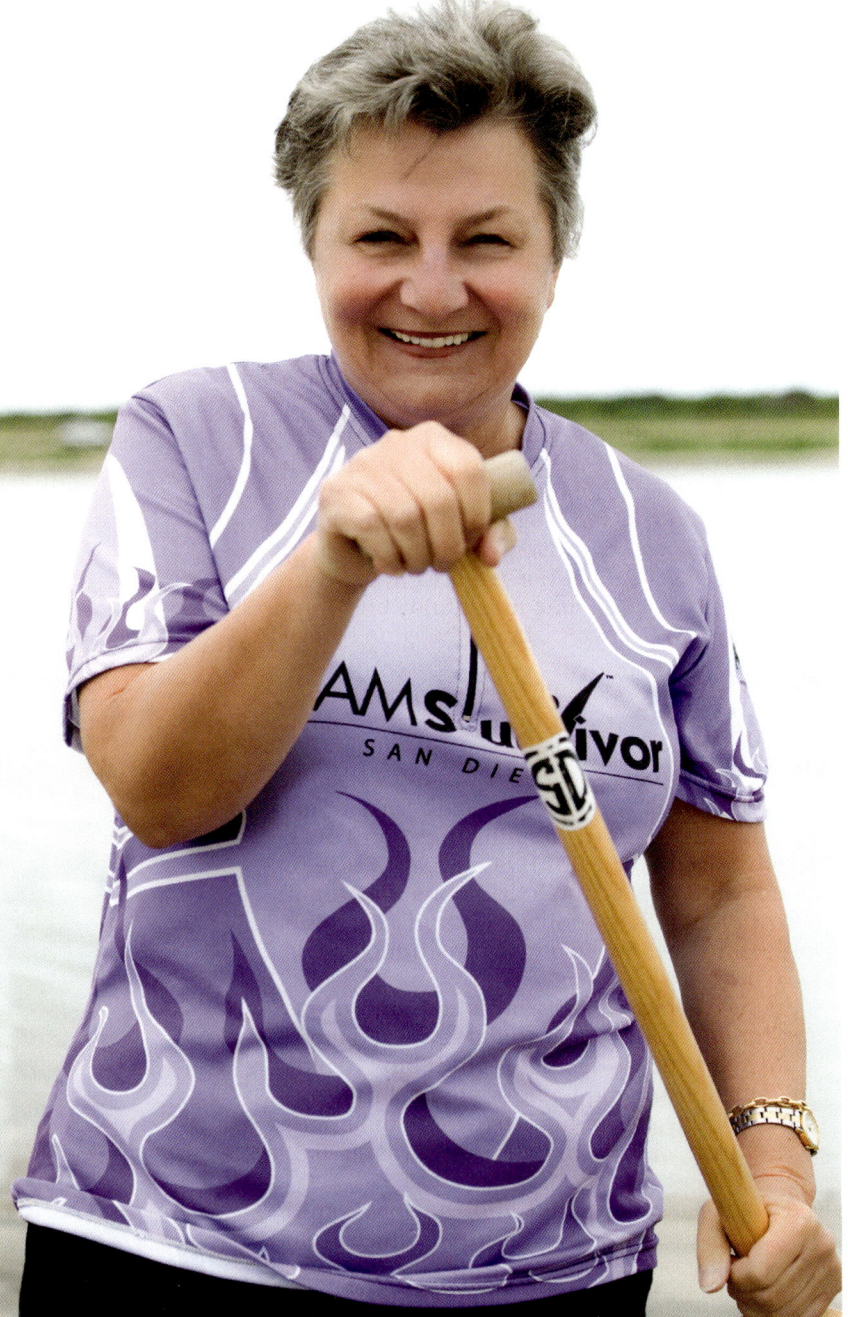

Laura

"Hidden Beauty"

My story with breast cancer started in May of 1976. I was a senior in high school when I found my first lump. It was a mass in my left breast. I don't have a family history with breast cancer, but I do have prostate cancer on both sides. I had the mass removed and spent the night in the hospital because I had difficulty waking up from the anesthesia. The mass was benign.

Since breast cancer was not discussed at this time, especially in high school, I told some friend I was out of school for a while and couldn't participate in gym due to a mole being removed from my back. Boy, how times have changed!

I had my first mammogram at 24. Ten years after my first lump, I found another lump in my left breast. Another benign lump. I did my monthly self breast exams as well as yearly mammograms. In March of 2000, I found another lump in my left breast. This time it was pre-cancer. After meeting with my surgeon and oncologist, I had three choices: Do mammograms twice a year, start taking Tamoxifen or have a prophylactic mastectomy. I decided to watch things by having two mammograms and doing monthly self breast exams. I removed all caffeine, sugar and artificial sweeteners from my diet and exercised on a regular basis. In June of 2000, I found another lump in the same area that was just removed in March. This was also pre-cancer. I met with my Oncologist as well as another Oncologist for a second opinion. It was decided that I could go on Tamoxifen. Tamoxifen is metabolized into compounds that also bind to the estrogen receptor but do not activate it. Because of this, Tamoxifen acts like a key broken off in the lock that prevents any other key from being inserted, preventing estrogen from binding to its receptor. Hence breast cancer cell growth is blocked. My body did not respond well to the Tamoxifen and I was taken off of it after 9 months.

In May of 2002, I awoke with a severely inflamed right breast. The Surgeon was unable to perform a mammogram or biopsy due to the inflammation. A few days later a Core Biopsy was performed and I had a severe infection. After several rounds of antibiotics, some of the inflammation was gone. The mass was surgically removed. In October, I found a lump in each breast. On October 28, 2002, both lumps were removed. The following day, I received a call from my Surgeon stating that I was out of time. I needed to have a bi-lateral mastectomy. After meeting with a Plastic Surgeon, my Surgeon and Oncologist, I had a Bi-Lateral Mastectomy on January 29, 2003. I was 44 years old when I was diagnosed. I was fortunate that my DCIS (Ductal Carcinoma in Situ) is a non-invasive breast cancer. I chose to have immediate reconstruction. I encountered some setbacks after my surgeries, however, I am truly happy with my choices.

Photography by Joanna Herr

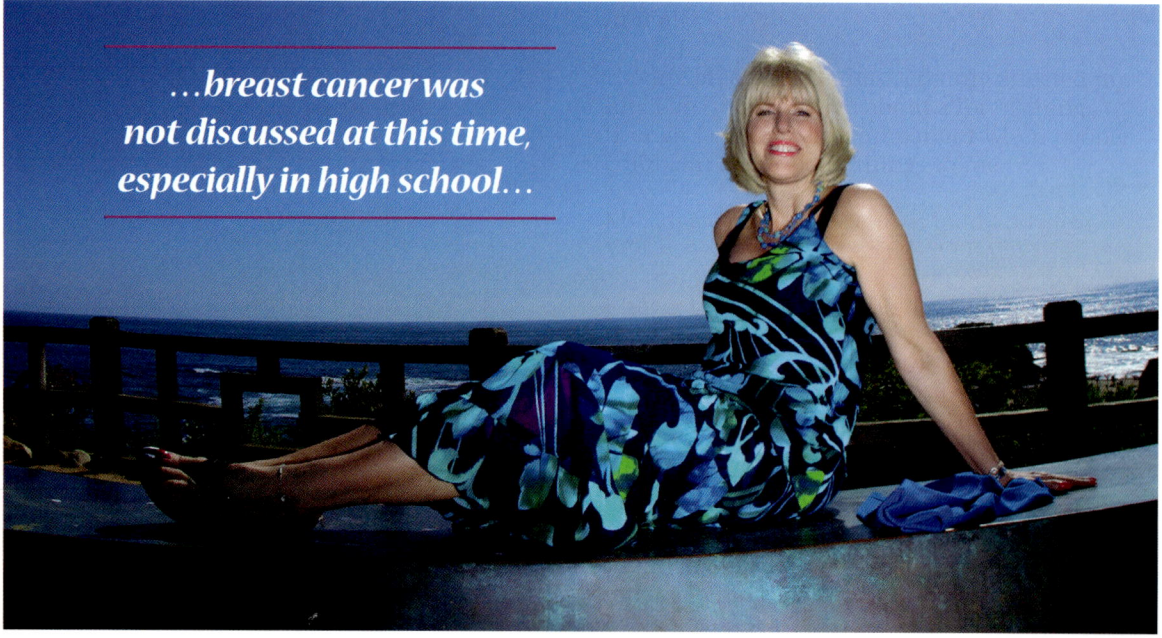

...*breast cancer was not discussed at this time, especially in high school*...

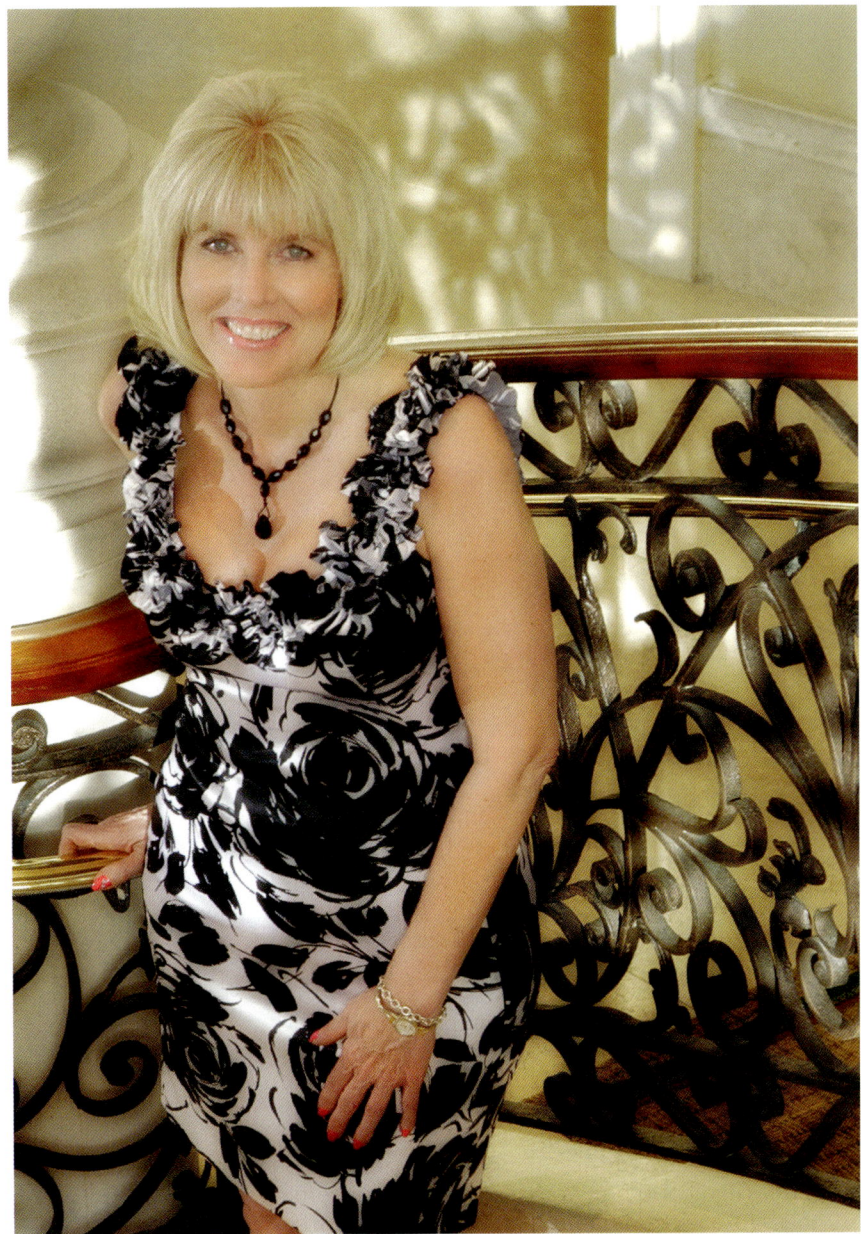

Photography by Joanna Herr

Jane Sussman and I met in Support Group in April of 2003. She was starting Pink Ribbon Clubs in local Orange County High Schools. The clubs increase teen and young adult awareness of breast cancer, provide community service opportunities and raise funds in the fight against breast cancer. Two years ago, I started helping Jane with the clubs outside of Orange County. It's so rewarding to work with these young teens who want to make a difference in their community and help in the fight against breast cancer.

I can honestly say that going through breast cancer wasn't a journey that I would have chosen. However, along this journey, I have met inspiring, courageous, compassionate women that I wouldn't have had the opportunity to meet and get to know had it not been for breast cancer. We've attended retreats with one another like Chrysalis to Wings. We felt it would be a nice get away and an opportunity to get to know one another better. During the retreat, we had an awesome time. While having fun and being pampered, something profound happened at this retreat, I was able to get to know myself better after going through breast cancer. During the retreat, I felt something changing within me. I acknowledged the change and kept on enjoying the beauty of my surroundings and the company of my current and new friends. I realized the changes I was feeling were from me as I was coming alive once again. That night, while participating in the Fashion Show, I realized that I had felt like a closed rose bud when I arrived at the retreat and now I was blossoming into a beautiful, glowing rose. Wow…what a feeling! After attending the retreat, I felt the true beauty, sexuality and the femininity that I had tucked away all those years. The retreat gave me back a happier self—a new emerged. I'm more self-assured, more feminine and ready to go back into the world. I continue to blossom each day. What a wonderful journey!

After my surgery, I volunteered at the Surgery where my Surgeon's office was located. I spoke to women who were newly diagnosed and answered their questions regarding reconstructive surgery. I was my Plastic Surgeon's "breast model". In helping other women with their breast cancer, I was also healing during this time. I volunteered at the Center for 4 1/2 years. My time there was quite rewarding. I branched out my volunteer activities to Susan G. Komen for the Cure. I volunteered at many of their fundraising events and for the last 5 years, my girlfriend, Jane Sussman and I have been Co-Captains for the I AM THE CURE educational piece at the annual Race for the Cure in Fashion Island. Recently we had 275 high school students from the area carrying the educational message during the race!

> *I have met inspiring, courageous, compassionate women that I wouldn't have had the opportunity to meet and get to know had it not been for breast cancer.*

Throughout my journey, I continued to have a positive outlook. I had moments where I would feel sad and throw a pity party for myself, however, I gave myself one hour to feel sad and then it was time to move on. Today, I still look at life in a positive way. I exercise regularly, attend yoga and Qi-Gong classes, share my time with family and friends and make crystal jewelry (a talent that surfaced during my healing process!). Life is good, and I continue my fight against breast cancer and give of my time to various breast cancer organizations.

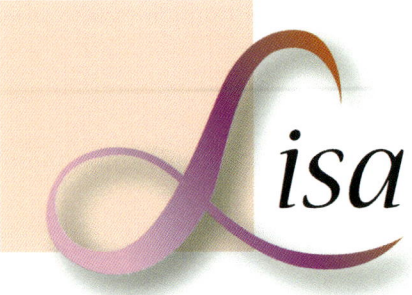

Lisa

"Next to Flossing"

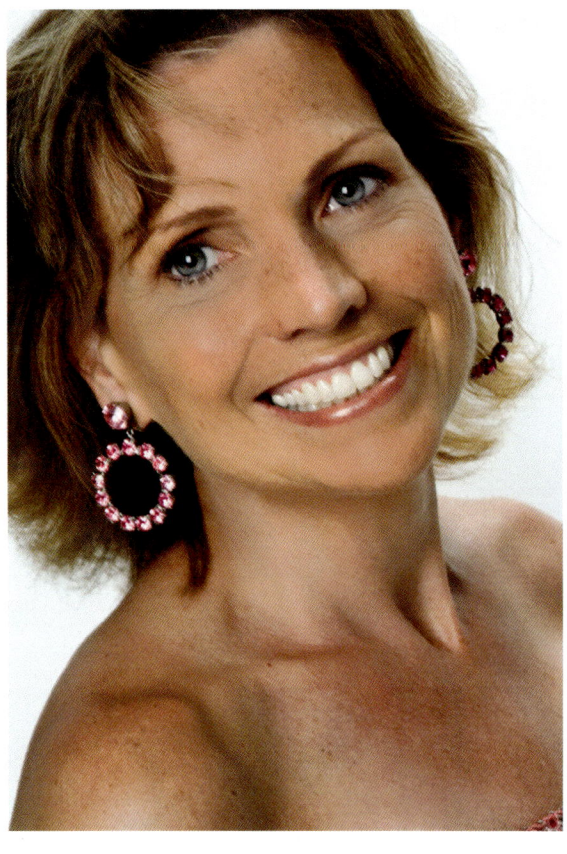

It's amazing what we make time for when we really love it. As a child, I can remember spending entire weekends on the floor building elaborate mountain chalets out of my Lincoln Logs. Fast forward to 2009, as a (reasonably) responsible single mother of three, I had learned to temper my creative passions with the realization that there are just some things we have to do whether we like it or not.

The most eye-rolling "have to do's" in my opinion were: a) flossing my teeth, and b) conducting breast self-examinations.

It was just two weeks after I received the form letter stating that my most recent annual mammogram was clear that I found my lump. It felt very small and round...just like a pearl. But I knew instantly it was not supposed to be there, and although the biopsy results were yet two weeks away—I knew it was cancer. My doctor's call to me on March 9, 2009 confirming the diagnosis was simply a formality. The tumor had not shown up on the mammogram earlier in the month as it was too close to the chest wall. I was 43.

Once the proverbial train left the station, I focused solely on getting the cancer out of my body. My mother had died of breast cancer. My father had died of colon cancer. My aunt had died of lung cancer. It mattered little to me what the cost would be physically or emotionally. I had three beautiful children I'd brought into this world and I had no intention of leaving them. Not yet.

Over the course of the next nine months, I placed myself in the trusted hands of those I will forever consider my dream team: the surgeons, nurses, oncologists, family members—and children—who saved my life. The kids and I dealt with my side effects with great folly. On the emotional days following my chemo treatments, I was referred to as "Chemo-Sobby" and of course, the bald jokes and fake boob references only increased in hilarity for us all. Four surgeries, three rounds of chemotherapy, and one bout with pneumonia later, I felt stronger in mind, heart and spirit than I ever had experienced. I had made it. I would go on.

> *I had three beautiful children I'd brought into this world and I had no intention of leaving them. Not yet.*

The greatest struggle for me did not present itself until weeks after my final surgery when I was happily told by my oncologist, "You're cured. You're done." I remember going into the bathroom as I was leaving the hospital that day and sobbing. I had a similar reaction when my surgeon later told me I didn't need to see him for another six months. What was I supposed to do now that the battle was over? I knew with every fiber of my being that I was not the same person I had been a year before, but who the hell was I going to be now?

What I slowly learned as the months passed was that I would never be the person I was before. I didn't have to be. And that was okay. I was on a new journey now; to define a new normal. One that reflects an acceptance of life on life's terms, and can be lived trusting that an inner strength of great capacity will always be there, if and when it is summoned. Most important is the

> **What I slowly learned as the months passed was that I would never be the person I was before. I didn't have to be. And that was okay.**

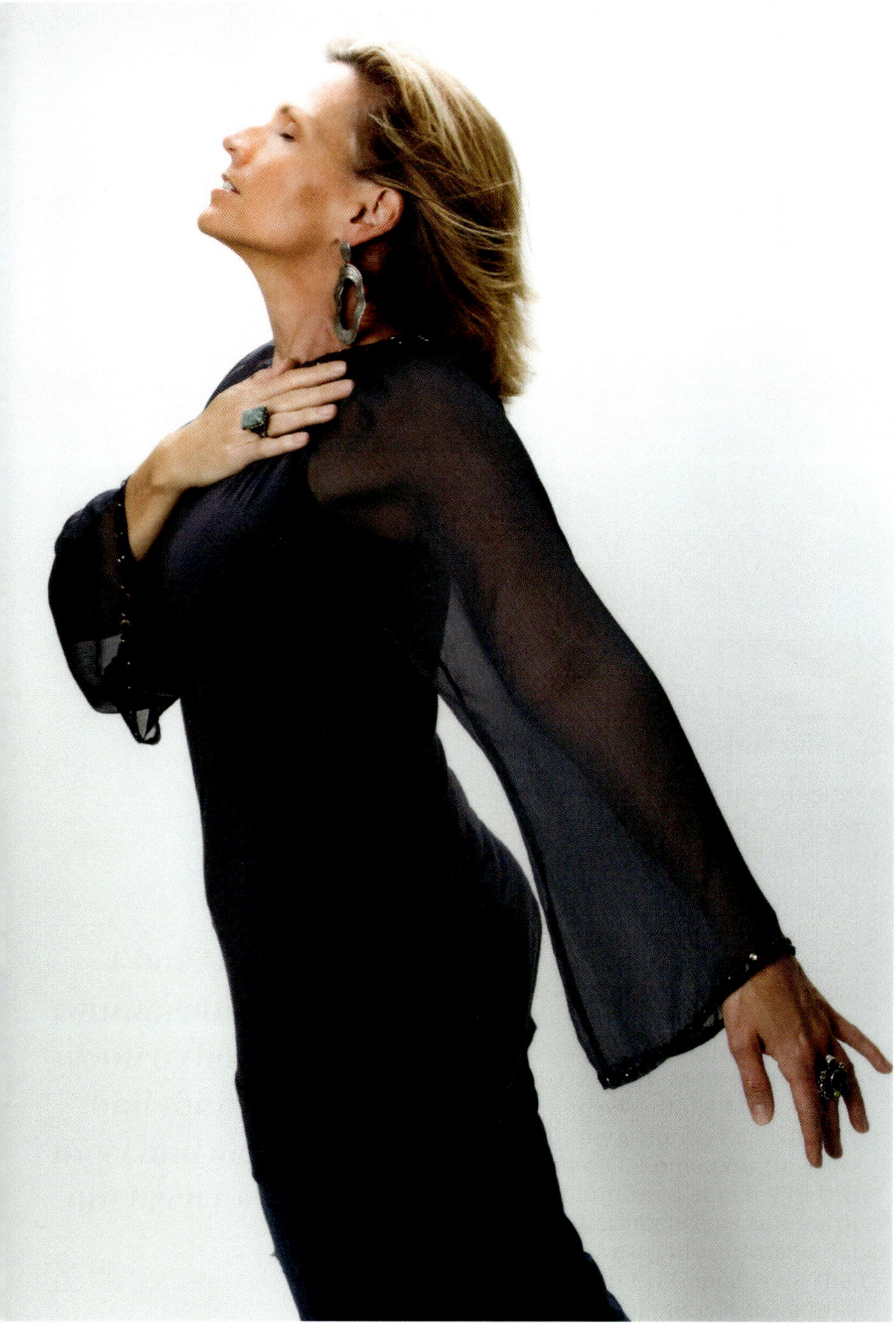

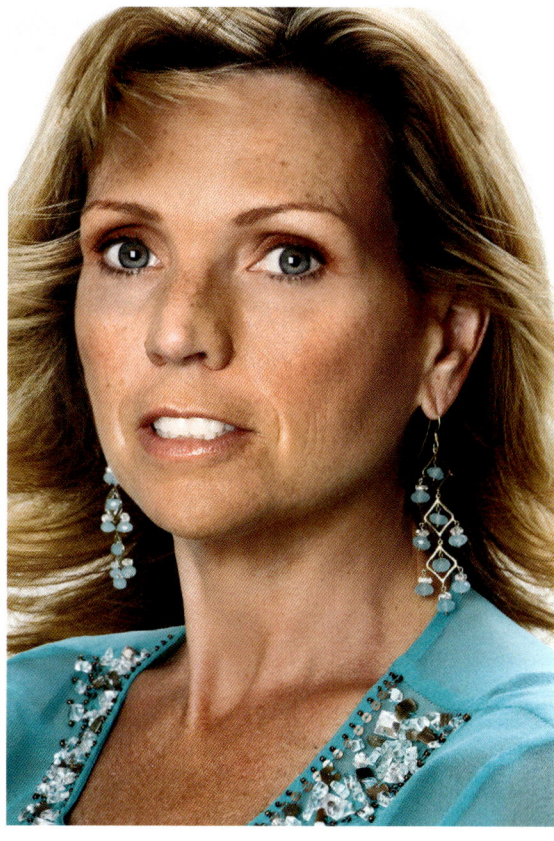

perspective gained as to what's truly important, what the tough challenges are, and specifically, what they are not.

When asked how I weathered my own challenges, my answer is always the same:

It was a journey I was meant to take. And through it, I gained so much more than I lost...

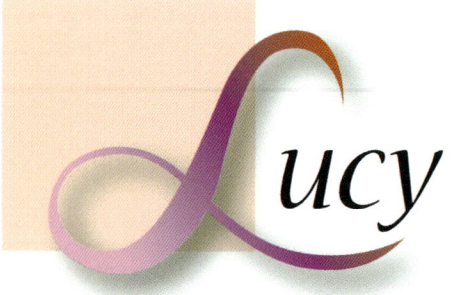

Lucy

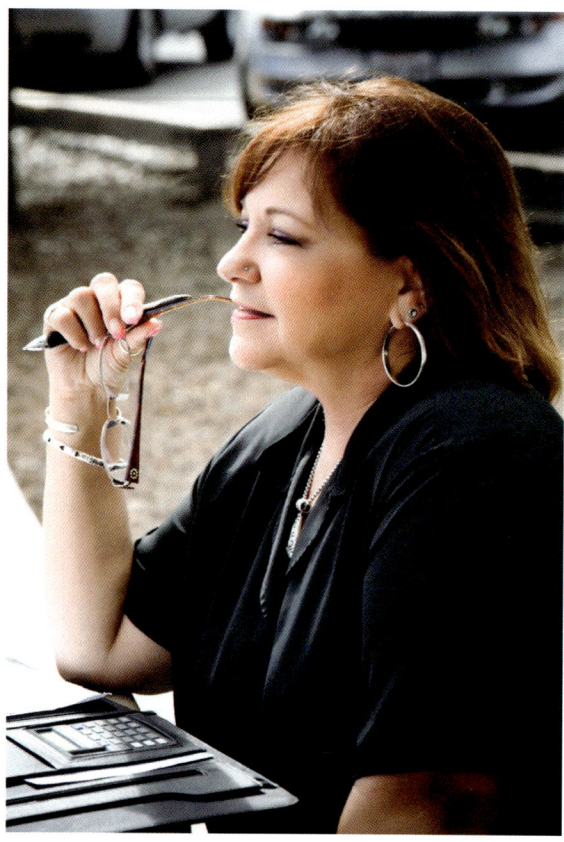

"1 in 8 Isn't Just a Statistic!"

My name is Lucy. I am currently 55 years old and I was 47 when I was finally diagnosed with Invasive Lobular Carcinoma, Stage 3B. I say "finally" because I had found a small pea-sized lump 15 months before my diagnosis and I was told it was a fibroid cyst. The problem being, I had had cysts before, only this one was different. It was hard as a rock and it wasn't painful. The doctors neglected to do a biopsy and I didn't know I was allowed to ask for one. Their neglect almost cost me my life.

My reaction, when I was first told, was complete shock. I had been confident that it wasn't breast cancer due to what I had been told 15 months earlier. So when I heard those words, over the phone, "you have breast cancer", I fell to my knees. My body started to shake uncontrollably. My mind was racing almost like having your life flash before your eyes. I was in school working on a new career, a career I was thrilled about. My children, who I raised on my own, were finally out of the house and making their own lives. The excitement of my new life came crashing down in front of me just by hearing those 4 words.

My family was devastated, but extremely supportive. One of my fears was it would be really hard for my mom and dad and I didn't want them to worry about me. My son, who was in the Navy at the time, flew home to be with me before, during and after my surgery. My daughter was in Boston and unable to come out, but called me almost every day. She would always ask how I was doing, but then would quickly tell me what was going on with her. I knew this was her defense system. She was scared and afraid that her mom wouldn't be around much longer.

> *I had many difficult times during this period, but I would say the most difficult was when I lost my prettiness.*

My treatment was very aggressive. Because my cancer was diagnosed at a late stage, my oncologist and surgeon thought it was best to treat it aggressively. My tumor was 7 x 6 x 3 cm. Due to the size of the tumor, a radical bilateral mastectomy was performed along with the removal of 19 lymph nodes. Out of the 19 lymph nodes, 7 were cancerous. The tumor was located in the lobes where milk is made. It wasn't detectable with a mammogram, just one of the facts I didn't know about breast cancer, and which is why, even though I had been having mammograms since my early 30's, it hadn't shown up in previous tests. My doctors also informed me that I had had it since I was about 40 years old, at least 5-6 years before feeling the actual lump. I choose to have reconstructive surgery two years later as well as a prophylactic, skin saving mastectomy of my healthy breast. I choose to do this after much research and discussion with my oncologist. She didn't think I needed to do it, but I decided to do it when I was told the chance of me getting the same cancer in the other breast was 80%. Along with the fact my cancer wasn't/isn't detected with a mammogram, I can now breathe a little easier knowing I have reduced my risk dramatically.

I had many difficult times during this period, but I would say the most difficult was when I lost my prettiness. For me, I had always been an attractive, pretty woman but after my surgery, and after taking the high doses of steroids, I lost my prettiness. I gained over 50 lbs during my treatment. Six months after treatment, I was diagnosed with Hashimoto's Disease, an auto-immune disease affecting the thyroid, directly caused by the aggressive chemo and radiation.

I had always been very active physically and took pride in myself. Now the only clothes that fit were baggy T-shirts and sweats. The beautiful clothes hanging in my closet just wouldn't fit me anymore. I went from a young looking, attractive woman to a matronly, obese woman. It was so very depressing and it would take me years to adjust. I sometimes still struggle with this issue. My mind thinks I look one way and the mirror tells me a different story. I'm not sure if it was the cancer that did this or just the fact that I'm getting older and don't want to accept it!! Therapy has helped!

Living with breast cancer changed my life forever. Have you ever had your palm read? I did years ago and my life line is split. The palm

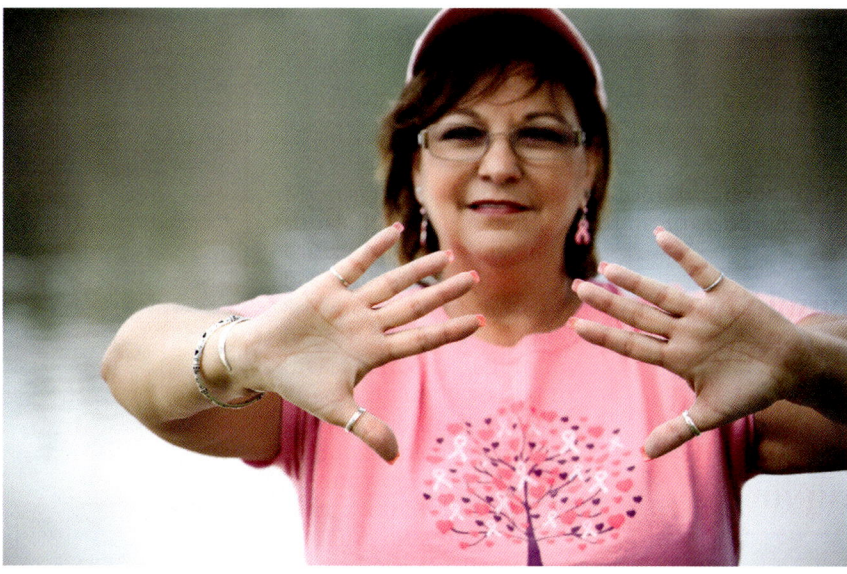

> *The palm reader told me that something was going to happen to me that would change the direction of my life.*

reader told me that something was going to happen to me that would change the direction of my life. I thought up all sorts of romantic, exciting life changing experiences, never dreaming it would be something as devastating as breast cancer.

I'm a "tell it like it is" kind of person. I have counseled newly diagnosed women, when asked. I tell each of them the same thing, STAY POSITIVE and LAUGH WHEN YOU FEEL LIKE CRYING. I also tell them to do research on their cancer as well as check out their doctor. Write about their journey because there are many sleepless nights during treatment. I was always open and upfront about how and what I was feeling during my treatment. I had such great support from family and friends.

I remember during a 60 mile, 3 day walk, I had just finished up chemo and had started my radiation treatments. A group of my friends started up a team, the "I love Lucy" team and we were going to walk 60 miles in 3 days. Seeing the sea of women with
friends or family members during opening ceremonies, I became very emotional. Some women had pictures on their shirts of women who had lost the battle. My friends and teammates hugged me and asked me what was wrong; I told them if I die, they better put a good picture of me on their backs for the next walk! Everyone started to laugh!

The thing I am most proud of and inspired by is the way I turned a devastating mis-diagnosis into a positive learning experience. After losing my lawsuit against the incompetent, neglectful doctor who didn't do HER job as she should have, I went into a deep depression. For a month, I holed myself up in my house. I only came out to go to work. Once I was home, I didn't answer the phone, I didn't want to talk to anyone. I wanted her life ruined as she had ruined mine. I felt that she had given me a death sentence and she was able to continue on with her life, no consequences for her neglect. One night as I sat on my pity pot, I received an email about a non profit organization looking for breast cancer survivors to do a workshop called "Just for Teens" in local San Diego high schools.

I filled out the application and a week later, I received a call from the Director. She loved my story and wanted me to attend their one-day training. Training was held one Saturday where I had the privilege to meet other survivors and listen to their stories. We all have a story. We were living our lives, minding our own business, when cancer knocked on the door; an unwelcome visitor, an intruder that would now take not only our energy to defeat it, but the energy of our family and friends.

My first school was Crawford High School in San Diego. There were 160 senior girls, dressed in pink and excited to hear what I had to say. My workshop consists of a Power Point presentation, a film, a hands on "How to do a Breast Self Exam" with silicone breast models, and my personal story. It was the first time I had shared my story with a group of girls and I knew I had to convey it in a positive yet serious way. When I began to tell my story, I started to cry. My voice broke but I kept talking. I noticed a few girls wipe their eyes. They were crying with me. As I continued, I got the strength I needed to compose myself, tell some funny stories to make them laugh and show them my tattoo. Afterwards, there was a line of girls wanting to give me a hug and thank me for the information I shared with them. On their evaluations of my workshop, they all loved it. They were so appreciative of the information as no one had ever spoken to them about breast cancer. I encouraged them to share this information with all the women in their lives. I encourage them to know their bodies and listen to their intuition.

I volunteered for the non-profit organization for two years. When they decided to end the program, I was motivated to start one on my own. This program is just too important and too close to my heart to not share this as long as I can share it. I call my new non-profit "One in Eight". When some of the students this past year asked if I had a book on this subject, I said no but I could easily get one written. And I started writing the book, "One in Eight—A Teens Guide to Understanding Breast Cancer and the Importance of Breast Health." I cover all the material in my workshops in a little more detail but fun and easy to read for a teen girl, affordable enough, for them to buy a few copies to give to their mom, or their best friend or their sister.

> **What inspires me today are the young girls. I believe if I had the education about breast cancer when I was younger, I may have had a different outcome with my disease.**

What inspires me today are the young girls. I believe if I had the education about breast cancer when I was younger, I may have had a different outcome with my disease. My mother asked me why I didn't tell her I had a lump in my breast when it was a small lump. I told her, I didn't know I was supposed to discuss it with anyone but my doctor. By telling my story, my hope is I will empower these young girls to take their health into their own hands. To insist they be listened to by their doctor and to not be ashamed because they know their bodies. With one in eight women being diagnosed today with breast cancer these girls are our future.

Today, I paddle on a dragon boat team with an amazing group of women, all cancer survivors. I work part time and spend the rest of my spare time writing the next great American novel. I walk 4 miles every morning. I garden and cook. Having cancer was a year of living hell, but it gave me a clearer outlook on the purpose and direction of how I should be living my life.

My mantra today…Knowledge is Power!

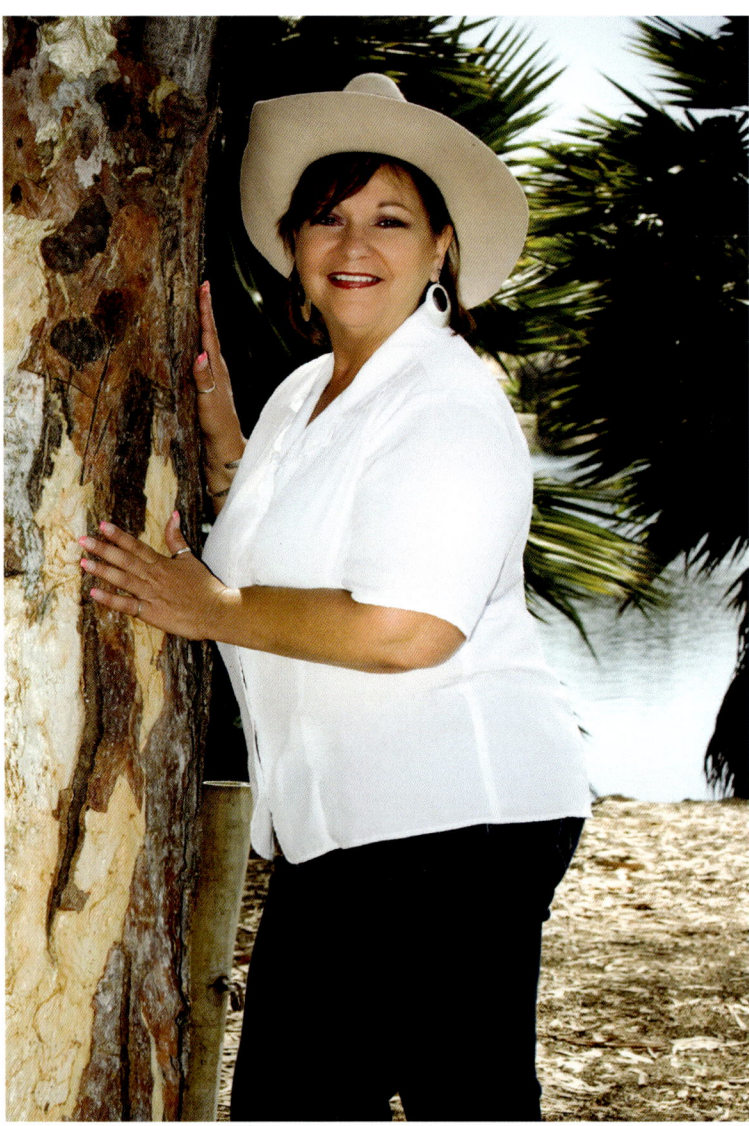

One in Eight—
A Teens Guide to Understanding Breast Cancer & the Importance of Breast Health

by Lucy Cafiero

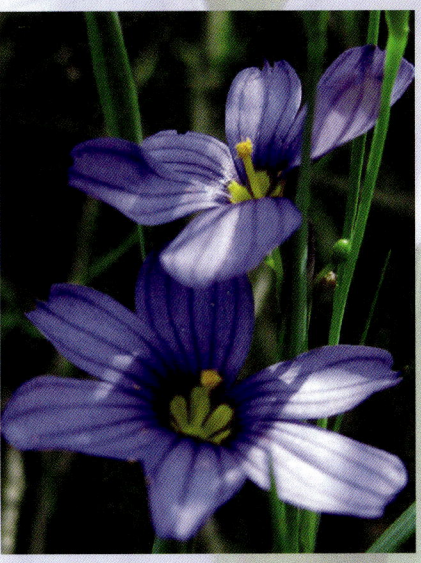

Photo: "LoveNoMatterWhat.com" by Petra

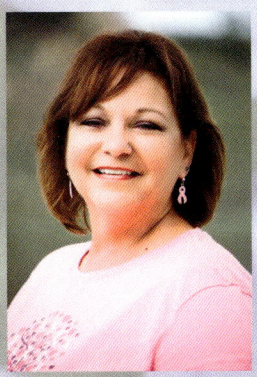

Having been misdiagnosed with Invasive Lobular Breast Cancer, a type of breast cancer that is not detectable with a mammogram, I was lead to develop a workshop and book entitled *"One in Eight—A Teens Guide to Understanding Breast Cancer and the Importance of Breast Health."*

My workshops are designed to educate and empower young teen girls and women alike. With 1 in 8 women being diagnosed today, these young girls are our future. We can not leave this to chance.

My goal is to have these workshops in every high school in the nation by training other survivors to give back in a positive way by telling their stories and bringing this information to our young women.

I am an advocate of breast self-exams and I teach the girls how to do one correctly with silicone breast models. Many women I have spoken with have told me they found their own lump while doing a BSE.

If you would like me to do a presentation at your high school, college or women's group, or if you want like to become involved in our training program, please contact me at:

One_In_Eight@yahoo.com

Or visit our Facebook page:

www.facebook.com/pages/One-in-Eight/133148596738808

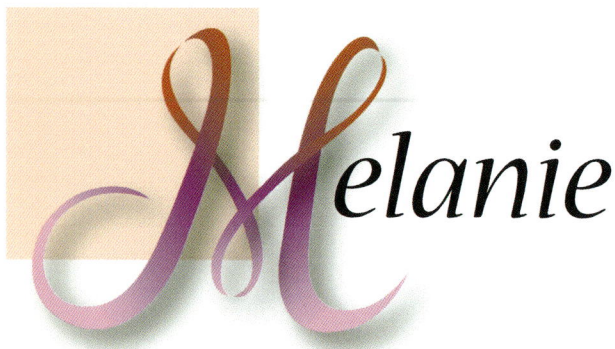

Melanie

"Don't Fight It Alone"

My name is Melanie Hansen. I am a 32-year-old woman surviving metastatic breast cancer. I also had leukemia when I was 19 months old. I was first diagnosed with breast cancer in July of 2008 when I was 29. I had found a lump on my breast around Mother's Day (May) in 2008. I was hoping it was not what I thought it was. I thought to myself, "Oh no, please don't let this be what I think it is. I don't want this to be what I think it is. I don't want to have to tell my mom that I found a lump on my breast on Mother's Day. I don't want my family to have to go through this cancer journey with me again."

When I did tell my parents, they went into action mode because our family has always stayed on top of health issues. My mom and I were convinced that it wasn't breast cancer and the lump was just a calcium deposit like I had had in the past. But indeed, it was breast cancer and it was already Stage 3. The lump appeared within about 5 months. I had been in for a checkup 5 months before and had also been doing self-exams. I was devastated. I was so upset and just kept thinking, "I can't believe I have cancer again, why does this stupid cancer have to keep interrupting my life? Why can't I just be normal and live a life with no health problems?" My family was also devastated because we all thought this cancer thing was behind us. It is hard to move on when you have this constant reminder and worry of being sick.

Since I had the cancer history of leukemia, and did not want to chance the breast cancer returning, I chose to have a double mastectomy. The mastectomy was done within a month of my diagnosis because I had the history of cancer, the tumor was aggressive, and the doctors were not sure how big the tumor actually was. After the surgery, I went for a consult from an oncologist but the doctor did not feel comfortable treating me with my health history, so I went to City of Hope. City of Hope was where I had received my bone transplant when I had leukemia. We got a second opinion and a doctor who would be willing to work with my treatment preference. I did not want chemotherapy or radiation if I did not have to have it.

My doctors kept a close eye on the progress and tried to chase down the cancer cells with hormone therapy but the cancer metastasized to the back in December 2009, and then to the liver in October 2010. In October 2010, I finally relented and went on a Phase 4 clinical trial chemotherapy drug called Abraxane. The cancer responded to the drug really well, exceeding the health care teams expectations, and within 6 cycles had decreased by 76%.

> "I can't believe I have cancer again, why does this stupid cancer have to keep interrupting my life?"

I am really pleased at the treatment I received from City of Hope and my doctor, Dr. Joanne Mortimer. She has really tried to meet my needs and create a relationship with me. Having a relationship with my doctor is important to me to reduce the anxiety of being in the hospital.

Despite my diagnosis and battle with cancer, I feel that I have grown as a person. I had to face challenges in the first 32 years of my life that

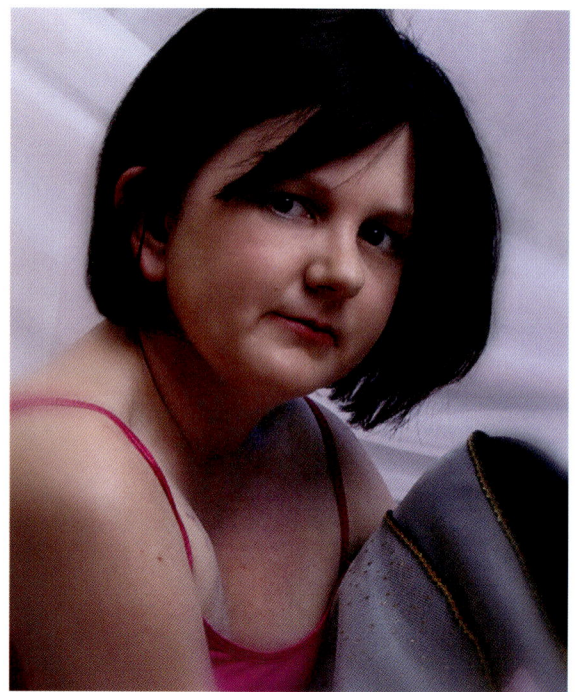

Photography by Joanna Herr

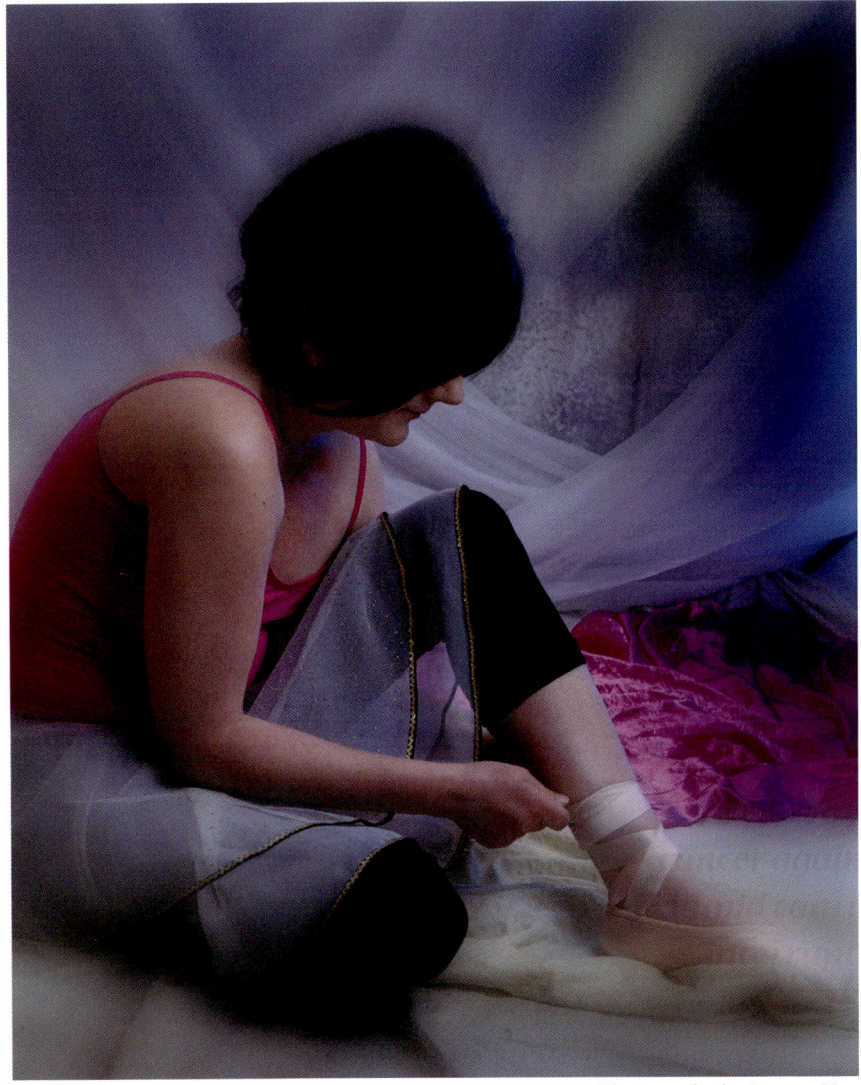

Photography by Joanna Herr

many people do not have to face in a lifetime. I overcame these challenges and gained a knowledge way beyond my years. This knowledge has helped me understand aspects of life that I never knew were possible. I realized that I was not living my life in a way that was healthy to me. I got caught up surviving and was full of unhealthy emotions. I found out what was important, what I wanted to do with my life, that I needed to find inner peace, and live a laid back lifestyle. The journey that I am on in my life has not been easy by any means, but I knew that I had hopes and dreams. I wanted to accomplish more than just existing. One of the major challenges was staying focused on these dreams and aspirations. I did get lost a time or two, but I did not give up and pushed on. I would like to let all of those people who are facing challenges in their life know to not give up because you can overcome more than you think and you will be a better person for it.

> **I learned to get outside of my head and just laugh and be silly so I was not thinking about the cancer 24/7.**

If you are having a hard time getting up, look to others who have gone through the journey to inspire you. I found my inspiration through meeting people who had different types of cancer that caused more health issues than I was facing and realizing that I was blessed. I was also able to be more compassionate because I knew that I was not the only one dealing with this issue. None of my family or friends had to face the challenges that I had to face so I would always hear how inspirational I was. I did not always feel inspirational but more isolated. I would always think if you only knew. When I started meeting people who faced the same problems, I gained a new perspective. One of these ways was going on the AWOL (a way of life) retreat. You meet people who have made breast cancer their way of life and are okay with it. The retreat helps a person explore themselves and learn to be okay with who they are. The people who organize the retreat, make every woman feel special. It doesn't matter if you are having issues with your body because of something the cancer did to you or something you had to have taken away. You are still you and the women at AWOL help you remember and cherish that fact.

To all those who are facing breast cancer or other type of cancers, do not try to do the cancer journey alone, let others help you because it is not worth giving all your time and energy trying to face cancer alone. I like to call the cancer journey a mud run because it is not a sprint or a straight shot down the road like a marathon. You get dirty along the way, you have to brave the elements, you face more than a couple obstacles, and you will need help to get back up or to be cleaned up. There will be all types of things that are happening in your life such as surgeries, doctor appointments, and health issues. You may have issues with body perception as I did because you think your body is deformed. I also faced grief and loss because I lost a sense of normalcy, control over what was happening in my life, and faced sadness due to everything that was happening to me. It was overwhelming.

Luckily, I did not face the journey alone. I went into it thinking I could and that I didn't need anyone because I had gotten so far on my own with what I felt was no one else to help me. I soon learned to rely on others. I had to have my parents help me financially and to take me to my doctor appointments. I realized that I was not going to be able to handle the emotions alone and that it would not be healthy to try to do so. I started going to laughter yoga which incorporates laughter exercises with yogic breathing. I learned to get outside of my head and just laugh and be silly so I was not thinking about the cancer 24/7. I then learned about different support groups in the area and tried different ones to see which ones that I liked the best. I ended up going to St. Jude's because they had different types of support groups and activities to help people bond and socialize. I also tried activities that were offered at City of Hope, like art therapy, music therapy, and yoga. St. Jude's ended up working out the best, location-wise for me and gave me the social connection that I needed. I did have to try different ones to find the best fit for me.

I hope that my story helps inspire you to find the strength inside yourself to persevere and overcome life's challenges.

> *To all those who are facing breast cancer or other type of cancers, do not try to do the cancer journey alone, let others help you because it is not worth giving all your time and energy trying to face cancer alone.*

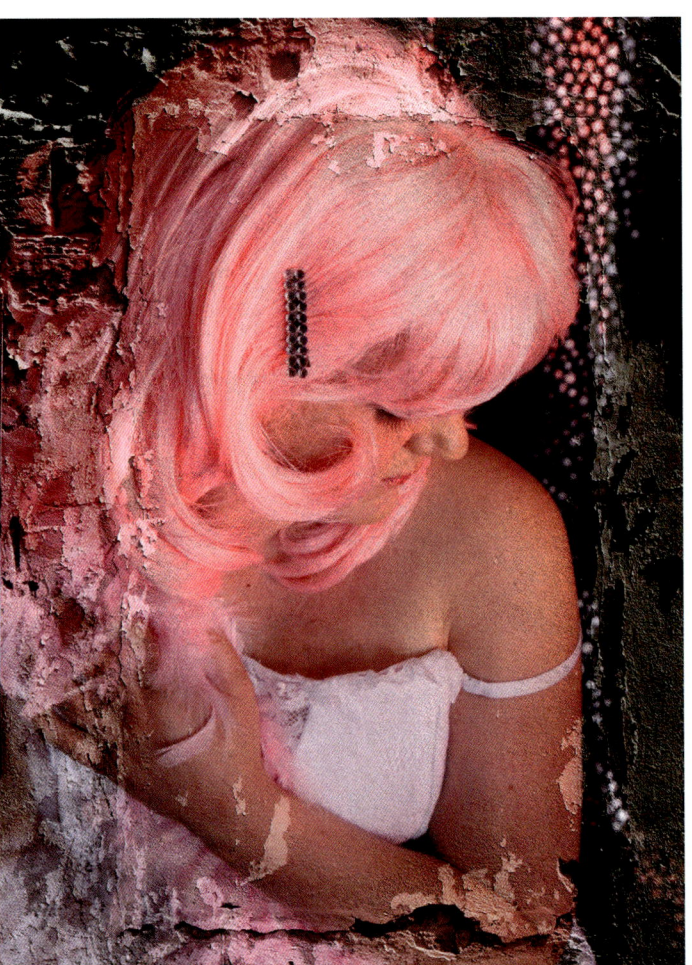

Photography by Joanna Herr

The 4 Stages of Cancer

Here is a brief summary of what the stages mean for most types of cancer.

Stage 1 usually means a cancer is relatively small and contained within the organ it started in.

Stage 2 usually means the cancer has not started to spread into surrounding tissue, but the tumor is larger than in stage 1. Sometimes stage 2 means that cancer cells have spread into lymph nodes close to the tumor. This depends on the particular type of cancer.

Stage 3 usually means the cancer is larger. It may have started to spread into surrounding tissues and there are cancer cells in the lymph nodes in the area.

Stage 4 means the cancer has spread from where it started to another body organ. This is also called secondary or metastatic cancer.

Heather

"Has Anyone Seen My Basket?"

Cancer changes lives. Last July, at age 30, my doctor diagnosed me with breast cancer. I can still vividly remember when I received the phone call, on a Tuesday afternoon, shopping in the book section of Wal-Mart.

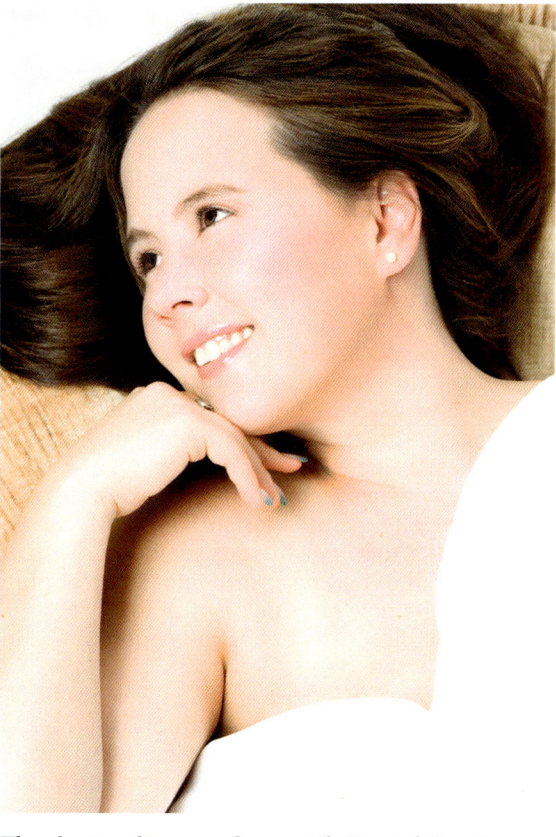

My doctor had just received the test results from my recent biopsy with detrimental results. After the phone call, I completely forgot why I went to the store. I left my basket and just walked out the door. My dad, unemployed at the time, was home when I arrived. I came in, sat down on the couch and cried briefly. Considering that I had reached my breaking point in life, my reaction surprised me as mild.

Apart from that one moment of vulnerability, I remained strong throughout the whole process. Although the situation seemed hard for my mother to accept, she stayed by my side. For the longest time she kept saying, "Why couldn't it have been me and not you?"

"Why couldn't it have been me and not you?"

The doctor diagnosed me with Ductal Carcinoma In Situ (DCIS) cancer. During the months that followed, my doctors performed three biopsies and several more tests. With luck on my side, the tests came back negative. The surgery to remove the cancerous cells took place at the end of September.

Deciding to go through with the radiation proved to be the hardest decision I've made. I didn't understand why my doctors deemed the radiation necessary if the surgeon had already removed the bad cells. My boyfriend explained to me that radiation treats the cells which could become bad, not for the cells removed. My doctor scheduled me with radiation for five days a week for seven weeks straight.

I owe a great deal of thanks to my family, friends, and the management staff at work. Without their help I couldn't have accomplished both the schedule and taking care of my son. Presently, in my cancer journey, I'm proud to say I'm cancer free!

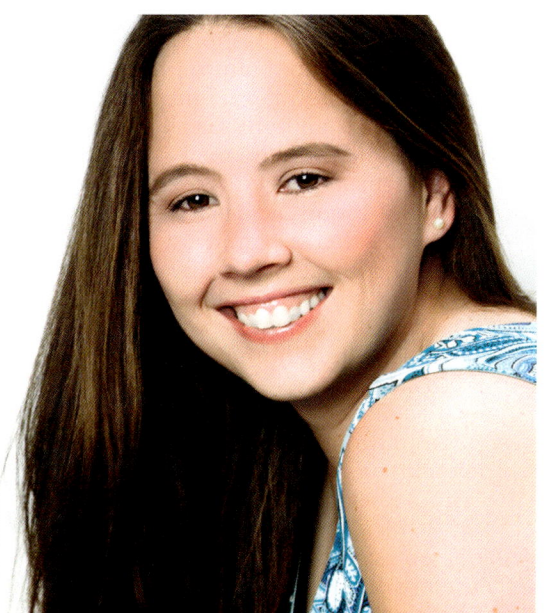

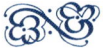

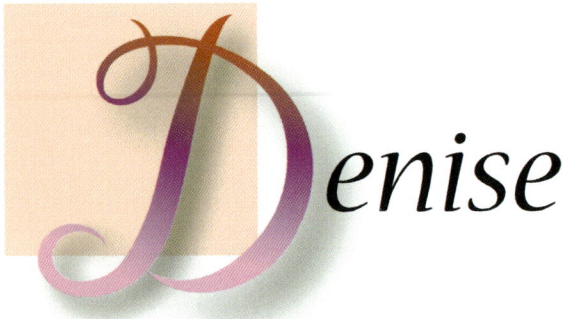

Denise

"From Moccasins to Stilettos"

My name is Denise Y. Lindstrom. I am 55 young years of age. I am an enrolled Arikara member of the Three Affiliated Tribes from the Fort Berthold Reservation in North Dakota, and also Turtle Mnt. Chippewa. I was diagnosed with Breast Cancer on May 13, 2011 which just happened to be, 'Friday the 13th!'

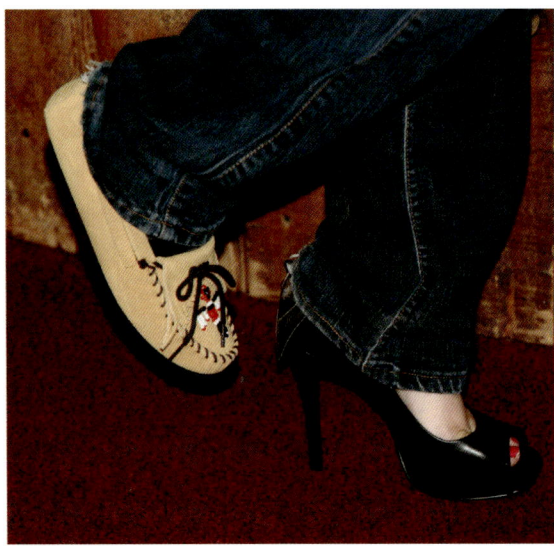

I have always jokingly said, "They Shoot Horses… don't they?" because I have had many health issues. Throughout my life and in general, I've always had something go awry with whatever it is I am doing, although none as serious as cancer.

But this time… this time something was different. I had been experiencing pain in my left breast, and have always made regular self breast exams. I knew about breast cancer from the work I have done with the Native American Research Corp., and was glad they were hosting the mobile mammogram van, so I made an appointment. The pain was sharp, but still not anything I would ever think would be cancer.

When I first got the call to come back in for another look at my left breast, a mass was seen from the mammogram. I still didn't think it was cancer. I have lumpy breasts, I told myself. Then when I was asked to wait following the mammogram follow-up, I got a little nervous. The doctor came in and went over what it showed, the mass was small, but suspicious and he wanted to do a biopsy.

The biopsy came within a few days, "it is happening all so fast", I was thinking. The next day the doctor gave me 'that call'! I was just numb; I really didn't think it was anything. The biopsy was difficult for me. I am startled very easily and found it difficult to stay very still during the procedure. Although small, it is cancer, I was told. I barely made it through the biopsy and now I had to have surgery for breast cancer…

I needed a margarita, and that's what I did! I found myself talking with strangers about my diagnosis, and I thought it was easier than telling my family and close friends. This way I was still the helper, promoting early detection. This took some of the fear away, knowing that my experience might help someone else.

Family, my loving family. I think I felt more hurt for them than I did for myself, especially the grandbabies. I reassured them everything would be fine. I didn't cry. I needed to be strong for them. The doctors gave me sincere hope for recovery and survival. I am the one who held the family together. I am the one that is always here to help you with your problem to a fault. I believe they all struggled with the idea of me being sick with cancer and they were not really sure of how to help me.

My oldest and only daughter didn't want to hear about my cancer, especially the word *cancer*. She would tell people, "I hate that word, don't even say it around me!"

Family, my loving family. I think I felt more hurt for them than I did for myself, especially the grandbabies.

You could see the worry in the boys' eyes. They both kept a stiff upper lip. The oldest Daniel has always been my rock he made sure I was comfortable while I am in recovery.

My youngest son Ricky, told me, "Mom, do you know how we are getting though this, it is because of you. Your strength, courage and sense of humor make us worry less. Your reassurance of "things will be alright, it will pass," with a smile makes us believe it too."

One of the most difficult times I had been to

have to depend on others, even if they wanted to help, *I have always been the caretaker of others!* I am very independent and in a blink of an eye, *I need help!*

> **I was so overwhelmed by life. I requested an increase in my depression medication which helps take a little edge off my attitude but did not take the feeling of loneliness… away.**

If I had to choose it would be the lack of money and the overwhelming bills, not the thought of death, but how to live in the here and now to fight back for some type of future. Another is all the doctor appointments, tests, questions…questions…questions, fill in another form! I feel myself becoming physically ill just thinking about this stuff.

Over the years I had developed depression and anxiety in addition to the health issues with cancer and changes in my employment situation. I have no health insurance and utilize the Denver Indian Health and Family Services for basic care.

I had to deal with cancer diagnosed Friday the 13th, and needed surgery for the kidney stones which was diagnosed April 1st, April Fools Day, and then a fall which effected my mobility. Do you see a theme here? lol

I was so overwhelmed by life. I requested an increase in my depression medication which helps take a little edge off my attitude but did not take the feeling of loneliness with my cancer away. I began reading about my diagnoses and knowing I was very lucky but still overwhelmed with all the information I had been given from the hospitals, social workers, and patient navigators.

I just hate it. I really wanted someone close to me, understanding, someone to wrap me up and hold me tight, helping me and focusing only on me, guiding me with every step. Selfish I know, but that wish stayed in my head.

To overcome some of the more difficult times, I cried. Just good old fashion crying alone mostly, but sometimes with family, patient navigator, nurses or a close friend, just enough to relief the stress of the moment. I have a crazy sense of humor and making light of the issue, and making others laugh brings me so much joy, so I try to laugh more than I cry.

One of the most important things for me was praying. My aunt had sent me some sage dried by a medicine man from the reserve. I pray to the four directions asking 'Grand Father' for forgiveness, understanding and courage.

How has living with breast cancer changed me? I have become more aware of my future. I am the type of person who wants everyone to be happy and will sacrifice my own happiness for others, especially the family. But now the cancer has made me think more about me, and my future. I have discovered I am lonely, more than I had ever thought. I have found myself in seclusion, knowing I had to make life changing decisions and I didn't want to do it alone. Everybody has there own lives to live and I feel like either this will give me just what I needed to get over the hump, or the thing that will take me down.

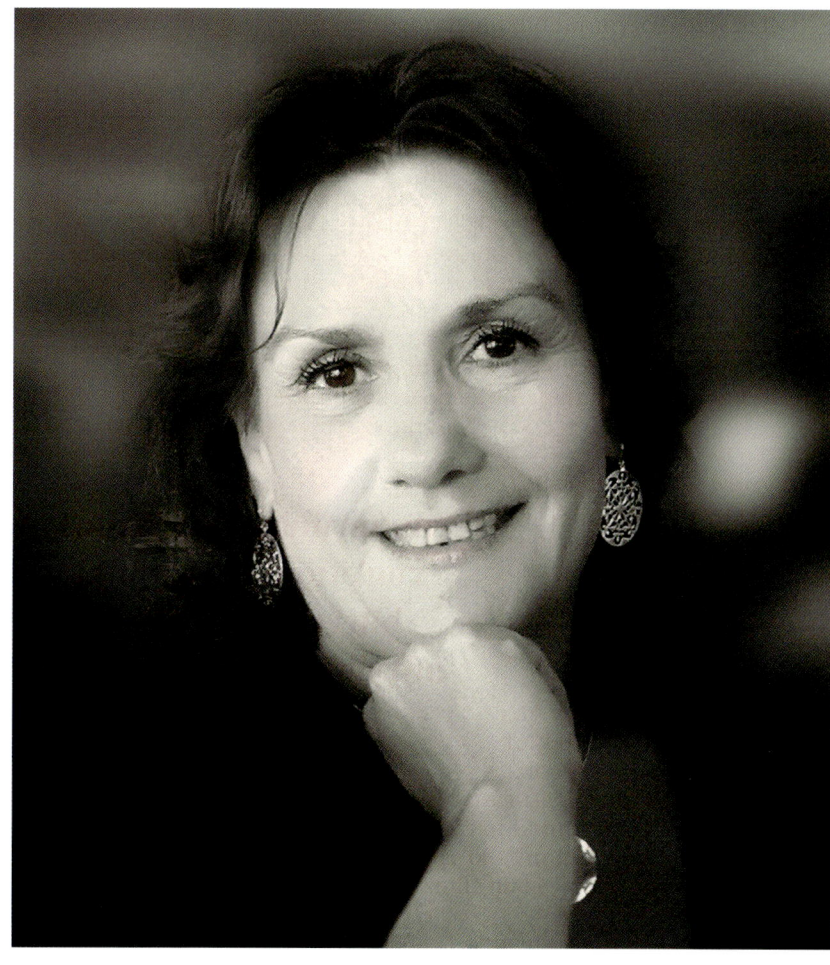

Oh and let's not forget the bra situation. I have found wearing a bra is so uncomfortable. Gone are the days of the French Push-up bra, or any type of under wire. Sweating is the worst!

My advice to new patients would be to not worry too much. Take one day at a time and live the best you can with things that will make you happy. Find that one or two special people that will help you. It is all so overwhelming at first, but you need to try to stay on top of things. Let life inspire you with the help of others. This will be one of the hardest challenges you may face, so try to face it with smiles and laughter. 'Be the leader in laughter, and watch how many follow.'

I am most proud of My Native Heritage. The most proud moments in my life is time spent with my aunty Peewee, her nickname, who helped me to know who I am and my Arikara heritage. She gave me the courage to have a ceremony to receive my Indian name, 'Red Paint Women.' The name was given to me by a relative and the name refers to the red paint worn by the Native women on their faces around their eyes, usually two red lines extending from the corner of the eyes. Also, that my great-granddaughter receive her name, which is 'Winter Star', and my loving children's support.

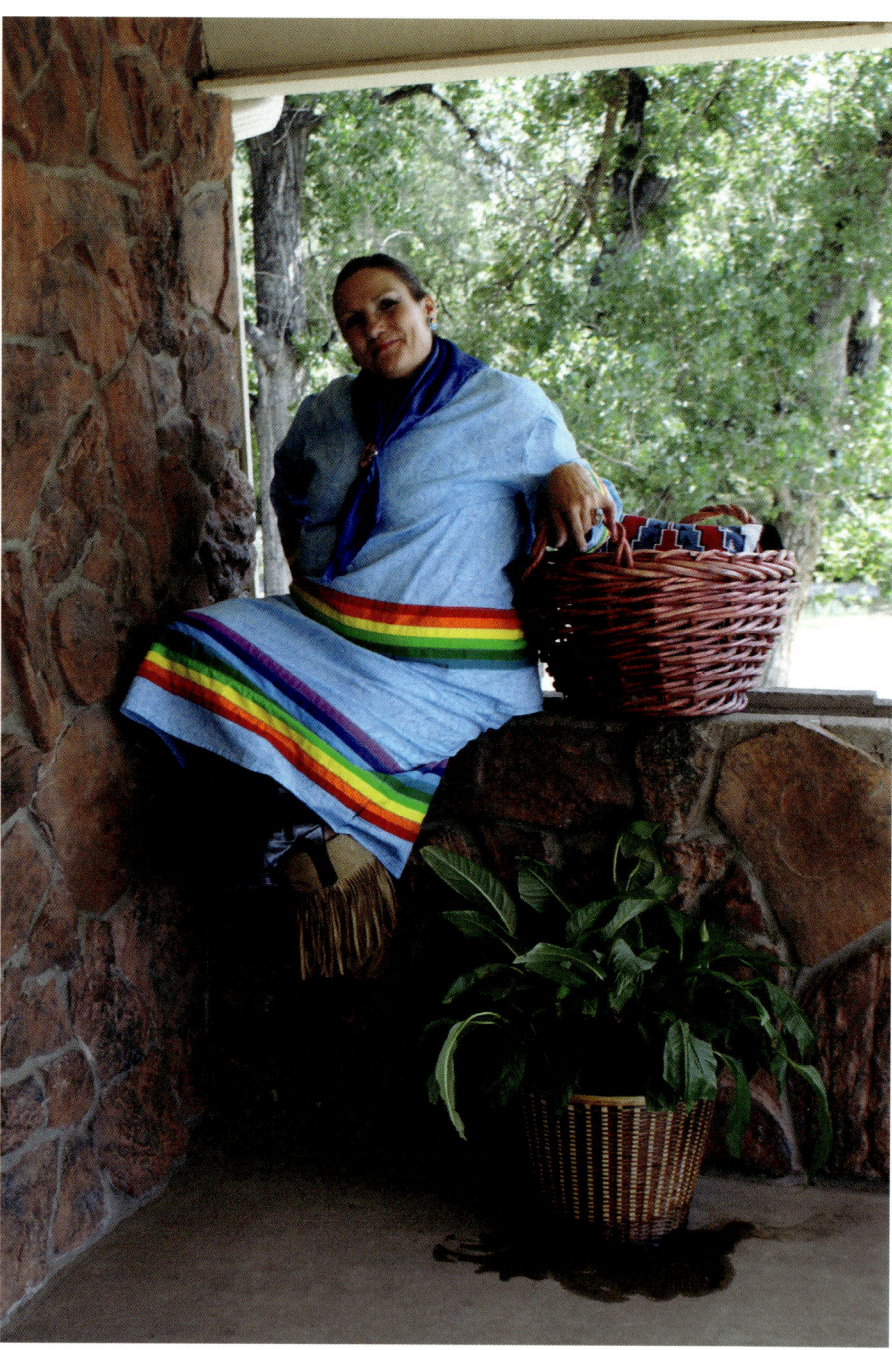

> **While in prayer, a voice in my head took over. The voice prayed for my health and body. I didn't know what to think, it surprised me…**

My inspiration came from usual experiences, and the kindness of others. One morning prior to my diagnoses, I was praying with sage, and was just beginning my prayer when I decided to invite my Grandfather, Ernest Redfox, to come and pray with me. His Indian name is "Many Horses". He is full blood Arikara. While in prayer, a voice in my head took over. The voice prayed for my health and body. I didn't know what to think, it surprised me, but I truly in my

> **Take one day at a time and live the best you can with things that will make you happy.**

heart believe that his prayer was heard and this is why my cancer was caught in such an early stage.

A Native Sister, and Navigator from the Native American Cancer Research Corp. made prayer ties to give to her Sun Dance sister who was participating as one of the Sun Dancers in Sisseton, South Dakota. Two of the prayer ties were for me and my family. "That she would be free of breast cancer and that she had all the support she needs to complete her journey in healing of her body". "The prayer ties are a special part of the Sun Dance which is placed in a sacred position at the Sun Dance. The prayer ties represent hundreds, even thousands, of prayers from the American Indian community.

My deep inspiration comes from my grandchildren not wanting to miss anything as they grow. I like to bring them little gifts and I love to make them smile it warms my heart. I have 10 grandchildren and two great grandbabies. I enjoy traveling and seeing new sights and returning home to North Dakota for Redfox Family Reunions, attending powwows, and a girls' night out every now and then!

It's not easy being *me-zee* and that's just the way my life is—chaos… Upon returning to the doctor's office from my surgery, she asked how I felt. I said, "not so good doc" She took one look at my breast and stated, 'Oh my! Your breast looks angry!' From then on when asked how I feel, I tell people it ranges from angry to cranky, and follow it with "It's not easy being *me-zee!*" And all those who know me agree.

'Have Courage for Good Health'—Early Detection It Really Works, it saved my life. Let it save yours!

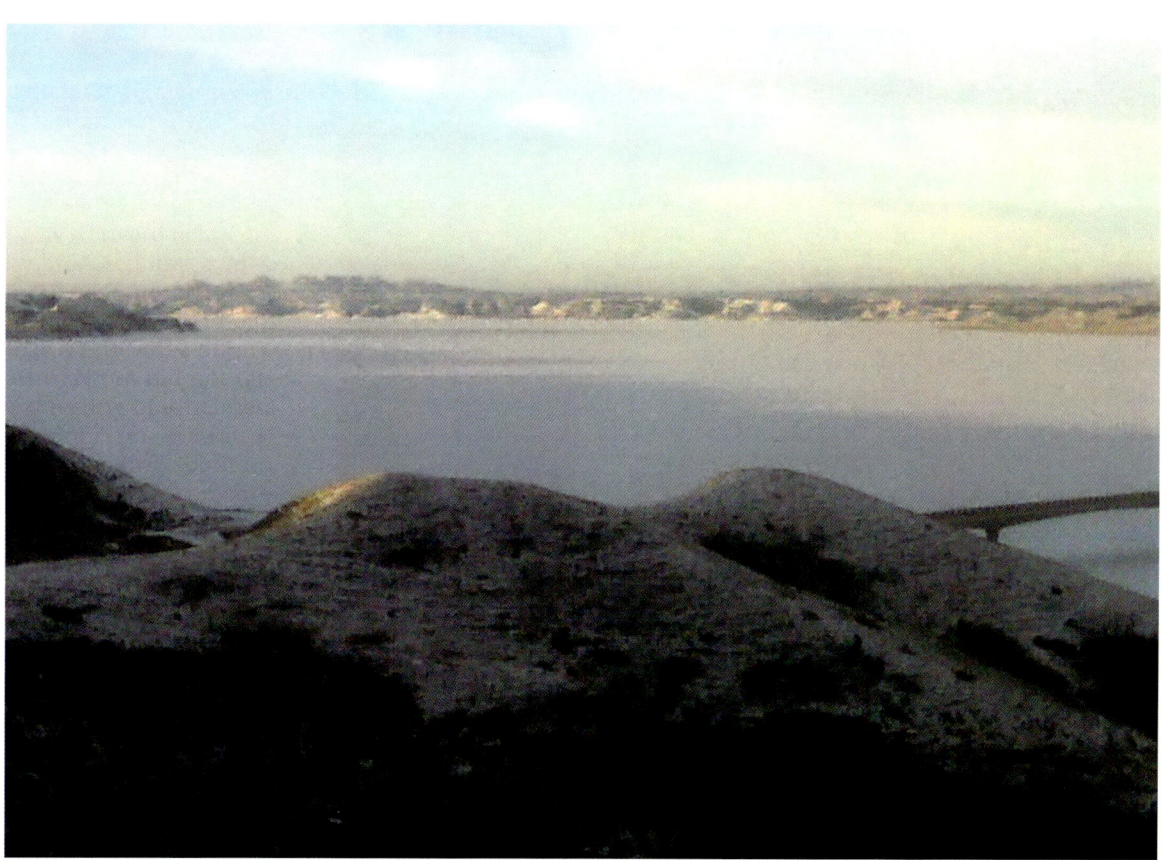

My reservation, overlooking Four Bears Bridge, west of New Town, North Dakota.

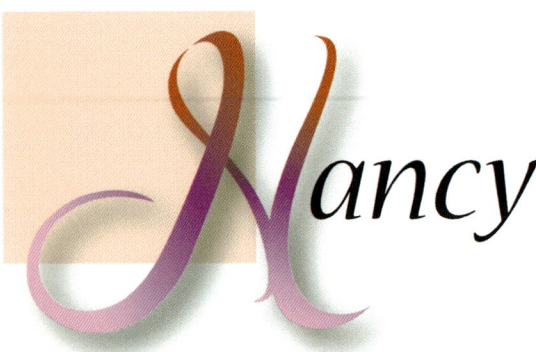

Nancy

"You Just Know"

Every woman who fears she has breast cancer will tell you the absolute moment she *knows* she has breast cancer. Mine was lying on a cold, stainless steel table during an 'ultrasound-guided core biopsy.' Despite annual mammograms that pronounced everything "normal," I tried to ignore the fact that something wasn't right. A small, numb disc I attributed to scar tissue from my underwire bra poking the same spot for decades seemed to be getting bigger. The fleshy spot had no exterior indicators; it didn't hurt, despite how much pressure I applied, and it was stationary.

You would think these facts would be comforting. To the contrary, they were alarming.

It wasn't long after graduating from training bras that I felt my first lump. When the family GP patted me on the shoulder and told me not to worry about it, I boarded a city bus and took off for my first, ever, visit to a gynecologist.

"Give me your hand," Dr. Bob said while I lie on the exam table. He placed my palm on the ball of my nose. "See how this feels?" he said, moving my hand in small, circular motions. "That's how a lump in your breast would feel if it was not a cyst. Cysts roll around and usually hurt when you push on them. The ones that don't move, that *don't* hurt, are the ones we worry about."

I took his diagnosis of *fibrocystic breasts* as one of my facts of life. I became deft at self-exams. Over the years, I had many cyst aspirations, even "chocolate cysts" drained. So the first time my fingers fluttered over the numb patch, I held my breath until the results of my annual mammogram arrived in the mail.

"Dear Mrs. Robinson: The results of your annual mammogram show no abnormal changes or signs of cancer. We will see you next year for your annual exam." I hushed the voice that kept whispering, "They're wrong," and filed the letter with the others.

A month later, the Friday before Memorial Day, was akin to me/Alice falling down the rabbit hole. A deep, debilitating pain in my abdomen began around 9 p.m., a pain so excruciating I opted to spend the night in the family room, close to a bathroom and far away from the rest of the family. Food poisoning? The stomach flu that was making its way around the kids' elementary school? The next morning my husband, Randy, insisted we go to Urgent Care. The attending physician suspected appendicitis and directed us to the nearest Emergency Room for a CT scan.

I waited hours in the ER, first to be seen, and then for the CT scan to be read. Finally, the ER physician bustled in, six hours later, said the scan looked good and I could go home. "Gas" was his official diagnosis.

"Gas?"

I delivered two children, one (at this very hospital) nearly *au natural*, when the OB/GYN nurse didn't think I was dilated enough for an epidural (I was over eight centimeters). I was familiar with pain. This pain was worse. Despite my protestations, the ER physician was unyielding and handed me my discharge papers.

> *I hushed the voice that kept whispering, "They're wrong," and filed the letter with the others.*

In retrospect, the following hours were surreal, in part because of the pain, in part because of the Vicodin prescribed for the pain. Randy was booked for a red-eye flight to New York to attend the wedding of a childhood friend's daughter. He didn't think he should go.

"Go," I insisted. "I'm fine." In all honesty, I was feeling somewhat chagrined that I went to the ER for "Gas."

The next morning I vaguely remember my 10-year-old shaking me, trying to wake me up. "A nurse from the hospital" was on the phone. I swam up from the bottom of a murky pond to take the phone. My films had been misread. My appendix ruptured more than 24 hours earlier. I needed to return to the hospital.

Again, I found myself waiting in the hospital emergency room waiting to be seen, trying to

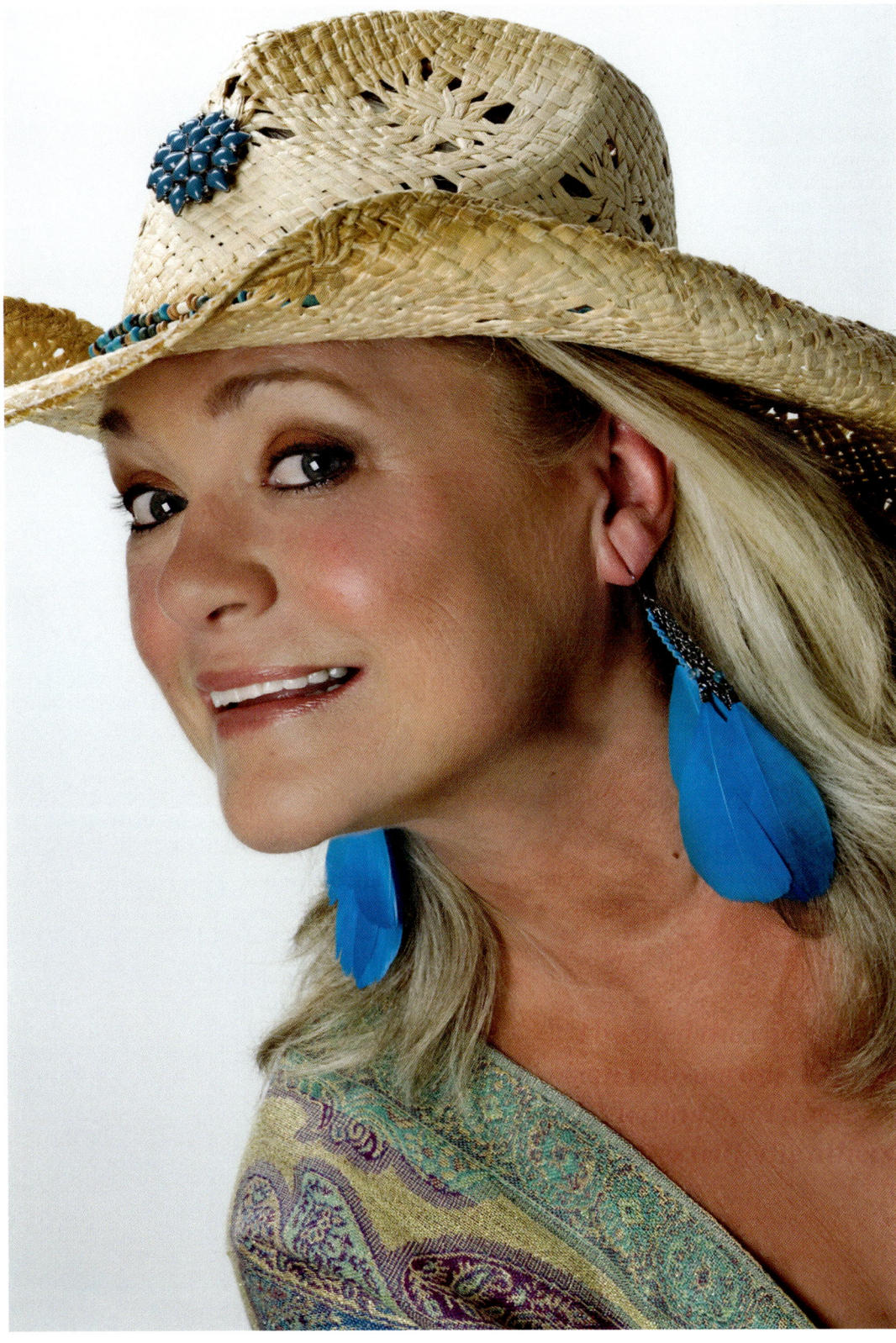

the poison that was dripping through my system, or all of the above, I contracted Sepsis, which, according to the Mayo Clinic, is "a potentially life threatening condition, in which your immune system's reaction to an infection may injure body tissues far from the original infection."

Things seemed to be going from bad to worse. Tests I insisted on, confirmed I contracted C-difficile, a hospital borne infection. It took four months and a switch to an infectious disease specialist at a different hospital system, before I was given a clean bill of health. It was the end of September. I was ready to be well. Randy and I decided to celebrate with a glass of champagne and evening in the Jacuzzi, which had been off limits because c-diff is highly contagious. As I pulled my t-shirt up over my head to put on my bathing suit I caught my reflection in the bathroom mirror. I was 15 pounds lighter than when this ordeal began, and the once flat disk on the side of my right breast was now bulging like a flat-bottom golf ball.

Two days later, I found myself, again, horizontal on a cold, metal table having an ultrasound-guided core biopsy. One technician usually assists the physician during this procedure, but this day there was an additional tech in training. Over and over a device punched into the tumor, extracting cells for the pathologist to examine.

And there it was.

> **Had I not been looking at that exact moment I would have missed the look exchanged between the two technicians just over my head.**

understand why I was waiting. Randy was frantic when he learned, somewhere over Iowa, that I was back in the hospital. It was a holiday weekend. Finding a flight back to San Diego was impossible. More than 48 hours after I first visited Urgent Care, I was wheeled into an operating room. Because of the initial delay, the misdiagnosis,

Had I not been looking at that exact moment I would have missed the look exchanged between the two technicians just over my head. Later "Debbie," the tech in training, met me outside the dressing room with a bag of ice chips to put on my bleeding, wounded breast. Her eyes seemed red-rimmed and she avoided eye contact. She mumbled, "Good luck Mrs. Robinson." It was barely a whisper.

So, yes, I knew.

I hated being the image on the screen that first showed her what breast cancer looked like.*

Life is unpredictable. It throws curve balls when you're totally prepared to bunt.

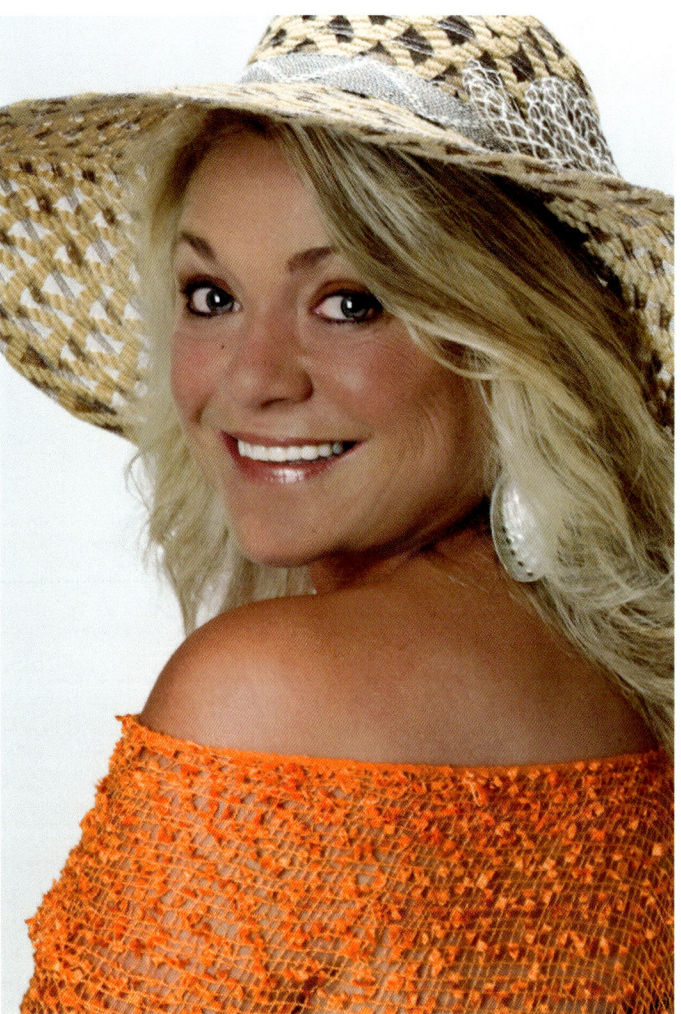

I was diagnosed with breast cancer on October 3, 2005. I was 49 years old, married, with two sons ages eight and ten. There was no history of breast cancer on either side of my predominantly female family. For the next two and half years I had three surgeries, three months of chemotherapy, a mastectomy, seven weeks of radiation, and TRAM-flap breast reconstruction. I lost my hair, suffered through MRSA following my mastectomy, and the chemo contributed to osteoarthritis and total deterioration of my knee, resulting in a full knee replacement.

I celebrated the end of chemo by skiing the following week in Utah, celebrated the end of radiation with a camping trip through the Dakotas and Canada, and in 2008 was able to take Alaska off the "Bucket List." We celebrated my five year "diagnosis date" by coupling it, three months after knee replacement surgery, hiking Diamond Head in Hawaii.

Life is unpredictable. It throws curve balls when you're totally prepared to bunt. It's easy to beat yourself up and ask, "Why did (or didn't) I...?" Or just, "Why?"

When I look at what I have been given in life, it's hard to be angered by these impositions. I am alive because Randy and my boys were always on the other side of that Operating Room door.

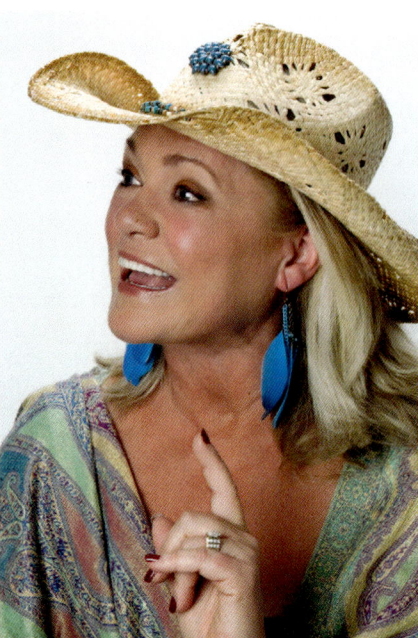

Of all the breast cancer patients and survivors I've met, I've not met one who used the word, "victim." Some have had a recurrence. Some have lost the fight. I cry, I get angry, I get tired of waiting for "the other shoe to drop." Until it does, I'll continue adding two items to the Bucket List for every one I cross off. Get mad, get angry, get up...celebrate the life you have, and keep on going.

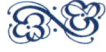

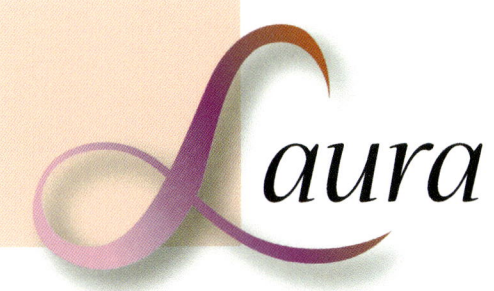

"One in a Hundred"

It was a typical morning about 3 years ago but it was a day that began the interesting journey to where I am today…

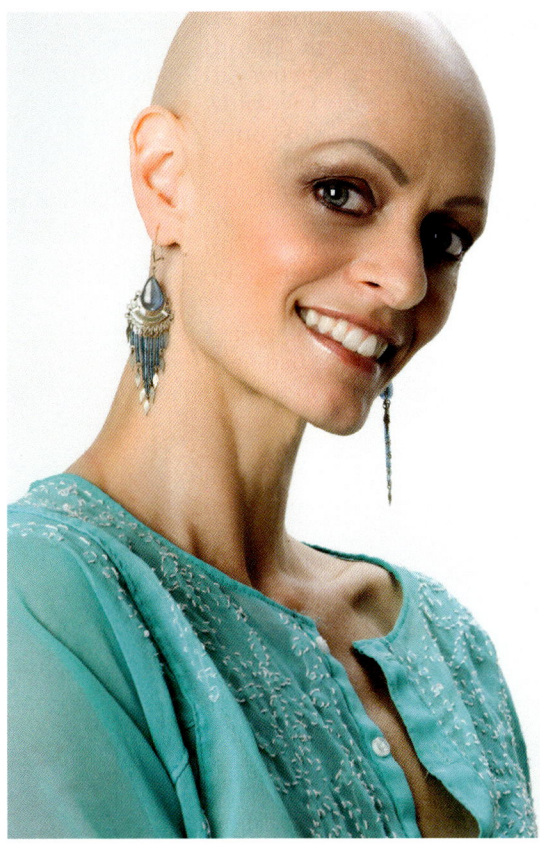

I woke up, yawned, stretched and rolled over. As I tucked my arm behind my head I felt it- a small bald patch, maybe the size of a quarter at the nape of my neck under my hair. "That's strange," I thought, but didn't give it much more consideration. A few weeks later when I went in for a trim my hairdresser felt it too. She took a look and said "You have Alopecia," (I hadn't heard that word before, yet little did I know it would soon become part of my nearly daily vocabulary). She told me I could get a few cortisone injections and my hair would grow back. Why bother? I had a head full of thick, long, wavy hair and one spot wouldn't be noticeable.

A few months later I began noticing other bald patches. Now I knew something strange was going on. So I made an appointment with my doctor and again I heard it: Alopecia. He told me it was an autoimmune disorder in which the body mistakenly attacks its own cells, thinking them to be foreign invaders. In this case the hair follicles are the victim. It affects about 1% of the population.

He also told me there are no known causes or cures and there was nothing he could do for me so he sent me on my way. Not satisfied with his answer I sought out another opinion. This time I went to a dermatologist who confirmed this diagnosis. There were now about a half- dozen bald spots on my head, some growing quite large, maybe 3 inches in diameter. I wasn't going to let this condition win so I waged a full on battle with my body. I endured the monthly cortisone injections (about 8-12 painful pricks per bald spot) and UVB laser treatments, slathered my scalp with Rogaine twice a day, gorged myself on vitamins and protein shakes. I was doing everything I thought I could to conquer this and grow my hair back. The cortisone worked, but only to a certain degree. Sure there was hair growing where I had the injections (kind of like a doll, whose hair is in neat little round plugs), but other bare patches were showing up. This went on for about 4 or 5 months.

> *I had become very creative in styling my hair or wearing headbands to hide my condition so I didn't look that different on the outside.*

I had become very creative in styling my hair or wearing headbands to hide my condition so I didn't look that different on the outside. But on the inside I was beginning to fall apart. I was essentially in panic mode but trying so hard not to show it. As a yoga teacher, I prided myself on being an exemplary model of perfect health. I ate right, got plenty of sleep, exercised and tried to maintain a positive outlook. How dare my body betray me? It was especially devastating given that I've been a performer for most of my life, often taking a great deal of time creating elaborate hair do's and makeup for various roles and shows, as well as taking pride in my appearance. Then there was the fact that as a woman, so much emphasis is put on our looks, with long, flowing locks symbolizing youth and beauty. I felt hurt, angry, scared, hopeless and ugly. I blamed myself a lot of the time, wondering what actions in my life, whether physical or karmic, I had done to cause this. I remember one horrible moment in the shower after washing

page 79

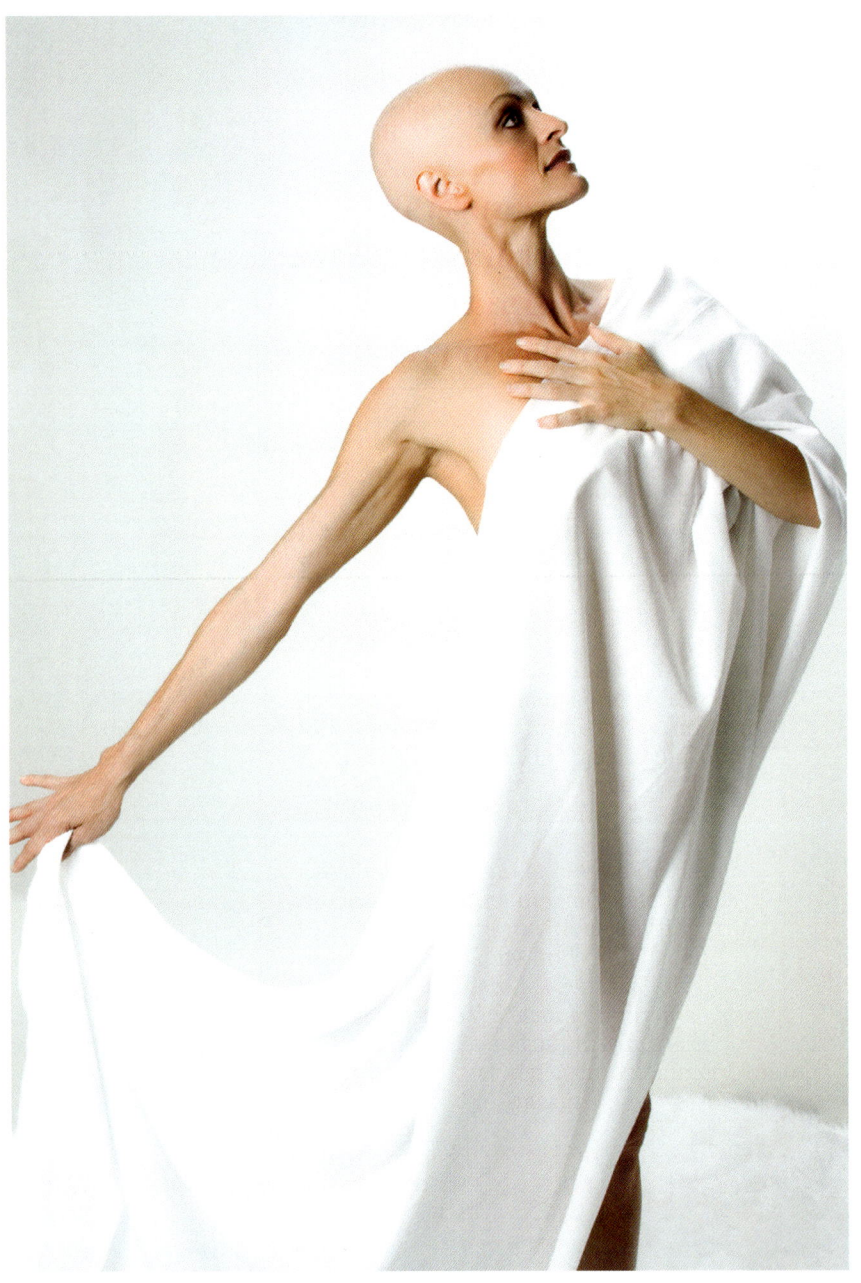

second thoughts about all the chemicals and hormones I was subjecting my body to and decided to look for a more natural, holistic approach. Ayurveda is the medical system that has been practiced in India for thousands of years. Like Traditional Chinese Medicine, Ayurveda treats the whole person, seeking to create balance and health rather than address only the symptoms. Through a Google search I found a doctor in India who had success in curing many patients of Alopecia. So I ordered his formula which consisted of daily herbs and oils to rub on my head and weekly mud packs. This treatment seemed much gentler and resonated better with my beliefs about well-being. And it was a lot less expensive! I became religious about applying these concoctions while stating mantras of my hair growing back quickly and profusely. I prayed to anyone out there in the Heavens who was listening to restore me to perfect health.

Four months and nothing. No new hair growing back, no slowing down of my hair loss. With the 10 or so scraggly strands of hair left on my head I felt like I looked sick. My eyebrows, eyelashes and body hair began to fall out too. My boyfriend had been very supportive through this entire process, telling me I was beautiful and he still loved me no matter what, trying to make light of it by saying "It's just hair." I didn't feel beautiful, feminine or even human. So with a feeling of defeat I told him "I'm done, cut it off. Cut it all off. It's gonna fall out anyhow". He chopped the flimsy bits of hair and I sadly watched them fall to the ground. This was the beginning of learning to surrender to this condition, but I still had a lot of internal work to do before I was ready to really accept what was happening to me.

By this time I had resorted to wearing wigs. "Wigs are only for old ladies," I thought. I felt ashamed, like I had to hide. It was frightening and embarrassing going into the wig shop, having to reveal myself, wondering what others may be thinking. In reality I was hiding behind this illusion I was trying to keep up, like nothing was wrong, nothing had changed. Once when I was teaching a yoga class and began getting quite warm, I started taking off my outer shirt and the wig partially came off with it. With a room full of students too! I panicked and scrambled to get it back on, hoping no one noticed. Though this moment was scary it brought me to an important realization: I can't try to hide anymore.

my (remaining) hair, heaving sobs of hysteria with huge handfuls of hair in each hand. At my darkest moments I even wished I had cancer so then at least I'd have an explanation for what was going on and could blame it on the chemotherapy.

But the fight continued. Since I am self-employed, with no medical insurance, my treatment was getting costly, not to mention emotionally draining since there was no real progress or change. In a moment of rational thinking I realized that maybe there was a better way. I began to have

> *I didn't feel beautiful, feminine or even human. So with a feeling of defeat I told him "I'm done, cut it off. Cut it all off.*

Shortly after this incident I showed up to teach class with my new do. A sexy, dark red and black bob cut, short in back, tapering to face-framing points around my chin. People were so surprised. They loved this new look! They asked me, "What inspired you to make such a drastic change?" "It's a long story," I said, "I'll tell you all after class." I had worn my hair long for my entire life (except that horrible perm back in the 80's when I was 12) and had never been daring enough to do something this extreme. I felt bold and flirtatious, the best I had felt in a long time. But this wasn't only from the stylish wig. It was from having the courage to be truthful and real about who I was and what I was going through. As my yoga students circled around after class and I told them about my disorder, I felt a deeper connection and understanding between us. As I continued to open up and share, others began to do so too. My compassion for myself and others grew.

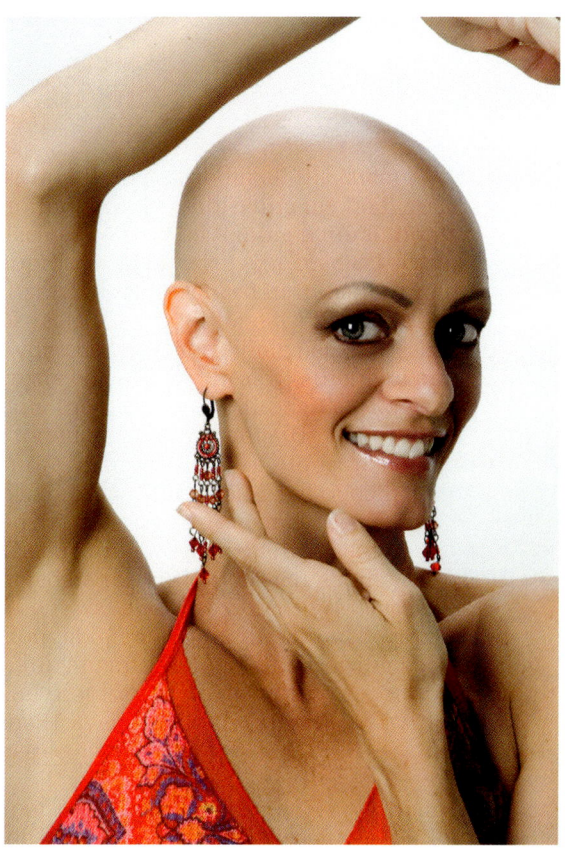

Often times I would look at myself in the mirror, completely bald with no brows or lashes and not even recognize my reflection. I was starting to get used to the new "me", but I didn't feel the outside matched how I felt inside. Before, while I was losing my hair, I would tell myself "My body is falling" apart and that's how I felt. I was weak and tired, physically and emotionally drained most of the time. Now that I had learned to accept that I was perfectly fine, my body was just choosing not to grow hair, I felt physically strong and healthy. The power of the mind truly is miraculous!

Growing tired of the mess and hassle of applying fake eyebrow tattoos every day I decided to get them done permanently. After that, at least I felt the image looking back at me in the mirror was human, not some strange otherworldly alien. I'd throw my wig on (with double sided tape for security!) and go about my day and those who didn't know me were none the wiser. They even asked, "Where do you get your hair done?" and here was a great opportunity to educate another person about Alopecia. So I would briefly explain my story and in doing so found more strength and empowerment. Not having to shave, wax or pluck anymore was an added bonus. I was beginning to look on the bright side, to see the gifts in this unique situation.

I now own about 10 wigs and my collection will most likely grow. It's fun to be able to change my look in a few seconds on the special occasions I feel like having hair. Although more often than not these days I go out in public without a wig and just wrap a scarf or bandana around my smooth, shiny head. I get looks of sympathy, some even asking me, "Are you going through treatment?" and although I don't have cancer people often think I do. My look represents a stage many go through after chemotherapy and radiation in their battles with cancer. My deepest sympathy goes out to those who are fighting that war and all the brave women featured in this book.

> *I've begun to use my unique look to challenge the stereotypes of feminine beauty. I am educating people about this autoimmune disorder.*

The most rewarding part of this journey has been my own growth and the amazing support of my loving family, friends and partner. I haven't let this condition run my life or stop me from doing the things I love. I've begun to use my unique look to challenge the stereotypes of feminine beauty. I am educating people about this autoimmune disorder. I've gained a greater appreciation of what lies inside, the beauty of the heart and soul. I've learned how to be at peace and accept whatever difficulties may arise in life. While I still hope my hair does grow back one day, it is anyone's guess whether or not it actually will. But regardless of that fact, I can say that I am strong and healthy, truly happy with who I am on the inside as well as the outside.

Christina

"A Journey to Remember"

First, let me start off this beautiful day by giving God his praise —Thank you Jesus, thank you Jesus, thank you Jesus. For it is by your Grace and Mercy that I am alive today. For only you are an awesome God you brought me through a trial that has come to take me out (OH!), but it has made me a lot stronger. Weeping may endure for a night but joy, but joy comes in the morning.

My name is Christina Marie Davis-Falls. I am 58 years of age and this is A Journey to Remember. At the age of fifty, I went in for my mammogram which was normal. Two months later I noticed a hard lump. I was first diagnosed with Breast Cancer on February 3rd, 2004. I had a biopsy and was told that I had an "Invasive Breast Carcinoma", the tumor was located in my Ductal lining. Tumor size 4.5 cm histologic grade was a 3. My margins tissues around the breast areas are free. My cancer was hormone-negative, "What a Blessing."

Looking Through New Eyes:

Depression is not just a case of the blues, it is a serious medical illness often caused by an imbalance of chemicals in the brain. Fatigue is a most common yet untreated side-effect of having cancer. It is a physical condition that causes you to "feel weak" or "wiped out". Cancer related fatigue extreme is the kind of tiredness, not relieved by resting or taking a nap. It causes depression, sleep problems and other medical conditions.

My thoughts were this emotional stress factor that "ME Tina" the strong and mighty was angry and has Breast Cancer". I will be sick, need surgery, need chemo and become very upset and unbalanced. Lose even my hair and go through some side effects. "God" gave me two choices "Keep the Breast and Die or Loose the Breast and LIVE". I remember how much faith I really have. How loved I really am and by all who has and will share my private journey. See in times like this, you need a spiritual guide, family, friends support. Stay close to your faith, somehow it makes everything alright and life looks clear after a while. My motto: I am too blessed to be stressed during this unclear mess.

I have learned not to worry, take better care of myself, even do some exercises, eat better (my chief "The Boss" does all the cooking). I have also learned from this experience how precious my family and friends truly are and I am grateful. I had to be honest with myself first...and then everybody else about my thoughts, feelings, and emotions that I was experiencing and I was a wreck. It is very important to have a support team that you can trust and remain transparent. Through this process you need a sympathetic listener.

My Feelings & Reactions when I first heard of my diagnosis:

I knew and realized the growing pains of life changing thoughts from crazy to sad to..."why me"...on February 3rd, 2004. Some of you sitting reading this recorded journey of my life, can share with this informational praise of testimony by the way of yourself or family member or even a close friend. But believe me, it is and was frightening as HELL! (The unknown). Sometimes we can get too comfortable in our state of life. If you are not careful, CANCER can and will cause you to lose your mind and cause you to forget your purpose and (destination) for God's will in your life. Because you'll forget how to live, love and laugh. That's why on February 4th, 2004, I was changed for a time such as this; I heard a soft voice; I was told Christina you have Breast Cancer, I cried and cried all day and sometimes, if I don't stay focused it tries to control me now, so I must control it. With each breath I realize I am a winner and a survivor. Deal with yesterday and forget it. Have pleasant thoughts of today for tomorrow is not promised.

You know at first, I wasn't going to tell anybody not anyone, not a single person, not a soul. I was going to keep this, my dark – ugly, medical secret to myself. I was scared and afraid of the unknown. I was shocked

> **Stay close to your faith, somehow it makes everything alright and life looks clear after a while. My motto: I am too blessed to be stressed during this unclear mess.**

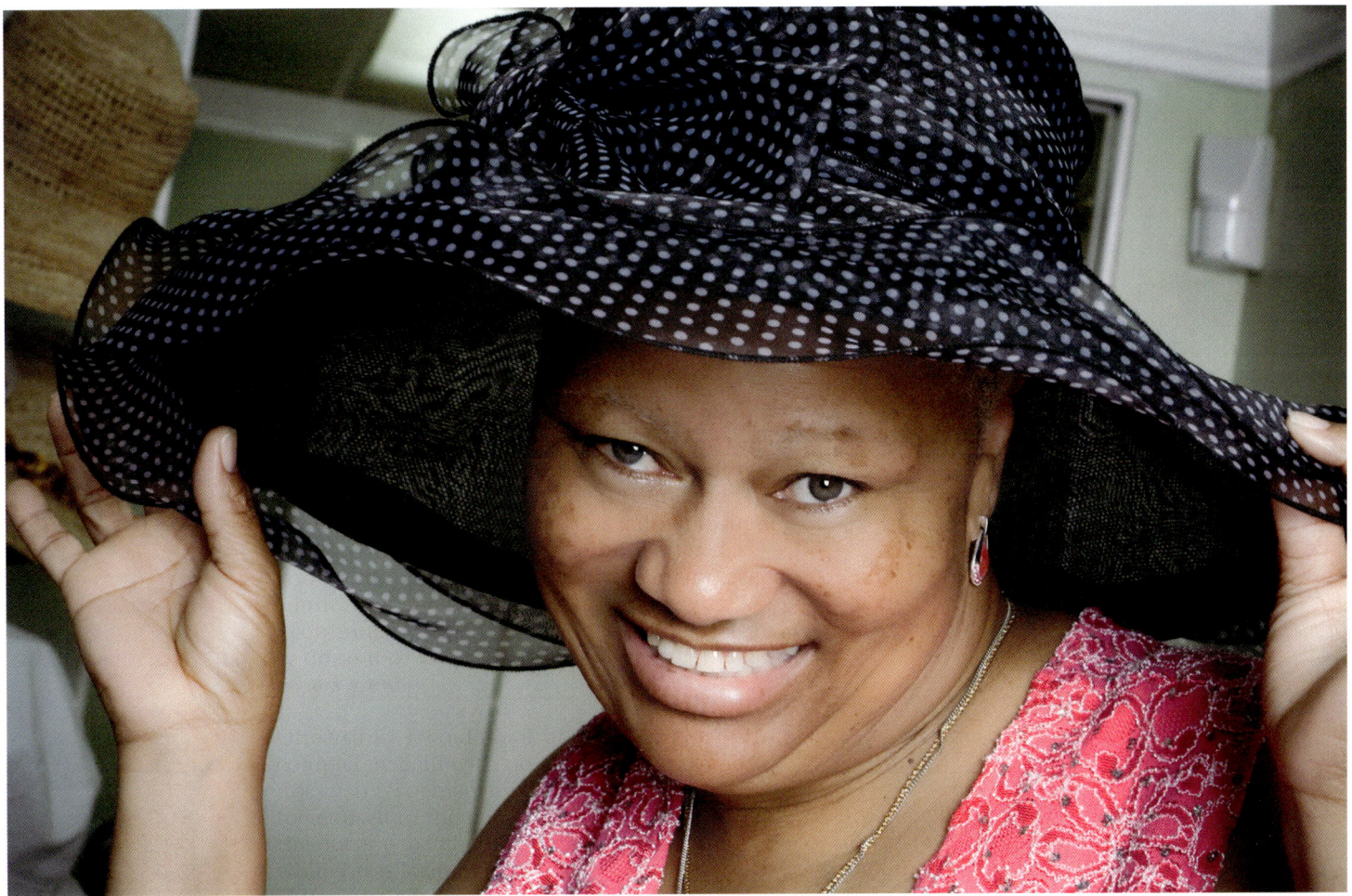

and overwhelmed. How was I going to tell my church families: Pastor William Exum of Mt. Sinai Baptist; Pastor Michael and First Lady Christina Page (daughter) of Liberty Temple Worship Center, (Son) Pastor Marcus and First Lady Jennifer Davis of Victorious Ministries in St. Robert, MO; my close friends and Professional Affiliations? My High School S.C.P.A. Students, where I teach American Sign Language for 12 years, then also the Special Education Students that I assist with at Lee Elementary for 25 years. Most of all, my loving and caring husband Ron Falls, who was and has been an Angel of Love, "The Boss", my two grown children, my six grandchildren and my four living siblings. My father and second Mother are still alive. My first Mother passed in 2007 and my brother passed in 2011, both of Cancer...

> *"don't worry Grammie, because you are the root of the tree and you won't die. You are our family's backbone."*

How my granddaughter reacted after hearing the news:

My granddaughter at age 16 said "don't worry Grammie, because you are the root of the tree and you won't die. You are our family's backbone." Your best is yet to come...Expect Great Things.

The Cancer Room:

On April 4, 2004, after surgery, I received 21 days of chemotherapy with the treatments lasting four to eight hours for 10 months. During my chemotherapy, I listened to Gospel Music and read books on cancer. I laughed at my head with wigs on backwards, so I decided to go BALD and LOVED IT. Soon after Chemo, I chose reconstructive surgery and later received physical therapy to enhance motion in my shoulder for teaching American Sign Language for City Community College, which I truly love.

Always ask millions of questions and get and keep all of your medical history reports from your team of doctors, which are as follows:
From Kaiser Permanente

Primary care physician—what is truly happening medically, "will I die?"

Surgeon—who does your operation (Biopsy-remove small sample of tissue).

Your Oncologist—who specializes in which treatment of cancer or both, i.e. Radiation therapy high-of energy rays to kill cancer cells.

Pathologist—doctor who identifies diseases by studying cells and tissues under a microscope

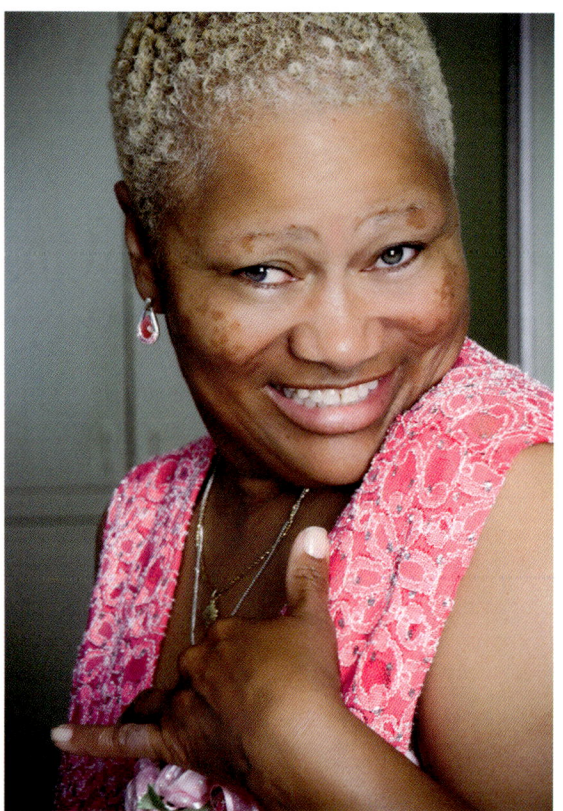

Plastic surgeon—who specializes in reducing scarring or disfigurement that may occur as a result of accident, birth defects, or treatment for diseases. (Such as Breast reconstruction)

Breast Care Coordinator R.N.—wonderful Sounding Board (My tears and my fears).

After much treatment, I was a good candidate for a mastectomy. I didn't want to take any chances so I had a Right R mastectomy. The surgery was April 4th, 2004, the Chemo was July 4th, 2004 through February, 2005, the implant was June, 2005, the expander was December, 2006, the nipple was July 2007, the areola coloring was August 2007. This was a 3 year Journey.

The Medical Terms Explained:

Breast Cancer: Is the most common type of cancer among women in the United States (other than skin, lung, colon, ovarian cancer). Each year more than 192,000 (one hundred ninety two thousand) women in this country learn they have breast cancer.

- *85% who have Breast Cancer have no family history of this disease*
- *One in eight women in the U.S. Will develop Breast Cancer.*
- *Forty thousand women will die from breast Cancer this year. You can help save a Life…*

— TAKE ACTION —

Men listen up this message is for you as well. A male friend of mine just returned to work after 3 or 4 months of having a double Breast Cancer Mastectomy. Breast Cancer affects more than 1,000 men in this country each year.

Lymph nodes: Small, bean-shaped organs located along the channels of the lymphatic system. The lymph nodes store special cells that can trap bacteria or cancer cells traveling through the body.

F.Y.I.: Clusters of lymph nodes are found in the underarms, groin, neck, chest and abdomen (also called lymph glands).

Chemotherapy: Treatment with powerful anti-cancer drugs, given by injection into the vein, or by mouth. Given in cycles, each followed by recovery period. Side effects: loss of hair all over your body, loss of weight, feeling nausea and vomiting, fatigue and infection, and sores in your mouth.

QUOTES I mediated upon daily:

Too Blessed to be Stressed…

Remember *"It Ain't my Fault GOD Choose ME Christina Davis-Falls!!!"*

The Physical Journey:

The most difficult time in my life was April 8th, 2004. Breast Cancer Surgery right modified radical mastectomy. Then the chemotherapy treatments August, 2004 (during this time I had (4) of my wisdom teeth extracted and (2) crowns, and going through physical therapy for my right arm for the swelling after surgery.

The Financial Journey:

Research and understand the mass of resources that are available to you in your city, state and government agencies. All of the aspects of your finances will be effected and hard.

Here are some resource services to contact:

* *African-American Breast Cancer Alliance (AABC);*
* *Women's Information Network Against Breast Cancer (WINABC);*
* *Y-me Breast National Foundation, Chicago IL;*
* *RA Bloc Cancer, Kansas City, MO;*
* *National Cancer Institute's Cancer 1-800-4Cancer;*

* *Sister Connection for Breast Cancer*, San Diego, CA 1-888-723-6722.

* *Community Organizations* (free wigs, beauty tips, support groups, etc).

* *The Brighter Side* (saved my life), Solana Beach, CA, Miss Sherre Cain

—STAND UP & REPEAT THESE WORDS—
(Must Yell Them Out So the Atmosphere Can Hear You)

*"I am a SURVIVOR"…"I am a WINNER"…
"I will never QUIT"…"I will KEEP on FIGHTING"*

*I may be knocked down, but I am not knocked out.
It is in me to keep on going…*
*"I CAN DO ALL THIS. I AM A WINNER;
I AM A SURVIVOR."*

— CLAP YOUR HANDS & BE THANKFUL —

A Journey to Remember:

"Why me?" but God says, "Why not you, Christina?" …ask your Questions after Questions. Take a family member or friend to each visit.

> **"Why me?" but God says, "Why not you, Christina?"**

"What is Cancer?"— A group of many different diseases that cells, the body's basic unit of life. The body is made up of many types of cells, normally, cells grow and divide to produce more cells only when the body needs them. This orderly process helps keep the body health. Sometimes cells keep dividing when new cells are not needed. These cells may form a mass of extra tissue, called a growth or tumor. Tumor's can be benign or malignant.

Benign tumors are not cancers. When removed, most cases they don't come back, do not invade other tissues and do not spread to other parts of the body. Benign breast tumors are not a threat to life.

Malignant tumors are cancer cells in tumors. Tumors can invade and damage nearby tissues and organs. Also, cancer cells can break away from a malignant tumor and enter the bloodstream. This is how breast cancer spreads and forms secondary tumors in other parts of the body.

In Summary:

Early Detection:
In most cases doctors cannot explain why women develop breast cancer. When breast cancer is found and treated early, the chances for survival are better. You must take an active part in your health. Women in general and Black women in particular, often do not touch our bodies, we don't examine our bodies, and we don't look at or like our bodies. Look in the mirror—we are beautiful.

* For self monthly exams, lie down on you back, close your eyes; take the pad of your 3 fingers; start at your collar bone in a circular motion press in on your tissue; few minutes of pain; to chest/middle bone; down to your waist/ribs; around your side, back up to you breast; press all around; squeeze your nipple; know your body; look for lumps, redness, size and shape changes.

* Annual physical exams (by doctor)

* Mammogram screening which is different that a chest X-ray

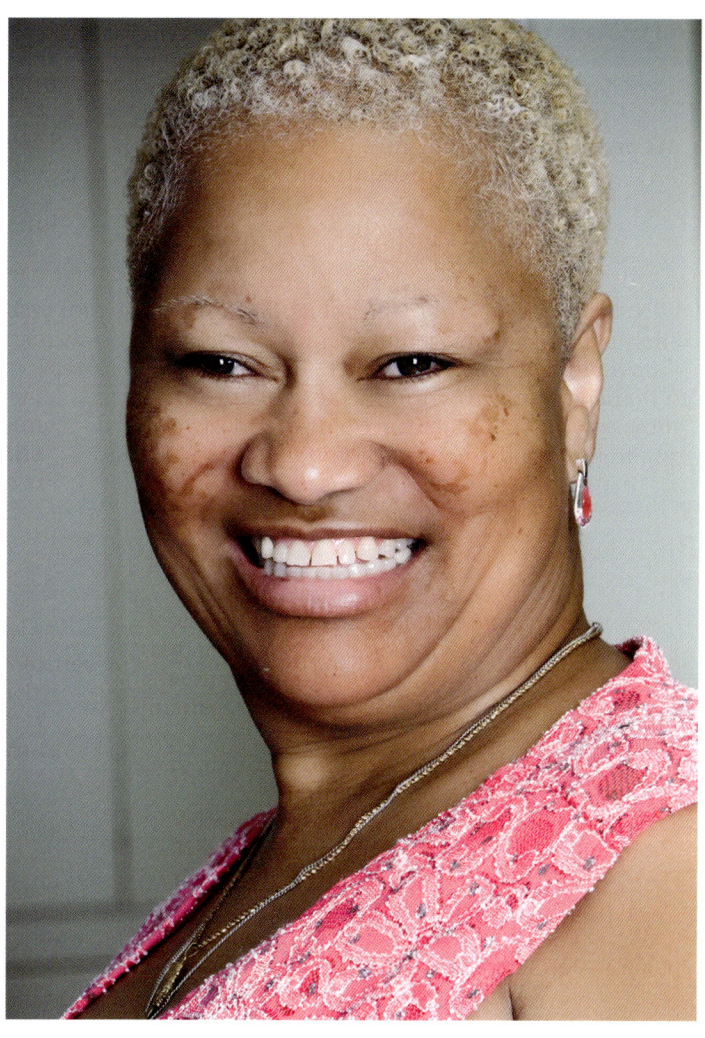

* *Request an Ultrasound (if you have to)*

* *Watch your diet...too much coffee, liquor, tea, coke, beef and pork, which stays in our bodies for up to 3 days. Drink plenty of water and exercise. Take better control of your new life.*

* *Keep your stress level down. It has depressed our immune system and made us open to diseases that really are preventable.*

* *Get plenty of rest and...*

* *If you find a lump **Get Moving**. Time is very, very crucial.*

Thank you for selecting and giving me such a wonderful opportunity to speak as a voice…
To share "**My Journey to Remember**" from Surgery to Chemo treatments to Reconstructive Surgery and Healing. It takes a lot of support to come through this type of Cancer experience. It causes you to step-up your spiritual connection which did strengthen my healing process. It caused me to think about what was and is "important" and what is "unimportant." Breast Cancer is not an end of the world sentence or a death sentence, but a platform for better health and for higher career and personal success. This disease is not contagious—it won't stop me from living my life.

…and today, **"I AM CANCER FREE, I AM A SURVIVOR AND I AM A WINNER"**

Today, I celebrate 15 years of marriage to "The Boss", as I always say.

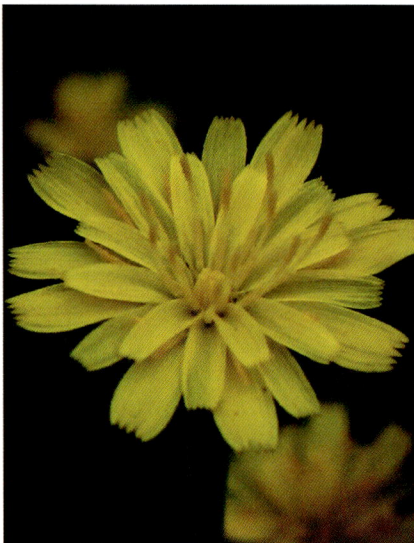

Photo: "LoveNoMatterWhat.com" by Petra

Since the beginning of my Journey to Remember I have started a Non-Profit Organization. Sister Connection for Breast Cancer—October 2005. I gave the first annual Cancer Awareness Fundraiser Luncheon. I pour from my heart my own experience with breast cancer. I feel I have a responsibility to my community. I believe I am a visionary and want to share with other breast cancer survivors and cancer survivors, their family, friends and those who have been touched.

From my eyes I see cancer as treatable, beatable and a survivable disease.

I see the total beauty within us and want to share my journey.

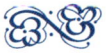

The Brighter Side
A BOUTIQUE FOR WOMEN WITH CANCER

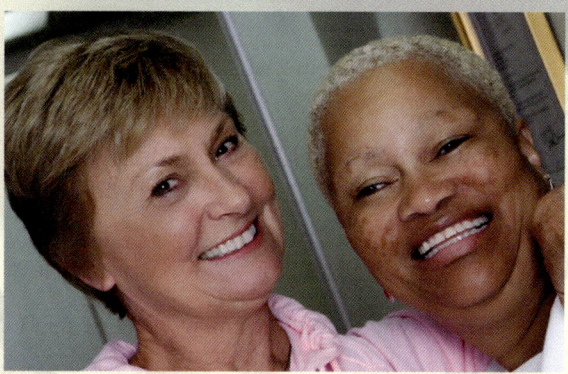

You've received a cancer diagnosis. Your treatment plan includes chemotherapy and you're told you are going to lose your hair. You're a breast cancer patient who has had a mastectomy and you have chosen not to have reconstruction. Your daughter has Alopecia, your income is limited and you have no insurance coverage. We can help.

The Brighter Side, a boutique for women with cancer located in Solana Beach is committed to bringing encouragement to women who are fighting cancer and the effects of cancer and women suffering from Alopecia. Our services are provided in a sensitive and caring environment. Services include wig selection, fitting and styling; mastectomy products—prosthesis and bras including fittings; head coverings and skin care products. The shop offers mail order throughout the country via its web site, www.mybrighterside.com. Phone orders are also accepted if client information is on file.

Our mastectomy products cover a broad spectrum starting with post-surgical drain containment garments, post-surgical bras and compression garments. Four to six weeks post surgery, our clients can chose from a wide variety of mastectomy bras and breast forms. Bra types include T-shirt style, camisole style and performance-style sports bras. Our silicone breast forms range from light weight to temperature equalizing and include full and partial styles. We also carry non-silicone forms. We carry a full line of bathing suits designed specifically to accommodate breast prosthesis. Our skin products include SkinCeuticals, Lindi and Jane Iredale Cosmetics.

The Brighter Side has certified mastectomy fitters on staff as well as a wig specialist who custom fits and styles our wigs for our clients. We offer women a supportive, feminine surrounding as well as comfortable, private fitting areas. One of our clients, Connie, is now a Brighter Side employee. Connie came to the shop in 2007 to purchase her mastectomy products and was so impressed with the atmosphere and our personal service she applied for a position and was eventually hired. "The Brighter Side is so different from any other store that I have been to that offers mastectomy products and other services for women with cancer. It's unique," says Connie.

The Brighter Side is also the administrator of The Virginia Ann Scheunemann Memorial Fund (VAS). The Virginia Ann Scheunemann Memorial Fund (VASMF), a 501(c)(3) non-profit, was established to ensure that any woman treated for cancer may have access to a wig or other head coverings, and/or mastectomy products at little or no cost to them. The fund is supported by donations and fund raisers.

The Brighter Side has been in business for over 15 years. Sherre Cain and Mari Muscio are shop proprietors. To learn more about us, contact us at

www.mybrighterside.com
or call us at **858-481-7565**
439 S. Cedros Avenue, Solana Beach, CA 92075

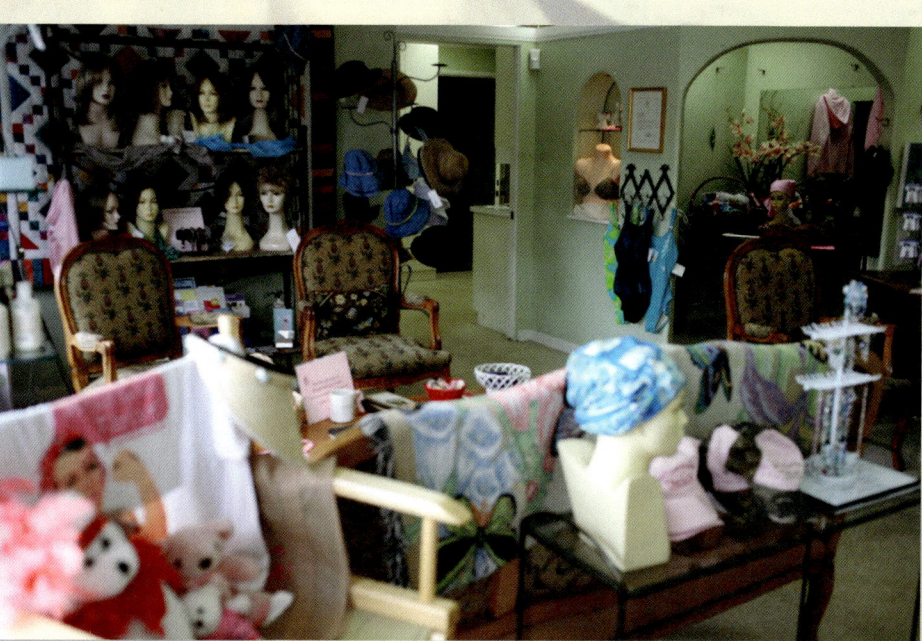

Chris

"Turning 60 Is Better Than the Alternative"

My name is Chris Eberhardt. At age 55 I was diagnosed with Stage 1 invasive ductal carcinoma and DCIS.

I'm a true believer on always seeing my glass half full, instead of half empty, so I waited a few months to call my doctor after noticing a small lump in my breast. After all, I just had a mammogram 6 months earlier without any indication for concern. My General Practitioner assured me that it was probably nothing since 70-80% of breast lumps are benign, but she still wanted to do another mammogram and also have an ultrasound done. The radiology department said they could fit me in at the end of the day, which was a Friday.

After the radiologist technician took the base mammogram, she came in and said that they did not see anything unusual, but that they had to do the ultrasound anyway because my doctor ordered it. I felt as if she just wanted to start her weekend and I was keeping her from it. With an attitude she asked if I could locate the lump for her so she could start the ultrasound. I watched the monitor as she began and she started taking measurements of the area. I asked her if that area was what I was feeling. She looked at me and said that she needed to get the radiologist in because she will want to see this. This time she spoke to me with a different tone and demeanor. The radiologist reviewed the monitor in the identified area and told me that I had a solid mass measuring just under 2 cm and asked me if I understood what that meant. I answered with, "It needs to be biopsied", still thinking the lump would be in that 70-80 percentile of benign lumps.

My family doctor called on Monday, after reviewing the radiologist's report, and wanted to set up an appointment to do the biopsy. I told her that I wanted to wait a few weeks because I was having company visiting from out of town. She said that the results would indicate that the lump was a category 4 and she strongly recommended that the biopsy should be done as soon as I could get an appointment.

So, a few days before my company arrived I had the biopsy done, still thinking that there was no way I was in that 20 percentile of biopsies that come back cancerous. Still, I did have the "fear of the unknown"… of the biopsy procedure, the pain (especially with company coming), but never fearing the results. My husband assured me that he would do all the chores and help with the company.

A few days later my Doctor called saying it was malignant. She believes in giving the results first over the phone and then with a follow-up appointment. She had cancer herself and knows what it felt like as a patient to be asked to return for the results, especially if they can't get back in for a few days because of their work or family schedules. She said it also gives them a chance to scream, cry, or get mad in familiar surroundings with family. Thank God my husband was home waiting for the call with me. As soon as my doctor hung up, my husband gave me a big hug and assured me that we would get through this.

> *I had the biopsy done, still thinking that there was no way I was in that 20 percentile of biopsies that come back cancerous. Still, I did have the "fear of the unknown"…*

A second later the phone rang again. It was my daughter calling from LA who was also waiting for the news. I told her that "it" was caught very early and was very, very curable. I felt so bad because she was crying and I was so far away and she was so scared because her close friend just lost her mother to cancer. I wanted to assure her that it was not going to happen to me.

The hardest part for me ended up being the easiest and best part for me…it was my first laugh. How was I going to tell my 80-some year old parents who had their own health issues? I had to tell them soon because my company visiting me was also family. How could I not tell my company? Although I hated to spoil their vacation, if I didn't tell them I knew they would somehow feel the tension and think they weren't welcome.

So, I had to tell my parents because I wanted them to hear it from me instead of my brother-in-law. My Mom answered and I asked her to get Dad on the second line because I had something very important to tell them. I told them that I had good news and bad news. The good news was that it was NOT a death sentence. The bad

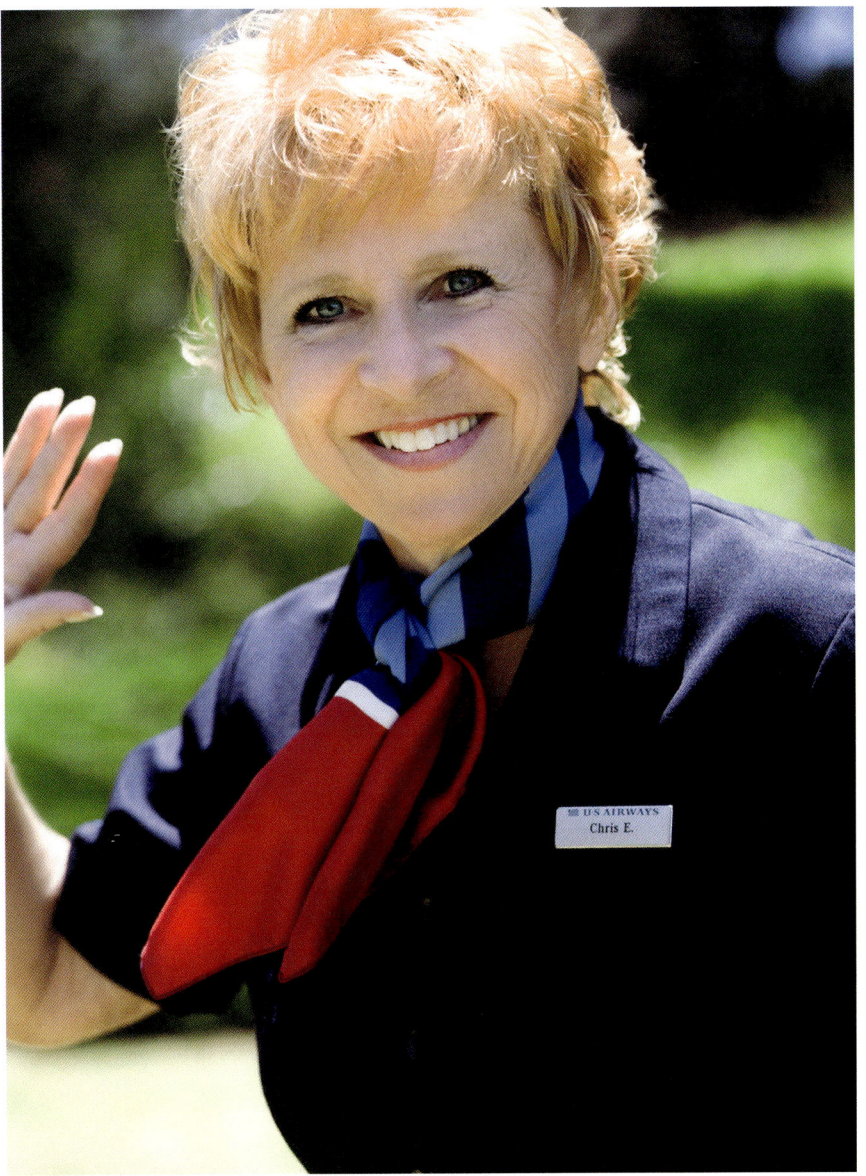

news was that I had breast cancer. It was the first time that I said "it" . . . the big "C" word, and it made me tear up. My Dad who believes he is not hard of hearing and doesn't need a hearing aid said "You have a can of soup???" "No Dad, breast cancer." "Huh, what kind of can of soup?" My Mom, not saying anything, yelled "Ray, can't you hear her?" He yelled back "I hear her; I just don't know what kind of soup." I just started to laugh and my husband asked what was so funny about this? I was laughing telling him that Dad thinks I have a can of soup. I tell my Mom goodbye and ask her to clue Dad in on what's going on after we hang up. A few minutes later, it's my Dad on the phone telling me that he beat cancer and so will I. And my Mom apologized for not knowing what to say and that she should have said something supportive instead of crying. I was soooo glad that it came off that way. I finally was able to say the word "cancer", I had my first tear, and my first laugh at the same time.

> *It was the first time that I said "it"... the big "C" word, and it made me tear up.*

The next stop on my journey was a visit with the surgeon. Again, always seeing my glass half full, instead of half empty, I could not believe what I was hearing. Listening to my surgeon give me two options: the first "package" as she called it was a lumpectomy with radiation, a lymphectomy and radiation. The second package was a total mastectomy and she explained the entire procedure from the incisions to the final tattoo of the nipple on the newly restructured breast that she would give me. WOW . . . I couldn't believe what I was hearing. I looked over at my husband for some guidance and saw disbelieve on his face as well. I quickly said "package # 1" and he agreed just as fast. Then the surgeon agreed with "Good Choice" but reiterated that the surgery must be followed up with radiation, or she would not do the surgery because the cancer would return. I asked her about Chemo treatment and she said that wasn't her department and I needed to see an oncologist and an oncology radiologist when the results came back after the surgery.

Even though all of my family support could not physically be here for me, I felt they were 100% "there" for me. My parents in Ohio could not travel due to health issues, and my sister offered to come. However, I felt less stressed knowing that she was back there for my parents and I would do just fine here. My daughter who just started a new job working on the TV program, Two and a Half Men, took two weeks off to come and help. My husband was wonderful. I was concerned about the financial ramifications of all of this. He would not let me look at one invoice and wanted me not to stress, but to focus on getting better.

The surgery went well and with not much pain. The really uncomfortable part was the drain. My surgeon told me the drain would stay in for a FEW days. 21 days in my vocabulary is not a FEW days. My husband was absolutely wonderful, draining it several times a day. My radiation treatment was a breeze. It lasted 5 days a week for 7 weeks. For most of the treatment, I would ride my bike to the cancer center. My last treatment was May 31st. Living in Arizona the weather became quite warm and my breast was getting totally burnt. I am not sure if it was the heat or the radiation treatment, but I drove in my air conditioned car the final week of treatment.

Now the real fun began. I wasn't prepared for the side effects from the treatment that followed the radiation. I was ecstatic that my lymph nodes were clean and I didn't need chemotherapy, but I still needed to be on a five-year treatment of

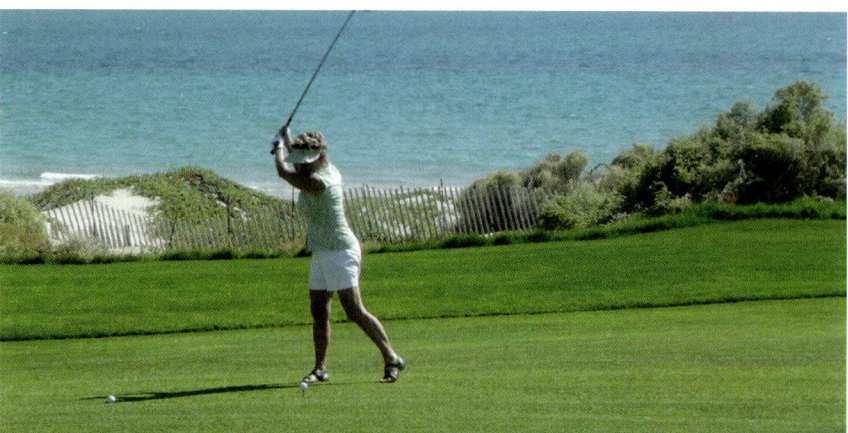

estrogen receptors. I started off with tamoxifen for several months, which has a big side effect of bone and muscle pain. I took it as long as I could, then I switched to aromasin, then arimidex, and then femara. All of these drugs gave me the same side effect. I kept loosing bone mass and now was diagnosed with osteopena, the beginning stages of osteoporosis and was put on medication that also causes more muscle and joint pain. Some mornings the pain and stiffness were so bad my husband would help me get dressed for work. I work at the airport, and normally take the employee bus to the terminal from the employee parking lot. I knew that I could not get on and off the bus so I would park in the short-term parking at my expense so that I could just walk into the building. As the day progressed the pain did lessen and I was determined not to give up. Then, three years into the treatment I finally told my oncologist that I wanted my life back to normal and was not going to take anymore medication. He said he wanted to try one more thing. It was monthly injections of Faslodex. It had the least amount of side effects of all the others, but comes with a high price tag. He checked with my insurance carrier and determined that most of it was covered. I still had the joint and muscle pain, but it was bearable and I completed my five-year treatment never even missing a day of work!

Six months after my surgery, with all my aches and pains, my husband and I participated in the Jimmy Fund walk and completed all 26 miles on the Boston Marathon route helping to raise funds for Dana Farber cancer research. We participated in this event every year that I was in treatment. Some years, I could only do half of the marathon due to the extreme joint and muscle pain. Without the cancer I probably would never have even attempted this. But, because of the cancer I became a more determined person to do things I only thought other, younger, more fit, more experienced people could do. Don't you believe it! You too can do whatever you put your mind, body, and soul into. Let the cancer be a catalyst to new and exciting adventures.

I am so fortunate that I found my cancer early and it was very curable. I finally have my life back and I am able to enjoy all of the things that I love and I can now do. I am semi-retired (work

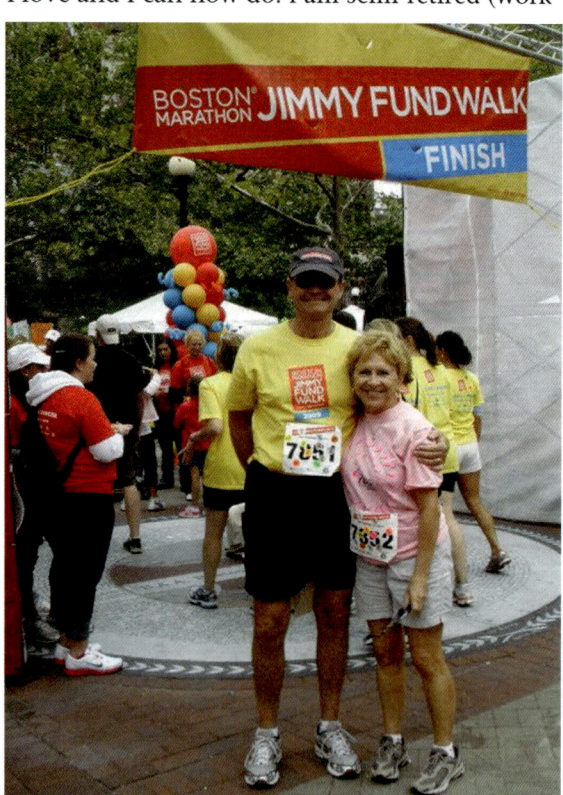

part-time) for a major airline. I still love to work, golf, hike, kayak and bike, and of course travel. I am a very active (almost) senior citizen... ouch, now that really hurts!

If I had to quote one thing that defines my experience, it would be that no one is invincible or safe from this disease, but together with the help and support of friends and family you can get through it. And surviving cancer will make you stronger, wiser, and a better person than before.

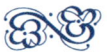

> ...because of the cancer I became a more determined person to do things I only thought other, younger, more fit, more experienced people could do.

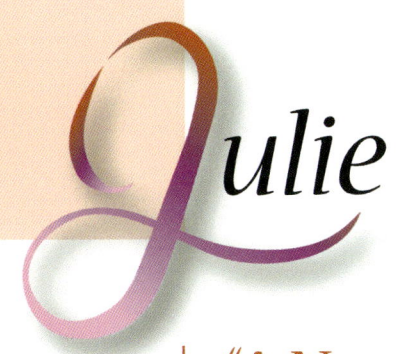

Julie

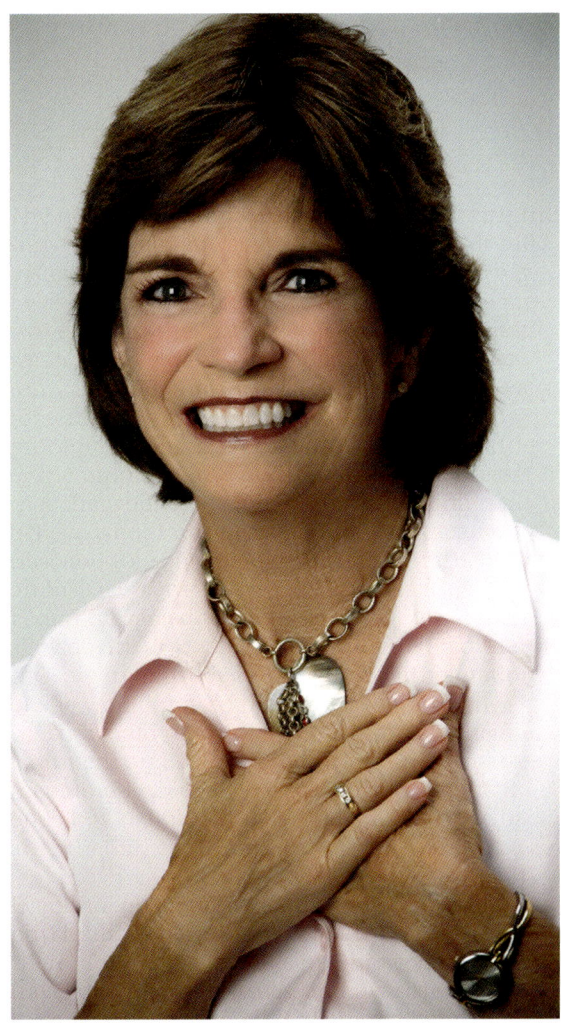

"A New Chapter Begins"

I have never been fond of the color pink even though it is perfectly fine for flowers and other parts of nature. So it is quite ironic that the color pink has become such a focal point in this new chapter in my life. A year ago, if you would have looked in my closet, which was arranged by color—red being most prevalent—you would have found most hues, except for pink. Whether it was just my skin tone, my mother's attempt to keep me in pink when I was young or my personal preference, I do not know. I just know that from an early age I was not a pink type of girl.

Just who is this lady that doesn't like pink? I am a 65-year-old semi-retired teacher who loves life and people. I am a mother, a wife, a friend, a learner, a cook, a shopper, a volunteer, an exerciser, a writer, an open-minded citizen and I just happen to be living with a breast cancer. My life is a happy one. I choose to find the positives within the challenges that develop in my life. And this is just one of those pesky challenges!

My story begins with a routine gynecologist appointment just like those I had done religiously year after year. On the patient's door was a poster that read "78% of all breast cancer occurs in women after age 50." That poster had probably been there for several years, but not until that day had it taken hold with me. After the exam, I went home thinking, "Wow, that is profound." But because the doctor didn't feel anything unusual, I thought I had slid through another year of blissful womanhood without a glitch. Wrong! A week later, I went to have my yearly mammogram thinking all was well, but that poster still was on my mind. Mammograms had always been so simple; boob in, boob out and repeat. Five minutes—done. No problem because I always had ample breast material—plenty to squeeze and squish.

Shortly after I got home, my concerned doctor called to let me know that all did not look well and that I needed to schedule another appointment for further investigation. Just another formality, I thought. Wrong again. An ultrasound, a biopsy, a pathology report, and Wham! I was now a statistic. I was the one out of 8 women diagnosed with breast cancer. Disbelief. There was no history of breast cancer in my immediate family. How could this be?

> *An ultrasound, a biopsy, a pathology report, and Wham! I was now a statistic. I was the one out of 8 women diagnosed with breast cancer.*

Throughout the next week, there was a trip to the surgeon, a call to cancel our Fall foliage cruise, and a call to my employer letting him know that I would be out of commission for a few weeks. I didn't want to talk about it—just push forward until the mass was gone. Get it out!

The diagnosis sounded manageable. The mass was about a centimeter, Stage 1 and well differentiated. No lymph node involvement. The oncologist and surgeon gave me choices. Should I treat the right breast only or the whole body? After days of pondering, I chose no chemo but instead a lumpectomy and radiation. Thank God for yearly mammograms and early detection!

The word cancer is loaded with powerful and emotional concerns and for my grown children, Jaime and Cory. They felt so helpless. They told me to stay off the Internet—just to listen to my doctors. What could they do to support me? How could they help? Jaime went directly to her writing mode using the Internet to get the word out to friends and family. Cory went to emotional mode and we cried and cried and hugged each other. My husband, Neil, was my usual Rock of Gibraltar. As the weeks flew by, we all settled down a bit and realized that there were so many women who were living full lives with breast cancer and so could I.

> *…it seemed like women came out of the woodwork to let me know that they too were breast cancer survivors, people I had known for years who had never shared their stories until now.*

All in all, I seemed to weather the storm quite well. My friends and family were there for me. I felt fine—no tiredness or unbearable pain. My teacher friends signed us up for the Susan G. Komen Race for the Cure under the team name "Jammin' with Julie" and 37 of us walked together, inspired by all those thousands of my breast cancer sisters and their family and friends. And yes I was wearing my survivor pink t-shirt. So much pink!

My life continues as usual, but there is never a day that goes by that I don't think about my

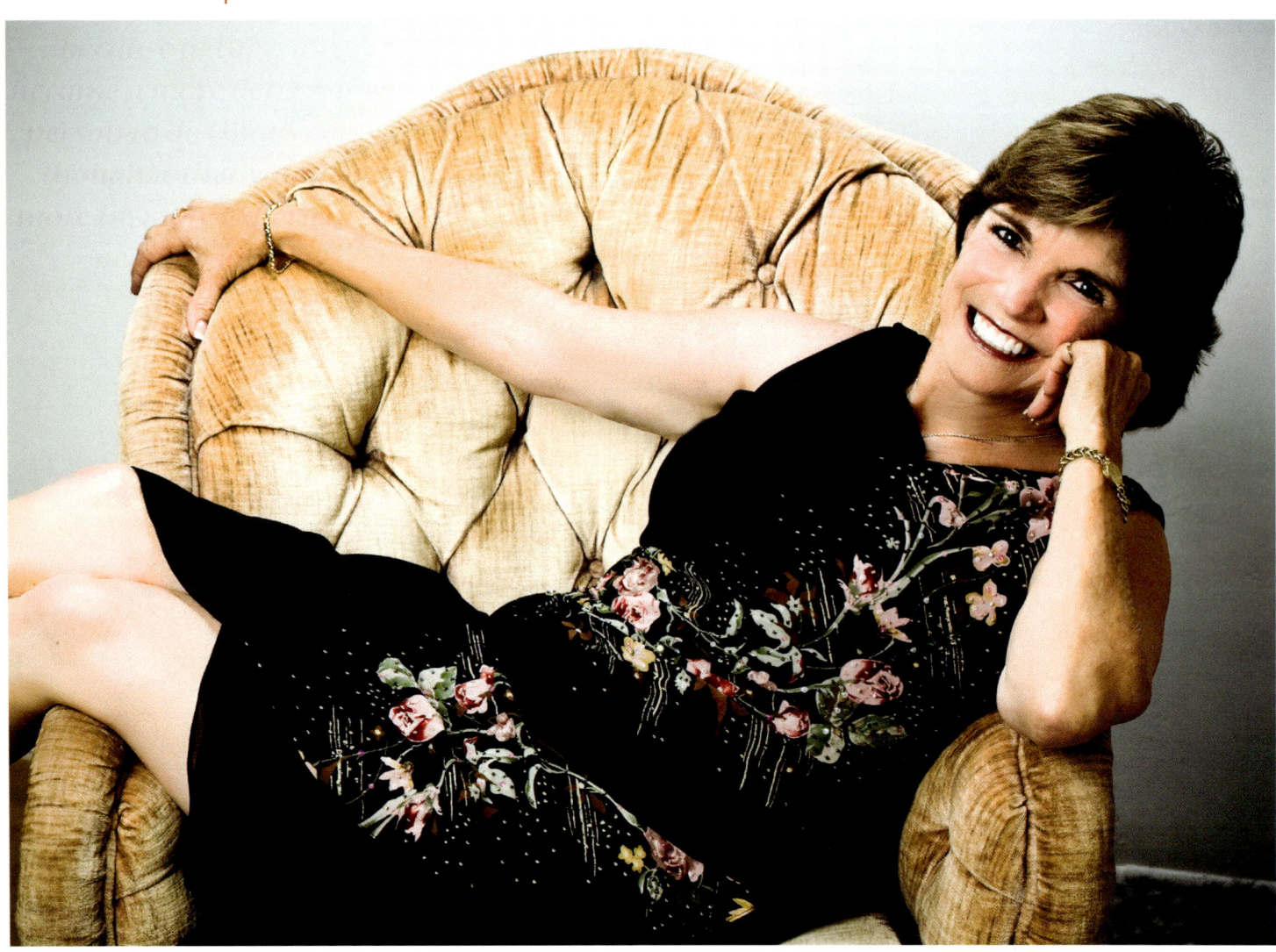

cancer. What does my future hold? Just because my cancer was Stage 1, there are no guarantees about what's ahead, but I keep a positive attitude and think about the many women in my life that are breast cancer survivors. In the beginning, it seemed like women came out of the woodwork to let me know that they, too, were breast cancer survivors, people I had known for years who had never shared their stories until now. I looked around and listened to what they had to say and realized that I was in good company and that a quality life does go on. The one story that really inspired me the most was that of my 91 year-old "aunt" who was diagnosed with breast cancer 54 years ago. When she came out of surgery after her

> *I have learned that it is our imperfections that make us unique; it is our challenges that build our character; it is our outlook on life that propels our spirit.*

mastectomy, the doctor said to her, "I just added 10 years to your life." Wouldn't he be surprised today at this remarkable women and how she proved him wrong!

In June of this year, I became involved in an energy study at UCSD. The focus is on exercise, nutrition, weight loss and maintenance. Although I had always been a bit chubby, I had never been overly concerned about my weight because I have always felt good. The study has changed my whole perspective on life. I am doing everything possible to make sure I stay healthy. Exercise, weight maintenance and caloric intake are foremost in my mind. I have some weddings, trips and grandchildren to look forward to and I plan on being there for these events!

Pink is still not my favorite color, but one by one, a few pieces of pink clothing have crept into my closet—even a couple of pink bras are in my drawer! I have learned that it is our imperfections that make us unique; it is our challenges that build our character; it is our outlook on life that propels our spirit. So here I am a senior citizen, full of energy and positive thoughts and I have a new color in my life that symbolizes hope. Breast cancer is now part of my life, but I am up for the challenge!

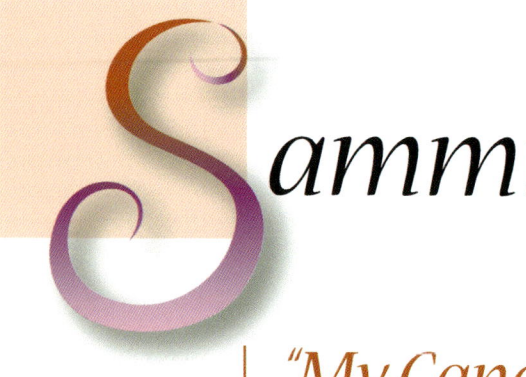

Sammi

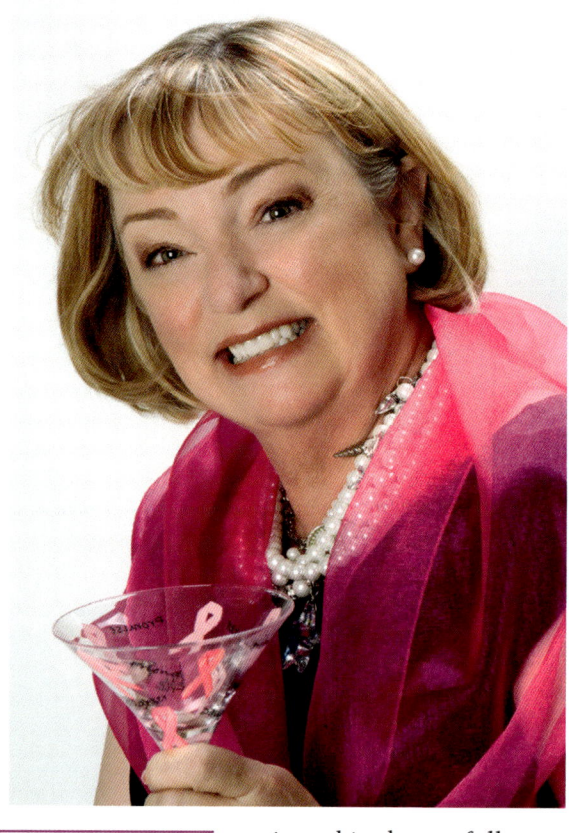

"My Cancer Is a Gift"

Hi. My name is Sammantha McDonald. I'm 61 years young (although I still feel like I'm 39) and I was 46 when I was diagnosed with very early stage breast cancer, DCIS. I knew absolutely nothing about breast cancer when I was diagnosed 15 years ago. And, the internet was in its early stages, too, so much of my research was done at the library via books.

When I received the phone call from my doctor, I was in shock. No one in my family had ever been diagnosed with any kind of cancer. I was the first, just like I was the first to graduate from college; the first to get a graduate degree; the first in my Irish Catholic family to get a divorce. I didn't know where to turn and I didn't know who to tell or how to tell them. I waited until I had all the facts and the dates of my surgery, etc., before I told any of my family members. My dad didn't want to talk about it. My mom was sympathetic, but didn't know what to do. My brother and sisters were loving and supportive. My daughter, who is much like me, wanted the facts and asked whether she should move up her wedding date. You see, everyone thought cancer was a death sentence. Although I feared the same at first, after doing the research, I was pretty certain I was going to be ok.

And then, I made my deal with God. I promised Him that if He got me through this, I would do everything I could to help other women making this journey. I would tell everyone who would listen about the importance of early detection via self-exams and mammograms. I would raise all the money I could to help those who didn't have health insurance and fund research to find better treatments and the cures for breast cancer.

So, on September 23, 1996, I had my left breast removed. I made that decision because I would not need to do any follow-up treatment and because there was so much non-invasive cancer, a lumpectomy would not have left me with much. Two weeks after my mastectomy, I got a call, asking me to talk with someone who was just diagnosed. I didn't think twice. I made the call and after I hung up, I knew exactly what I was to do with my life. Breast cancer had changed my life and given me a whole new direction.

> *I made my deal with God. I promised Him that if He got me through this, I would do everything I could to help other women making this journey.*

I become involved with the American Cancer Survivor where I received their first Celebration of Life Award for continuing to exceed in my work with my community and my career after my diagnosis. I served as a legislative ambassador both in Sacramento and D.C., lobbying our legislators for programs and funding, I was also an honorary spokesperson at the Making Strides Against Breast Cancer Walk and Relay for Life. Susan G. Komen for the Cure honored me by appointing me as their Honorary Survivor in 2000. I've continued to volunteer with Komen holding positions from Race Volunteer to President and am now holding the prestigious title of President Emeritus. I've raised nearly $200,000 for the Race and the 3-Day. I was able to secure nearly $1 million in sponsorships for the Race. And I'm still talking to anyone who will listen about the importance of early detection.

15 years later, I'm still nervous when I have my annual mammogram and blood work. I actually look at the mammogram to see if there are any changes. Usually, I just scare myself because I really don't know how to read them. But I'm learning a lot about cancer. I was lucky to be chosen to participate in the Scientist–Survivor program with the American Association of Cancer Researchers. I learn from scientists and medical personnel who attend these sessions, so that I can be a better advocate, whether I am attending a doctor's appointment with a newly diagnosed patient, or I'm on Capitol Hill, asking for more money for research. It helps me keep "abreast" of all the technology that is going on. I've also reviewed research grants that are proposing some very exciting projects that may find the cures for breast cancer.

> **Keep hope in your heart. Never stop laughing. Allow people to help; they really want to DO something for you.**

If you are reading this because you are newly diagnosed and you've read all the magazines in the doctor's office, take this bit of advice. Keep hope in your heart. Never stop laughing. Allow people to help; they really want to DO something for you. Rest. Snuggle a baby or a puppy dog. Dance. Hold hands with someone you love. Learn to do something new during your recovery. Make a new friend. Help someone. And most of all (and I know this is going to sound odd), look at your breast cancer as a gift. A gift that makes you look at life differently. A gift that inspires you to do good things. A gift that really changes your life for the better. Cancer changed my life for the better, honestly. And it will change yours, if you let it.

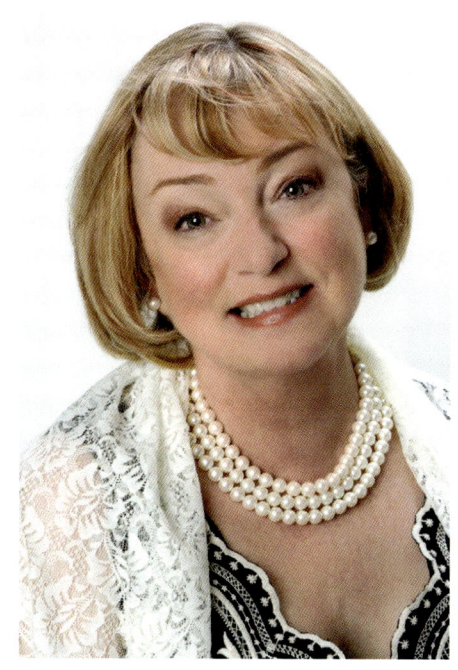

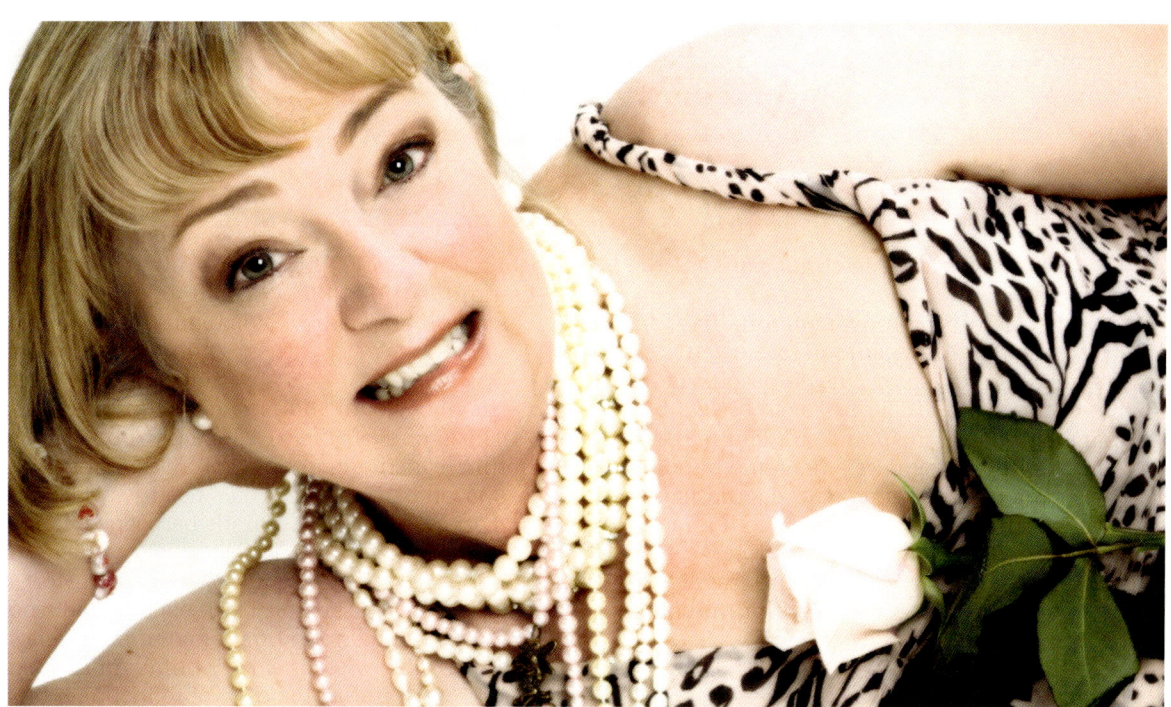

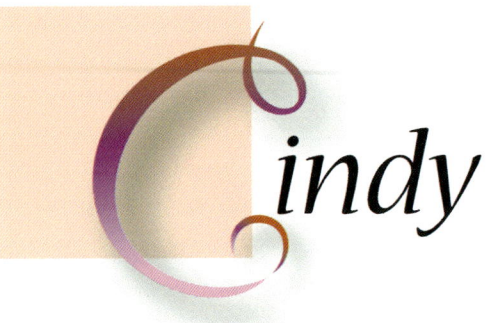

Cindy

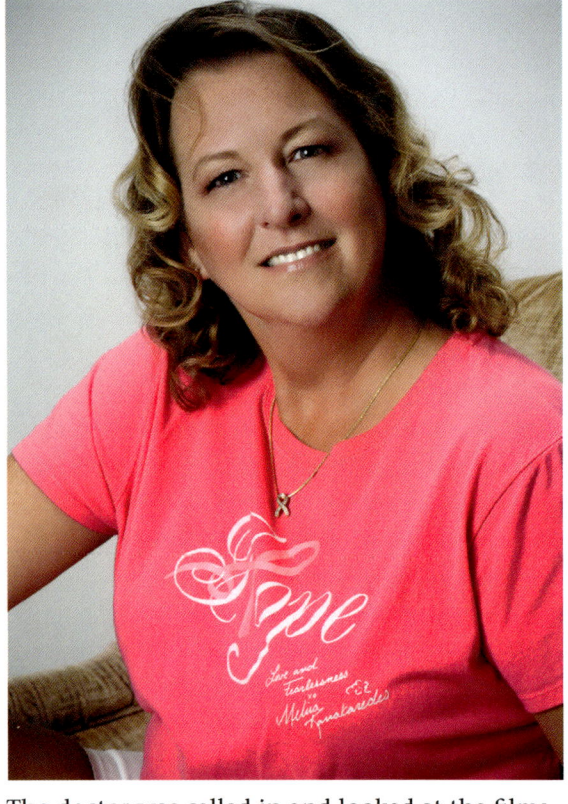

"My Daily Journal"

Friday, September 26, 2008

Hello Family & Friends,

I've decided to start this blog to keep everyone informed so you know what is going on with me. Please know that I'm not asking for pity whatsoever. Again, this is to keep everyone informed. Some may think it's saying more than it should, but this is where my heart is. It's to give informational facts and honesty of what I'm feeling, I hope not to say something that hurts anyone…so please take it for what it is.

Pre-September 2008

I found out that I had a polyp on my cervix so I called Chris, I was crying, scared of what it meant. Then I called my mom and my mother-in-law, Tina. After talking with them I then scheduled myself to see the nurse practitioner to find out where to go with this.

September 2008

My appointment was on 9/3, what I now call my trifecta day. The nurse practitioner decided to do a full exam. She saw the polyp and felt a fist-sized mass above my uterus. She also found a lump in my breast. This is when my world turned upside down.

I went home and called a select few, of course my husband, then my Children, then my mother's, and a couple of girlfriends. Before I knew it, I had doctors calling me. My first scheduled mammogram was on Monday, 9/8. 16 different x-rays were taken. They did not like what they saw and sent me immediately to get an ultrasound. In the ultrasound room, Tina joined me and sat patiently (and didn't speak much at all), and all of you who know my mother-in-law, that's unusual. She always has questions and firmness within her, but I could see in her eyes something was wrong (even though I didn't let it sink in at that time).

> …this was a time when my husband and boys scattered. They didn't look or talk to me, I felt like I had the plague, but I feel it was fear.

The doctor was called in and looked at the films himself and ordered biopsies. Tina was told that too many people would be in the room and it would be best if she waited outside. So she left with phone in hand to call my mother. I still at that time did not know what she was feeling inside (she later described it as a big spider body with lots of legs).

The doctor took four biopsies and also put in a titanium clip to assist later in the surgery, if needed. During the biopsies there was a new intern in the room. She could not handle the needle and biopsy procedure and passed out. I still left the office with hopes that nothing was wrong and everything would end up fine.

My next appointment was on 9/10, Wednesday, with the module director of OB/GYN. He did his exam and removed the polyp and said he did not feel a mass above my uterus, but just to be safe, he ordered an ultrasound.

Later that day, at 2:22, I couldn't handle it anymore. I called to find out what my results were, and that's when I was first told that I have INVASIVE DUCTAL CARCINOMA. You all know that my family has always been very close, but this was a time when my husband and boys scattered. They didn't look or talk to me, I felt like I had the plague, but I feel it was fear. As soon as Kathy (my sister-in-law) heard, she rushed to be by my side and spent the evening with me.

Monday, October 20th, 2008

So it comes Monday now. I get up and get to the hospital to have my Double Mastectomy, and at the hospital right away I met with my sister-in-law Kathy, and my niece, my boys are there, my mother and father, and we're ready to go and we sign in.

> **I hurt off and on in different ways, but I don't show it and I don't want to show it. I want to be as normal as possible through this road that has been given to me.**

And everybody else is told to go up to the third floor. I had to have a mini procedure done on the first floor, and so Kathy joined me. It was where they put a radioactive material into you, and I'm not going to get specific. It is quite painful, the location of how they did this, and I will just say that each shot that they did felt like lightning to my breast, and that's all that needs to be said.

After getting into my room, and was changed into my pre-op clothes, three people at a time came in to say good luck to me until all the family and friends had said hello. Before you know it, they said, "Okay, it's time." And I was out. I don't even remember being put under.

So we left the hospital at 8:30 at night and came home, and a lot of people were hungry. Chris didn't even eat at all during the whole day because of his being worried about me. We stayed up until about 11:30 at night, talking and me sitting in my recliner and just winding down from the whole day's events.

Saturday, November 8th, 2008

This was the first day that I would get to take a shower because I had to wait until the holes from the drains sealed up. So it was my first real shower. Boy, was I excited. The thing is, when you go to do things that you're so accustomed to doing, you don't realize when you can't do them, sometimes until it's too late.

So today I tried to relax most of the day because it seems like every time I would go out, my body would lose all its energy and the next day I'd pay for it. So I kind of relaxed because I knew that Saturday evening was my girlfriend Jill's son's 18th birthday party and was really looking forward to going and sitting around their fire pit.

Everything was going great, and then something happened. And, Jill, when you're reading this, I hope you understand what I'm saying. Let me get through it all before and I hope you don't get hurt feelings. She had made mention to a gentleman that was there at the party that I was the one that he had donated money to help us, and he gave her a look of "She is?" Now, I don't know how I was supposed to interpret this, but the way I interpreted it is I didn't look ill enough or sick enough, and I felt guilty.

I then turned and thought what a nice person to have given to our family, donated some money to help us with all these different costs that we have. We have never taken a handout and never felt the need until now, and I wondered, should I go just sit down and not move around and not be so happy, but I can't live my life this way. And for all of you friends, I need help with this. I know that this person was probably just thinking good thoughts for me, it is just my self-esteem.

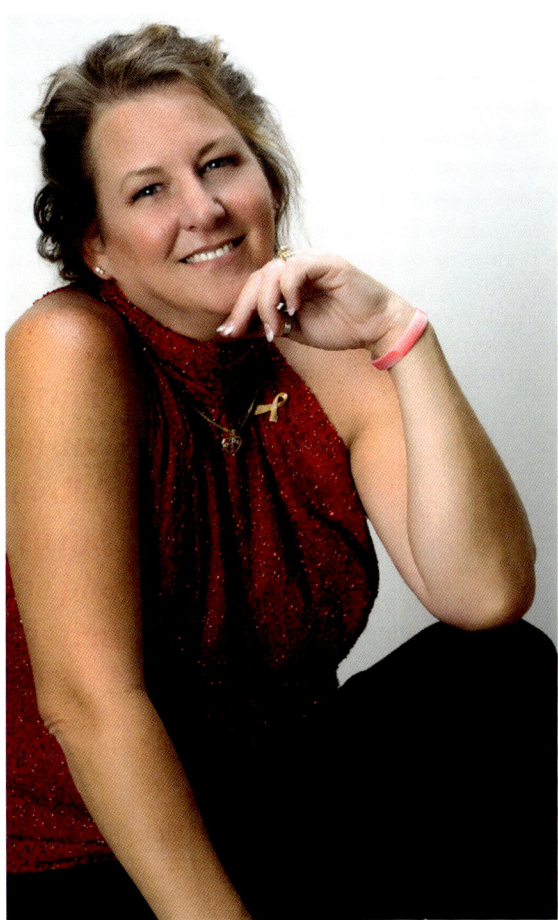

I want to act as normal as possible so I don't feel sick. I believe I'll feel better if I keep a positive outlook and don't struggle with the illness that's been given to me. I don't want to show signs of defeat, but I felt so guilty, thinking that because I'm out or not looking sick that someone's giving to me was not needed.

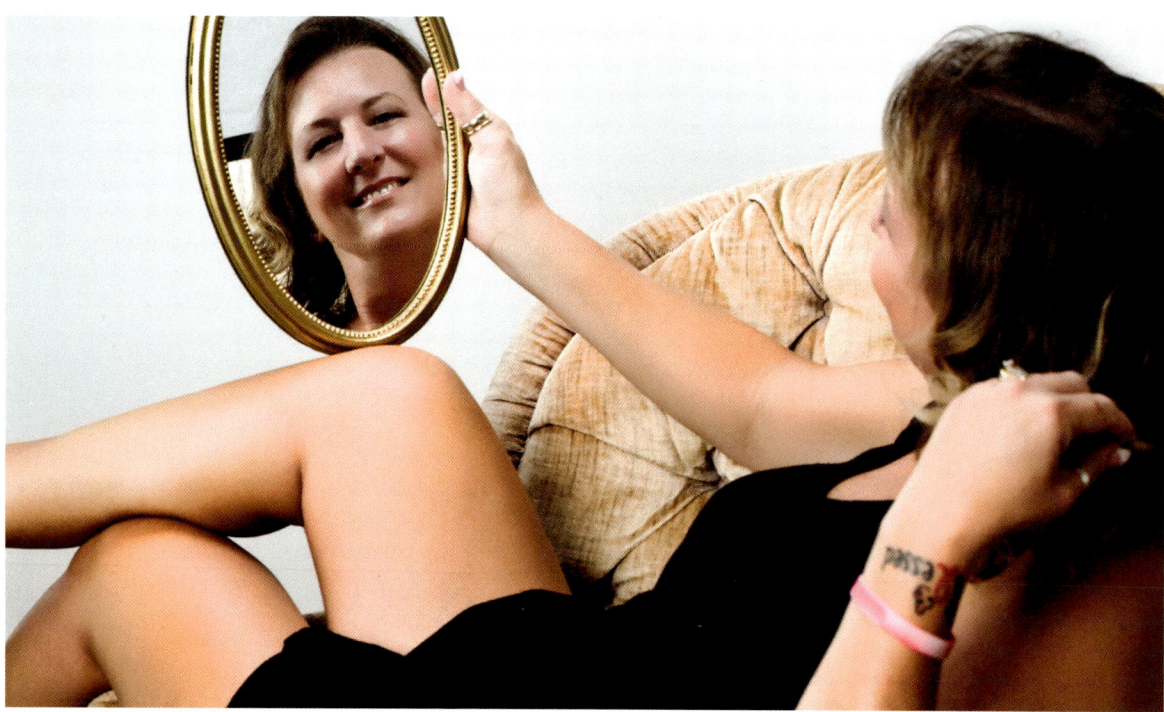

I hurt off and on in different ways, but I don't show it and I don't want to show it. I want to be as normal as possible through this road that has been given to me. And maybe I shouldn't have taken it the way I did, but I don't want this person to feel that he wasted his money.

I don't know what better way to explain it, and maybe I'm not even explaining it correctly, but I hope that anybody that's reading this that was so kind to help us through this would know that I'm not being frivolous at all, that this donated money is covering so many things, from me getting a few button-down blouses to getting mineral makeup to paying for the doctors' appointments to paying for my pharmaceutical meds to paying for the post-surgical bras, and it will pay for the wig that I'll need to get soon, and it's paid for gas to get me to and from my far-distance appointments that I have to go on a regular basis. It has been a blessing more than you can imagine.

Tuesday, November 18th, 2008

Urgent! Urgent! Urgent!...My girlfriends decided a while back that we wanted to do a big hair night before my hair is gone (I love the idea and would love you ALL, Men and Women to join). I wanted to forward this info so that you would receive it after my blog was completely up-to-date now, but it's going to be brief so you know about the plans now.

> *My girlfriends decided… that we wanted to do a big hair night before my hair is gone.*

It's this Saturday, November 22nd, at Patrick's II, downtown. It will be my last day of having my hair. On Sunday, my boys will be shaving it. The theme for the party is "BIG HAIR." I'm going to "Farrah Fawcett or 80's" up my hair. Aunt Pattie, I'd love to see that magenta streak back in your hair that I was used to when we were growing up in High School. Hopefully you can find the Halloween spray to do that! Since hats and head covers will be in my future, Guys...or ladies...feel free to wear a funky hat or unique covering. There are no rules to the Hair theme!! And if you don't want to do your hair, that's okay too. Really, I'd just love to see you. You all have given me so much hope & spirits & love. I look forward to Saturday.

Tuesday, December 23rd, 2008

So I end this with a thank you to my friends and family. I know we struggle with hard things ahead, but we are blessed by YOU and without your strength and belief, I don't know where we would be. I love you all, you make me stronger because I know you care and are there for me. So thank you, with much love.

Have a Very Merry Christmas and a Happy New Year.

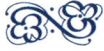

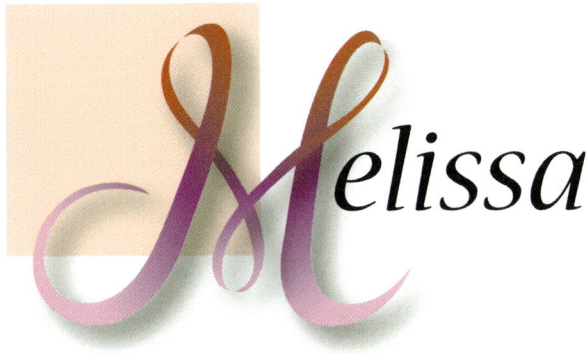

Melissa

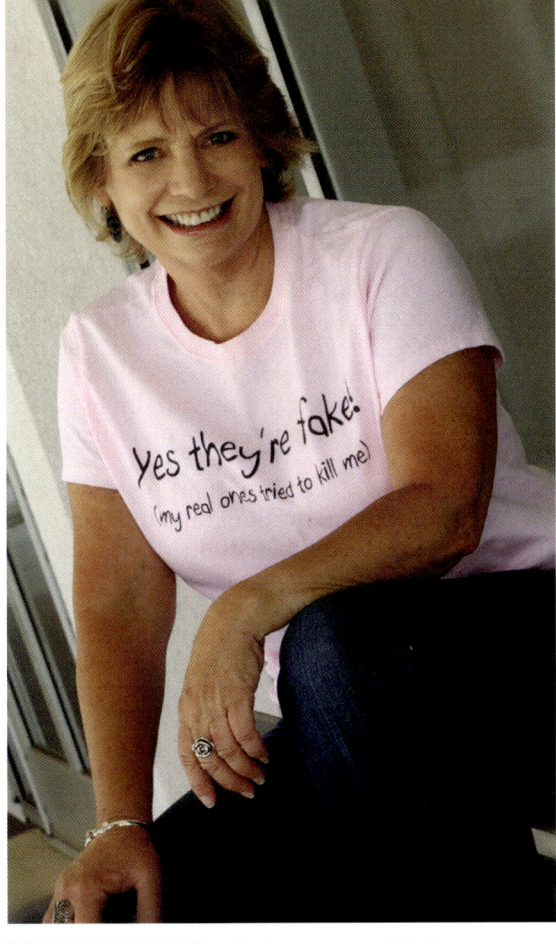

"Never, Ever, Give Up"

My name is Melissa Maki. I have been married to Bill for almost 24 years. We have one daughter, Mallory, who is 21 years old. I wasn't sure I would even see her graduate from middle school. I am happy to say she will graduate from San Diego State University in the spring of 2012.

I was diagnosed with stage 3 breast cancer in August of 2001 at the age of 42. After having a mastectomy with TRAM-flap reconstruction we found out that of the 11 lymph nodes removed, 7 tested positive for cancer.

So began chemotherapy. I hated watching that poison being pumped into my veins. I was so sick; I slept on a piece of foam on the bathroom floor for the first 5-6 days after treatment. YUK!! If that wasn't bad enough I lost every bit of my hair, even my eyebrows and lashes. Radiation followed 5 days a week for 6 weeks. Then another round of chemo. I often thought I was going to die.

I am so happy that I survived! Life is good!

My greatest concern through everything was leaving my daughter. How would Bill raise Mallory without me? I am so happy that I survived! Life is good!

In June of 2006 I attended a retreat for breast cancer survivors. That weekend changed my life. I finally felt pretty! I actually felt good emotionally for the first time in my life. I met so many incredible, strong women who are so inspiring. I am better for having met them. I know the medical team saved me physically, but the retreat saved me emotionally.

My advice to newly diagnosed women—never, ever give up, and try to laugh everyday.

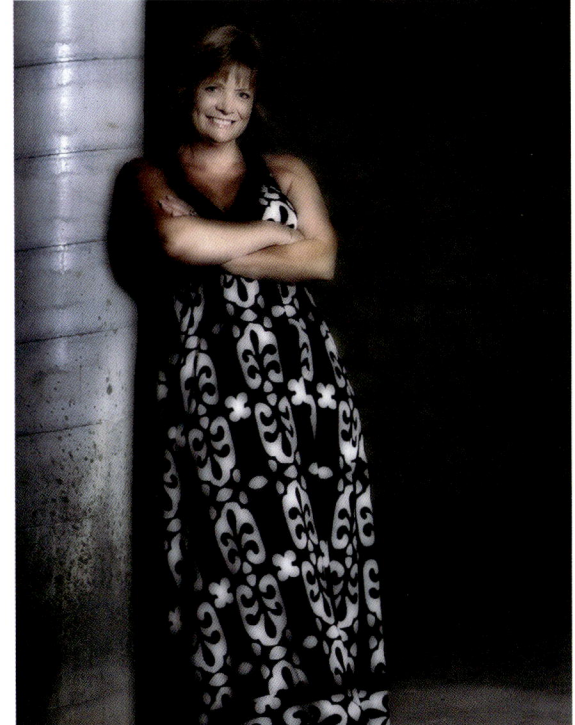

Photography by Joanna Herr

Ana

"Case of the Flying Prostheses"

My name is Ana Maria Montes de Oca, I'm 56 years old and was diagnosed my first time when I was 34, with stage one. I didn't have medical insurance at the time and had gone for a physical or health appraisal and one of the questions was, "when you squeeze your nipples do you have any discharge"?

I had never done this before, but I tried and although very hard for me to do, I had some fluid come out from both of my breasts. I made an appointment, thinking that I was going to see a doctor and instead saw a NURSE PRACTITIONER. When I explain to her my concerns, she said I was starting an early menopause and wanted to give me hormones. I said "no I want a mammogram" and she said "no, you are not at high risk and don't qualify because you are too young". At that point I said I want to see a doctor and finally she said OK and arranged for me to see one.

> "…I want a mammogram" and she said "no, you are not at high risk and don't qualify because you are too young".

The results from my left breast were abnormal and I was sent to a surgeon. It was explained that there were calcium deposits that looked suspicious and a biopsy showed it was cancer. I had a lumpectomy and radiation for 6 weeks. At that time my girls were 9 and 13 years old. My 9-year old didn't know what was going on, she only wanted Mami to be good. My 13 year old was very quiet. One of my most difficult times was that Christmas in 1989. I remember wrapping gifts when the kids went to school and cried thinking that maybe this would be my last holiday. I asked myself the question over and over again, "why me"? During my first radiation treatment, I saw so many people with cancer and some of them were very ill and sad. At that point I said to myself, "stop asking, why me, Ana" you don't even look sick.

Seven years later, after having my regular mammogram, I found a small lump in the same breast while doing my monthly breast exam. The cancer was back again. My doctor said we'd have to do a mastectomy, that was my only choice. I said okay, take both and give me two new ones. Laughing for me is the best special medicine, if you can laugh at yourself. While waiting to have my reconstruction, I went to Magic Mountain with my kids, my youngest at that time 16. She wanted me to ride with her like always and I said I couldn't because my prostheses will not stay on and what would people think if my breast popped up to my shoulders or flew out? We both looked at each other and started laughing.

I became a volunteer with a group of survivors who help women who have just been diagnosed. My best advice for every woman is that mammograms are only 70% accurate and the other 30% is your monthly "check yourself," which is how I found my second cancer. My lump never showed up, not even in the special mammogram. If you find a lump, don't wait and if you need to change doctors do. Go for a second opinion and don't be afraid to ask questions. I was very fortunate to have a very good and caring doctor.

I'm now celebrating my 22 years of surviving breast cancer. Three years ago, I joined an exercise boot camp and love it. But my favorite hobby is cooking.

I come from a family of 6 girls and 1 boy. I'm the youngest and the only one with breast

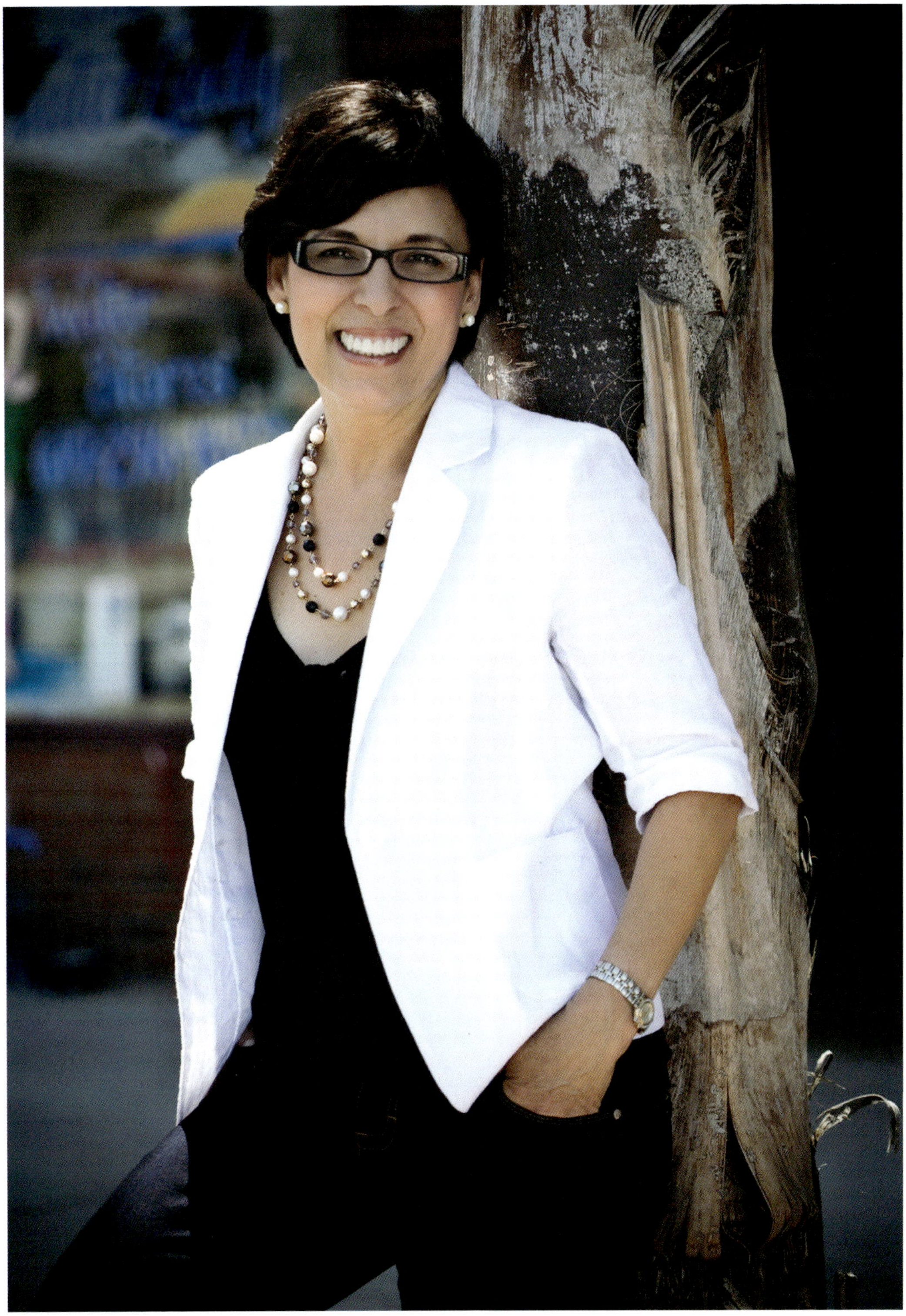

> ...don't wait and
> if you need to change
> doctors do.
> Go for a second opinion...

cancer, until 2 months ago when my second sister was diagnosed with the same kind of cancer. But we both are planning to live very long lives like our mother who this year celebrated her 97th birthday.

P.S. I'm from Peru and my first language is Spanish, so I hope you understand my English.

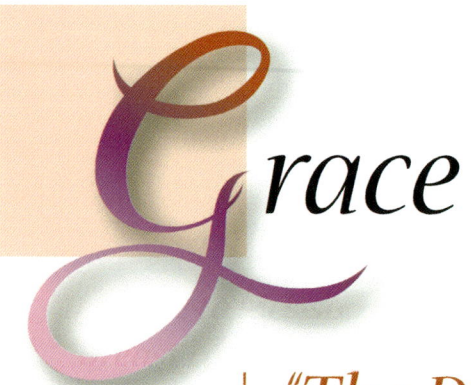

Grace

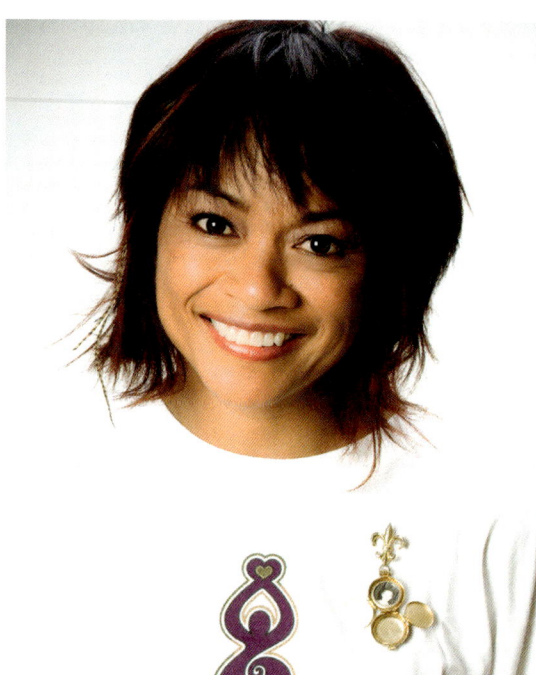

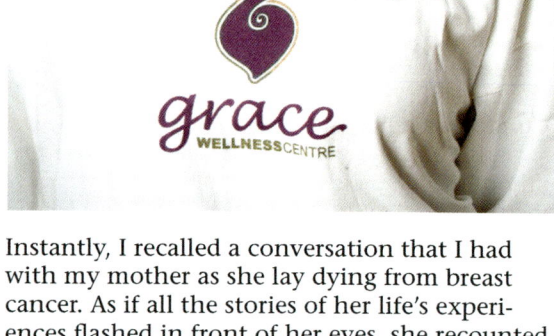

"The Delivery"

"You have breast cancer." Dr. Levine delivered the news. The air in that few seconds that hung in silence was thick. I almost wanted to laugh in disbelief. "I'm sorry, who are you calling?" I sat in my room at the Optimum Health Institute. I think it was the 3rd or 4th day of my "cleansing" visit in this raw and wheatgrass food based institute. When my doctor and I hung up, I lied back on my bed. "What am I supposed to do now?"

I took a deep breath, exhaled, scrunching up my face, burrowing my eye brows, clenching my fists and summoning deep inside me the tears that I thought should flow. None came. I tried it again and again until finally I realized the futility of my efforts. Silence. With my eyes closed, I looked inward- the dark emptiness began to fill with images. A question mark floated by.

"The Question"

"What would I tell my family?" Each of their images floated by me; all my family's beautiful faces looking at me...no emotion betrayed them at the time in my mind, and it is then, in retrospect, that I believe that I may have begun my "denial" by not looking each of them in the face, in their eyes. I could not even utter the words, for surely the mere utterance to say something so devastating to many would make it true, because I was supposed to believe a voice on the other end of the phone receiver. I looked around at my family. All is well..? Taking another deep breath to go even further inside myself, I searched for my parent's faces. It was the thought, the very image of having to tell my mother, that my eyes began to sting.

"Mmmaammmaaa! Please forgive me! I am so sorry! I didn't listen to you! I created this, I created this, I bought in, I created this?"

> *I could not even utter the words, for surely the mere utterance to say something so devastating to many would make it true...*

Instantly, I recalled a conversation that I had with my mother as she lay dying from breast cancer. As if all the stories of her life's experiences flashed in front of her eyes, she recounted to me her experiences with her eldest sister. (In my mother's own unwillingness to budge, she gave her energy away to her sister, her anger away to things that she did not know would affect her living the rest of her life the way she did, with anger in her heart and her unwillingness to forgive the things she thought so cruel as suffered under her eldest sister's rite in the hierarchy of her birth order in a Filipino family.)

My mother told me before she passed away that my sisters and I did not have to die of cancer. That cancer did not run in our family, that forgiveness was the key to being healthy, remaining healthy, Always...my mother was a very intuitive being. She had a deep sixth sense. I believe that some of my siblings and I inherited that sense.

"The Discovery"

I felt I had failed my mother. I was just told I had breast cancer. Then something interesting happened. I gave myself two minutes to cry about it; about everything I had done to get to this place. I was mourning the passing of my parents, my Godfather, brother-in-law, too many too quickly, when my beautiful husband of 20 years asked me for a divorce. I saw the faces of the forces that I had allowed to cause me to go deep into the abyss. I looked into their eyes, I felt their energy. And while I did not like their behavior, somehow I understood. I have known since I was an infant that we are, all of us, special in the eyes of the creator. No matter what. The Source that loves, the Source that forgives. In my gratitude, I began to forgive them, asked for forgiveness, and more importantly, forgive myself. I vowed NEVER again to let anyone or anything have my joy, my spirit. And in the abyss that I had been living in, suddenly, after many dark months, there was light. I took three very deep cleansing breaths reenergizing my spirit and said out loud, "It's time to kick some breast cancer ASS!"

> "It's time to kick some breast cancer ASS!"

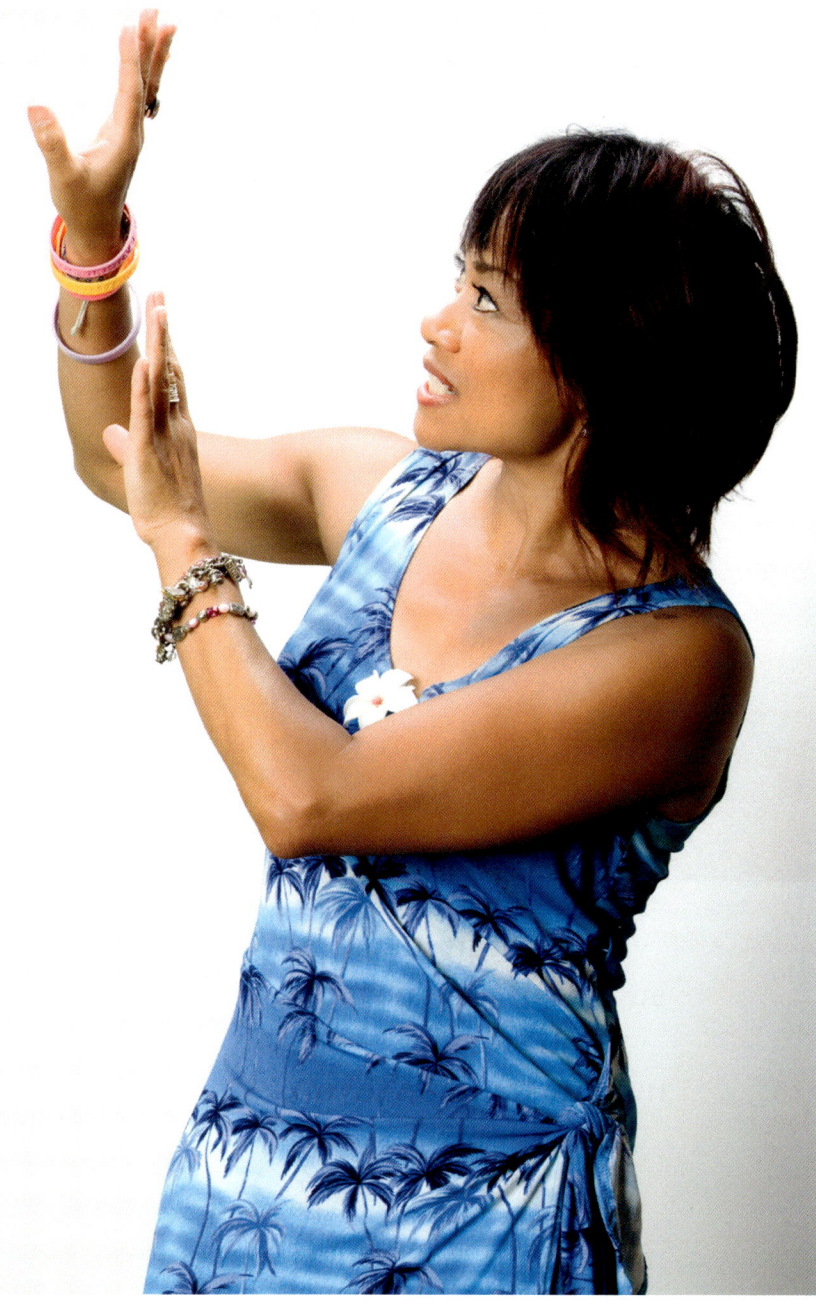

"The Belief"

"If people say it, is it true? If I say it, is it true? What's true for you?" he would ask. So forth go I. In my truth, knowing I have something to conquer, a light to step back into, a light to go forward in, a path unknown by experience, but clear in my knowledge of its possibilities.

I believe that a healthy mind and attitude is the first line of defense in most confrontational situations. That, followed by a healthy way of eating and living. I believe that the body in all its miraculous ways can reproduce healthy cells. Before, during, and after my right breast lumpectomy, and auxiliary lymph dissection a week later, I ate a raw food regimen and drank several ounces of wheatgrass juice and other various homemade organic juices and smoothies. This lasted into a year beyond my radiation and included practices in meditation twice daily, and exercise. I didn't miss work, and enjoyed a whole new way of living and literally, breathing.

"Lymph not Gimp"

A few days after my lumpectomy, Dr. Levine informed me that I would need an auxiliary lymph dissection. I listened in disbelief at first, and told him I couldn't do it the following week. He insisted we would have to and I began to cry. Stanley told Dr. Levine that I had been training for my first marathon. It was scheduled for June 1, 2003, the surgery was scheduled for May 13th. Dr. Levine said, "June 1st? Well, we'll see about that." While I kept silent, my head was screaming, "YES! WE WILL SEE ABOUT THAT! YOU HAVE NO IDEA WHO I AM!" The surgery was about my lymph nodes, not about me being a gimp. As Dr. Levine contemplated me for awhile, he suddenly said, "If you can raise your arm above your head after the surgery, maybe you'll be able to run the marathon." A sudden glint of light became brighter with those words. There's a Jewish saying, "From your mouth to God's ears," I didn't have to say it to Dr. Levine. I knew he had already been heard.

"Trail to Treasure"

"What's your name? Birthdate? What procedure are you getting done today? Which side are you having the procedure on? Please take this pen and write on the side you're going to have your axillary lymph dissection.

I took the red marker and with my left hand drew an arrow that said, "This way to treasure." Underneath my armpit I drew a smiley face. I said a blessing for the steadiness of Dr. Levine's hands and gave thanks to the miracle of my body, thanked it for its perfection, and said good-bye to it as I knew it.

"Eyes Wide Open Times Four"

I woke up from the surgery with eyes wide open and announced through the tube in my throat, "I'm hungry!" The nurse quickly came to my side, and with her eyes wide open said, "Hey, you're not supposed to be awake for another 30 minutes! Look at you!" I was so excited and hungry that she smiled broadly and acknowledged how different I was to the previous week's recovery time and attitude. We laughed in amazement at both. As she wheeled me out to the waiting room, I could see and hear Stanley and my sister Meg talking quietly. The nurse said, "Look who's here and she's hungry!" We were both smiling at Stanley and Meg and both their faces were frozen with surprise. With their eyes wide open and mouths dropped, suddenly my sister jumped up and said, "Ok, what are you hungry for?" and I said, "Sushi!" After Stanley snapped out of his amazement to my quick departure from the recovery room, he said, "Ok, let's go! You look GREAT! WOW!"

"From Wheatgrass to Sushi!"

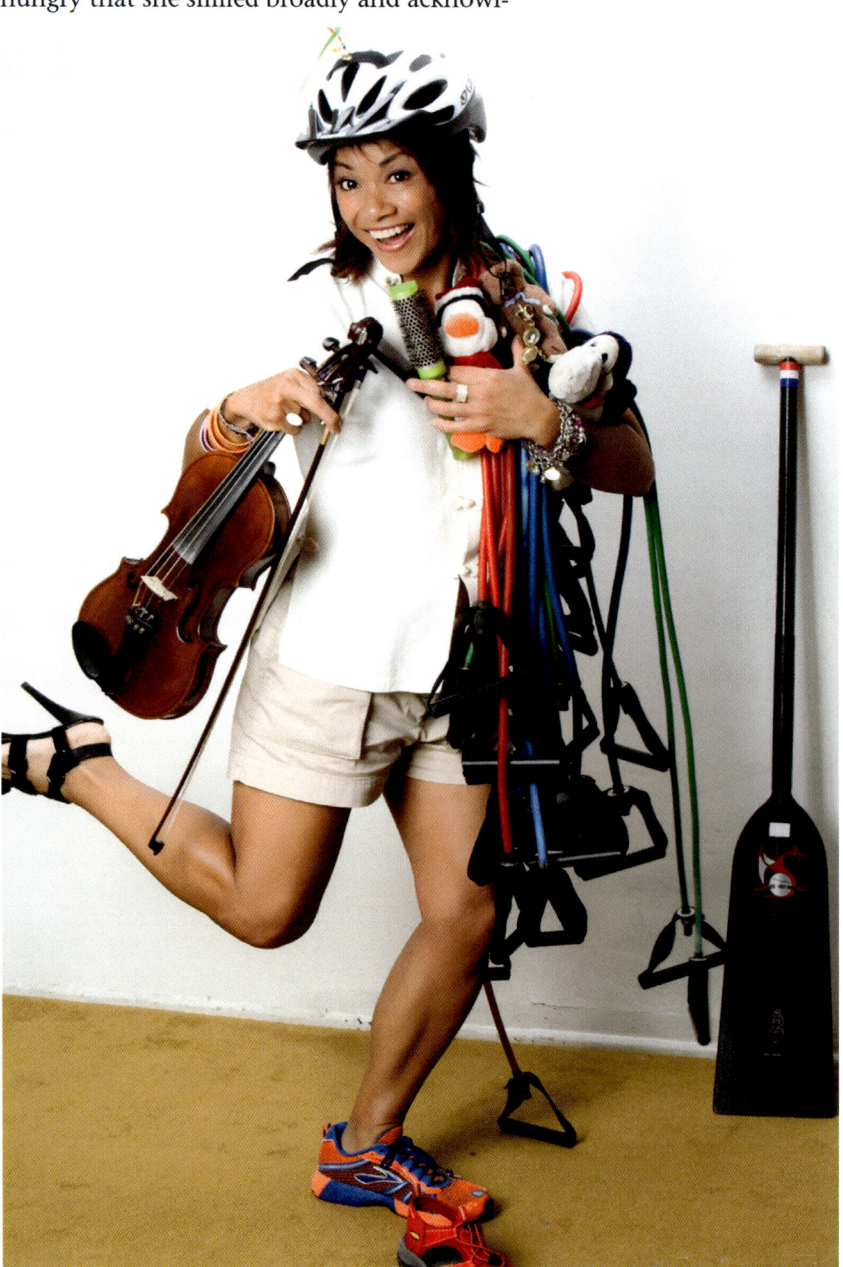

Kazumi San welcomed us into his restaurant and after he and my sister became reacquainted, asked what she and Stanley would like. He never asked me but simply looked at me and said, "I know exactly what you need." I looked at him in amazement and checked myself to see if there were obvious signs that I had just come out from the hospital. No one said anything to him about that. Kazumi San fed me all the fish that he thought would help me to heal quickly. He was like an all knowing Health Ninja Angel serving me up exquisite healing cuisine from the sea.

Stanley and Meg began to contemplate my quick recovery. How different I was from the previous week. As I thought about it for a minute, it occurred to me that the night before, the anesthesiologist rang me to remind me about the "nothing after midnight and just before surgery rule." As I listened to him recite the do's and don'ts of the pre-surgery list, I was especially interested in the "Okay to have 1 or 2 ounces of water, coffee, or tea 2

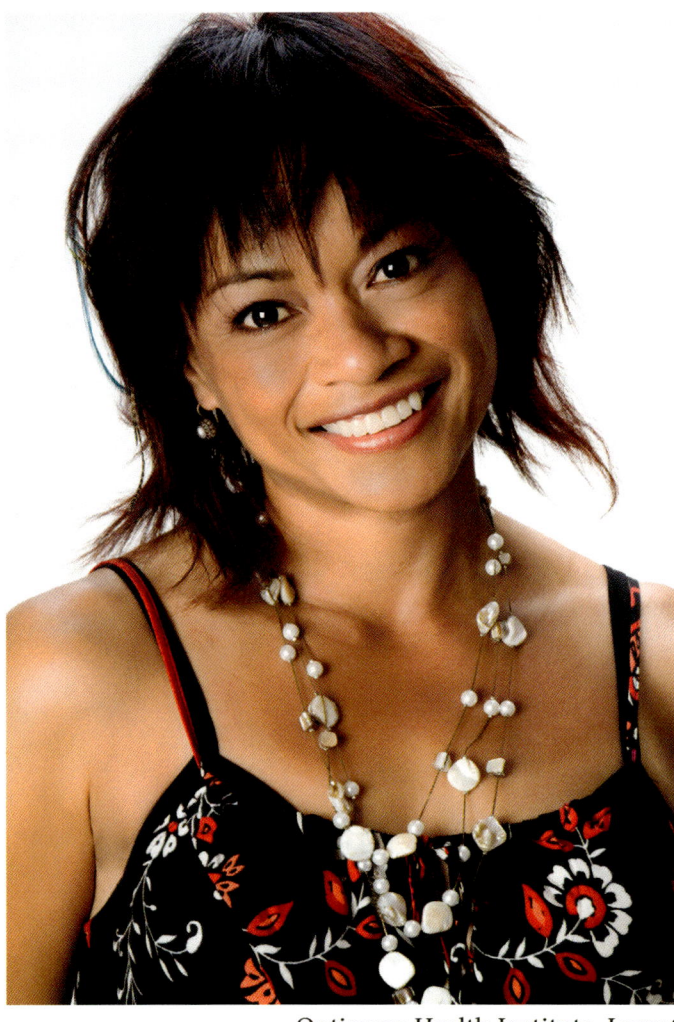

hours before the surgery." I asked him if it was okay to have 2 ounces of wheatgrass juice 2 hours before the surgery. After some silence, he finally said, "Yes, I think that should be alright!" A big fat juicy smile crept onto my face as I knew I would be better off being able to take this special elixir that I had been training with on a daily basis since I was in The Optimum Health Institute. I went to bed happy even with the impending change to my body.

"You Will…"

Two days after the surgery, I went back into Dr. Levine's office. He examined me and was pleased with me and his work. Ha! Then he asked me to stand perpendicular to the wall and walk my arm all the way up the wall until the side of my body was touching the wall and my hand was well above my head. I did this with no problem what so ever. Dr. Levine said, "Uh huh," and nothing else.

After Dr. Levine told me about the findings, "One of the 7 lymph nodes taken out had a little bit of cancer but we got it. Everything else was clear…," he walked Stanley and me out of the office. Just before he opened the door to the outer room, Dr. Levine said to me, "Oh, and by the way, YOU WILL DO THE MARATHON!" I looked up at him as he said those words and it was if he had been pumping fresh oxygen into me, inflating me with the confidence and drive that I had lost in the many months before I was diagnosed.

> *The road the year before my diagnosis, to the day I was diagnosed, and from that day until now has been paved with so many extraordinary life's experiences.*

I felt like I grew a few more inches. I thanked him with a hug and silently cried as I turned to walk away from him and toward the marathon that would be one of the great contributors to start me on the road to my successful survivorship!

"The Marathon"

When my friend Christy asked if I would be interested in training for and running the 2003 San Diego Rock n' Roll Marathon, I immediately said yes. I didn't even know when it was or how far it went. I was just happy that we had 10 months to train for it. I believe that that drive and tenacity to stay by Christy's side, no matter how much I didn't want to get up to run, was the true training and also, on an ethereal level, would be the impetus for me to get up and go after my diagnosis.

The morning of the marathon, (equipped with a double sports bra even though I didn't need much support) found Christy and I at the start early, excited and ready to go. As the gun went off I began to hold both my breasts to keep them from bouncing too much. But after mile 5, I began to wonder why my arms were getting so tired! I relaxed my left arm at first and slowly, and with trepidation, relaxed my right arm. I soon realized that my natural running posture was the way to go. The double bra was doing its job and I could suddenly enjoy my natural movements more. At many points throughout the marathon, I was struck by the many supporters along the way. I saw faces of old friends that my former husband Joseph and I had known. I saw people and children in wheelchairs cheering us on, I saw signs on the backs of people that read the names of people they were running for.

When Christy and I came around the corner from the 163 to Friars Road, there was a friend of ours from our gym that had a large banner sign she and her daughter and husband had made that said, "Go Christy and Grace!" At some point, Christy ran ahead of me as I had many bathroom stops that I made along the way. At one point, there was a man with a bull horn yelling, "Go! Go! Go! You all look great, relax, and smile!" We would turn a corner a few more miles down the road, and he'd be there again! I wondered how he did that throughout the whole marathon!

At mile 17…"Did that sign say mile 17?" I asked the runner next to me in disbelief. She said, "Yes!" As I looked around at the many people on their phones calling friends and family saying they were at mile 17, I suddenly wished I too had a phone. And then I remembered that Stanley insisted I run with my phone. I was

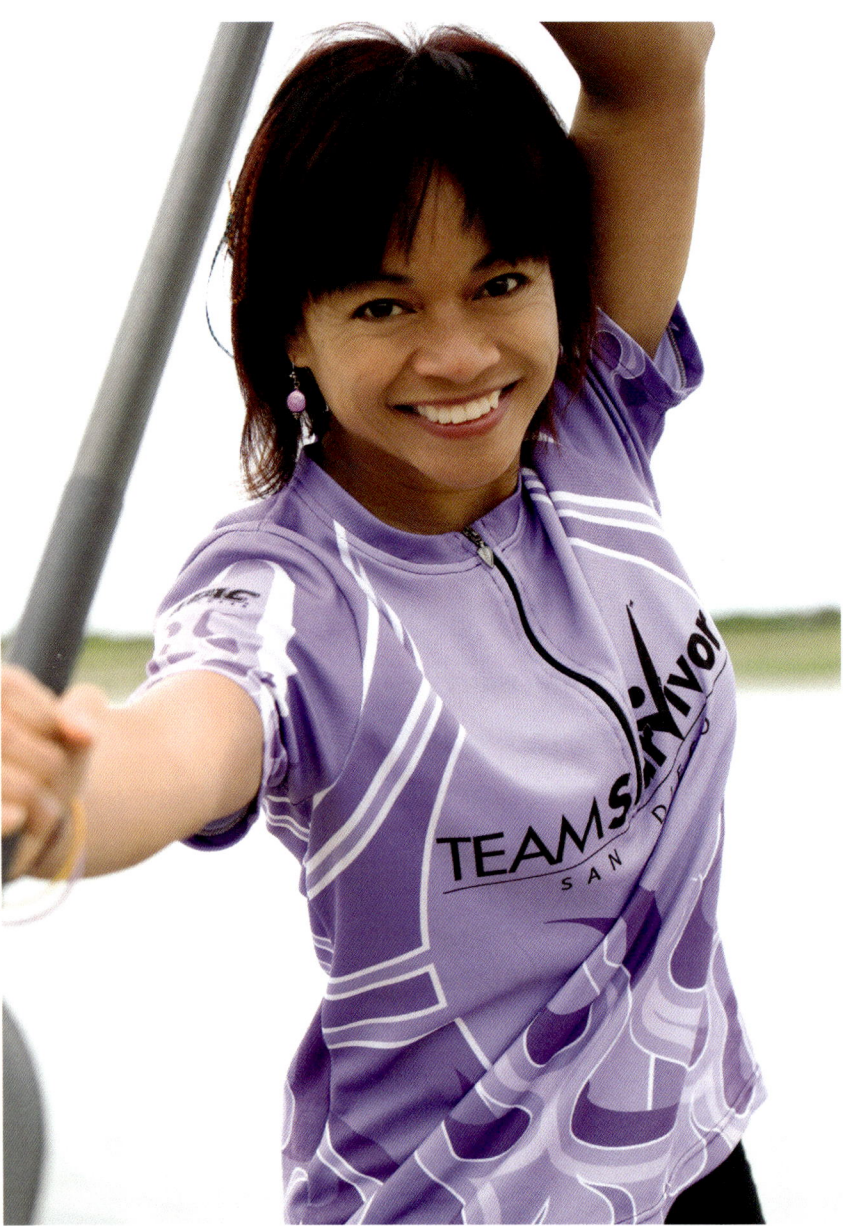

loons? That's where the finish line is. OK girl, it's you and me, let's bring it in, let's get us across the finish line!" and I grabbed her hand and ran with her to the finish singing, as I do upon crossing all finish lines, the 'Theme From Rocky'.

Tears flowed for me throughout the entire experience of my first marathon, although none had flowed as much as at the finish line. I had done it, I had finished 26.2 miles!

Days and weeks later when people asked me how I was doing after my surgery, I said that I was doing fine. I never missed a day of regular work cutting and styling hair. I continued to do my work outs albeit modified. But when I would hear Stanley speak to people who were checking in on me but were afraid to be a bother, he would exclaim, "She's doing great and she just ran her first marathon right after her second surgery!" I didn't think much about what he was saying except to say that he seemed more excited about coupling the two events as though it was a great feat. Many people would acknowledge that accomplishment and I searched for the awe in it but could feel none. To this day, they are two complete and separate feats that happened to be so close together. I know it sounds strange but both were things I HAD to do.

In truth, I have cried many times since, crossing many more finish lines whether they be on land or sea. As I get further and further away from my original diagnosis day, I have to work harder to shake the fears of possible recurrence. Every time February rolls around, I am reminded that it takes a minimum of 90 days for the body to regenerate many of its reparative cells. So from February to April when my annual check up comes around, I take on a mostly raw food regimen with a daily dose of wheatgrass juice. In April I remind myself to breathe extra deeply as I embark on the annual check up date. When it is all over, I walk taller knowing I've lived another successful year and pray it continues this way for many, many, more to come.

adamantly opposed but Stanley said he was so worried about me that I acquiesced and put it in the pocket in the small of my back. I didn't feel it as I ran. So, I called my sister, my brothers, my friend Brad, and no one answered their phones! Ha! Not even Stanley! But no doubt I left winded, (yes, a double entendre!) and excited messages for all to hear!

Just before the finish line at the Marine Corps Recruit Depot, I spotted a young Asian girl I had seen from time to time along the route. She had been running with a very tall Caucasian woman and was now alone. I ran up and beside her and asked, "Hey, how are you?" She said, pointing to her waist and up, "From here to here, I'm fine," and pointing to her waist down to her feet she said, "From here to here, I'm numb." I said, "OK, so the good news is, do you see that arch of bal-

"The Finer Points"

The road the year before my diagnosis, to the day I was diagnosed, and from that day until now has been paved with so many extraordinary life's experiences. There is a sense of grey, then black in the lead up to the day I was diagnosed. That darkness opened my eyes to the understanding of people who are in a deep depression.

My Family, My Friends, My Loves

When I came out of surgery the first time, the

nurse told me there were many people in the waiting room who love me. She wasn't kidding. The room was packed. I felt so blessed!

Gratitude

For each day I wake up and give thanks for all the miracles that abound and to have so many people make a difference in my life. I am grateful!

Meditation both in prayer and quietude was literally a saving Grace for me. Running, exercise, and Qigong were all apart of my meditation. A complementary holistic healing regimen is paramount to my whole healing process. Raw and Wheatgrass! Woo Whoo!

Being questioned about and have it recommended to stop my running and exercise for awhile was the impetus for me to keep going in that direction and enroll and consequently graduate with a degree as a Fitness Specialist.

Finding Team Survivor San Diego and paddling dragon boats with them has brought me the greatest of joys as a survivor! What an awesome group of all cancer survivors! It's a sisterhood to be reckoned with, especially on the water! I have vied for and won a position on Team USA—the United States International Dragon Boat Championship Team. The first time was in 2009, held in Prague, Czech Republic. The second time was in 2011 in Tampa, Florida. In each experience there was a time that crossing the finish line after "leaving everything I had on the water" was met with a deep sense of catharsis. Like many of the other finish lines I have crossed, "Because I can!" has been a resounding cry in my life since I have become a survivor.

> "Because I can!" has been a resounding cry in my life since I have become a survivor.

Fear and Loathing

I read that Lance Armstrong could take the challenge of thousands of feet of climbs on his bicycle or give him several days to ride hundreds of miles in a row on terrain he had never been on, and he would be able to handle it. But tell him he had to go see the doctor for his annual check ups and he would instantly break out in a sweat. When I read that, I cried with relief knowing I wasn't alone.

Although it took a few times for Dr. Levine to really get a sense of who I am in my early stages of diagnosis and survivorship, I believe our relationship is something that we might not have expected it to become over the years. A deep respect for each other and I hope, lessons unspoken but shared that were learned. In the oxygen that Dr. Levine breathed into me when telling me I WILL do the marathon, there existed the birth of many ideas that would lead to the inspiration for The Grace Wellness Centre; the byline which is "Movement of Body is Movement of Mind."

Many people would argue that it is the other way around, but to me, had I just sat down to take the breast cancer diagnosis and didn't listen to my body, listen to what it was feeling, I may have simply assumed a seated position to all that would be handed to me. I may have just continued in the framework of the darkness that enveloped my being that led me to awakening breast cancer in me. By standing up to it, and continuing to move forward in motion, leaving it behind and discarded in the pieces of my body that were removed, I was able to move my mind away from what is possible in the darkness, to what is possible in the light. And I never want to turn back. I never want to hear "You have breast cancer" again.

"bright ideas" © grb 26 August 11
ramblings for Tom Denlick's book

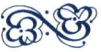

THE GRACE WELLNESS CENTRE IN SAN DIEGO
was founded by Grace Bernal

"Movement of Body is Movement of Mind."

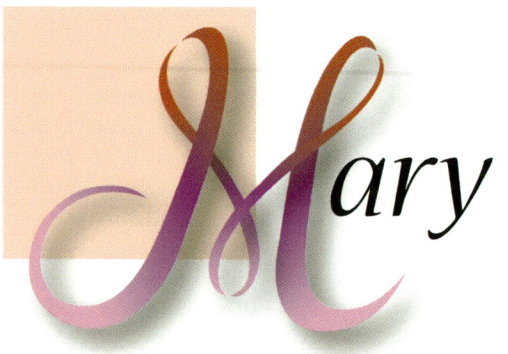

Mary

"I Will Survive!!!"

My name is Mary Brewer and I am a survivor of breast cancer for almost eight years now. I was 53, physically active, working full-time, and caring for the needs of three dear aunts when the big "C" hit me. My husband had been home on disability, so I was the only breadwinner in the family.

With so many people relying on my strength, I had no time to be sick. I also did not take the time to do monthly self-examination of my breasts. As a result, when I finally DID check myself after one of my aunts died of, guess what, breast cancer....I could actually see the mass when I looked at myself in the mirror. It was 5 cm by July 31, 2003. My previous mammogram done in 2001 showed nothing.

> …when the surgeon told me that he had NOT gotten a clear margin on the breast and BOTH nodes were positive, I went into shock…literally.

Still hopeful that God would not take me right now with family counting on me, I agreed to a lumpectomy and sentinel node dissection. This would be followed by radiation therapy and I would be done with cancer. This did not happen according to my plan and when the surgeon told me that he had NOT gotten a clear margin on the breast and BOTH nodes were positive, I went into shock…literally.

An excellent nurse came in and tended to me, made me an appointment with the head of reconstructive surgery, and just generally did what the doctor had not done…think about how this diagnosis was affecting ME. The surgeon DID connect me with a special Breast Care Coordinator who was wonderful!! She gave me the best advice which I am passing on to you… **Educate yourself!!!**

With a list of websites and stacks of articles to read I felt that I was more in control of my treatment. When the oncologist told me his plan I knew that this was the Gold Standard treatment for breast cancer because I had read it in an article by a Johns Hopkins oncologist at the **breastcancer.org** website.

Another amazing resource I had was a group of women in my book club. When I announced to them what

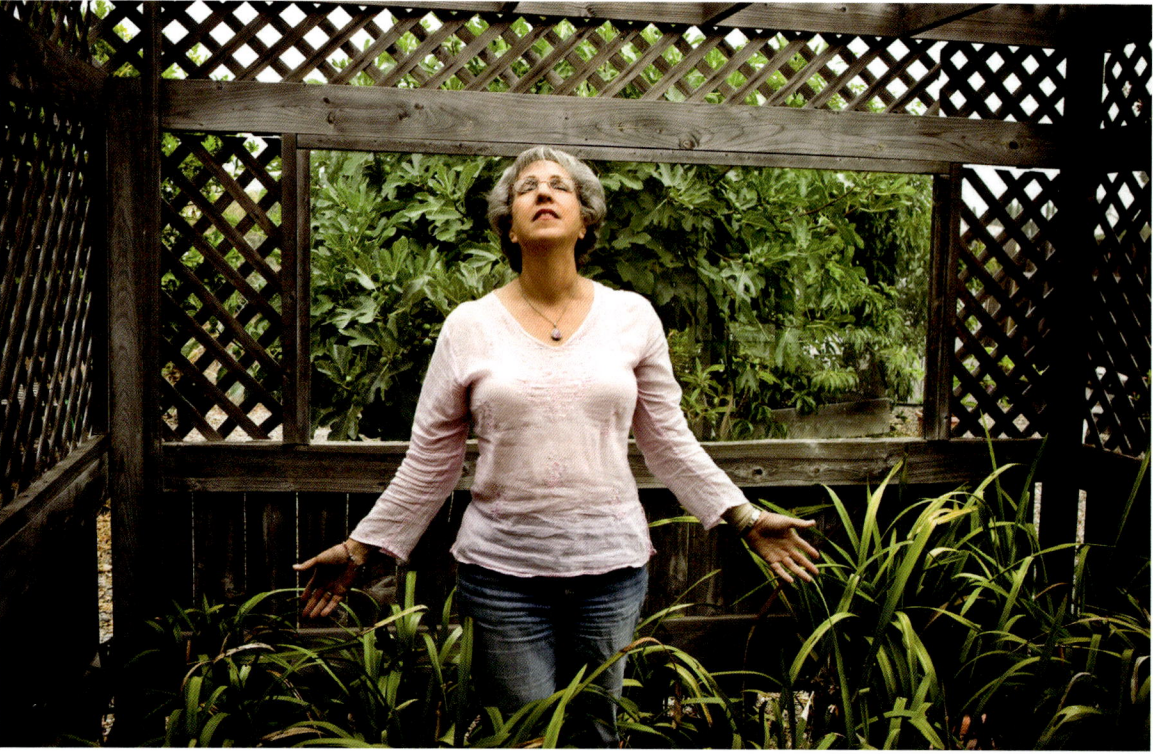

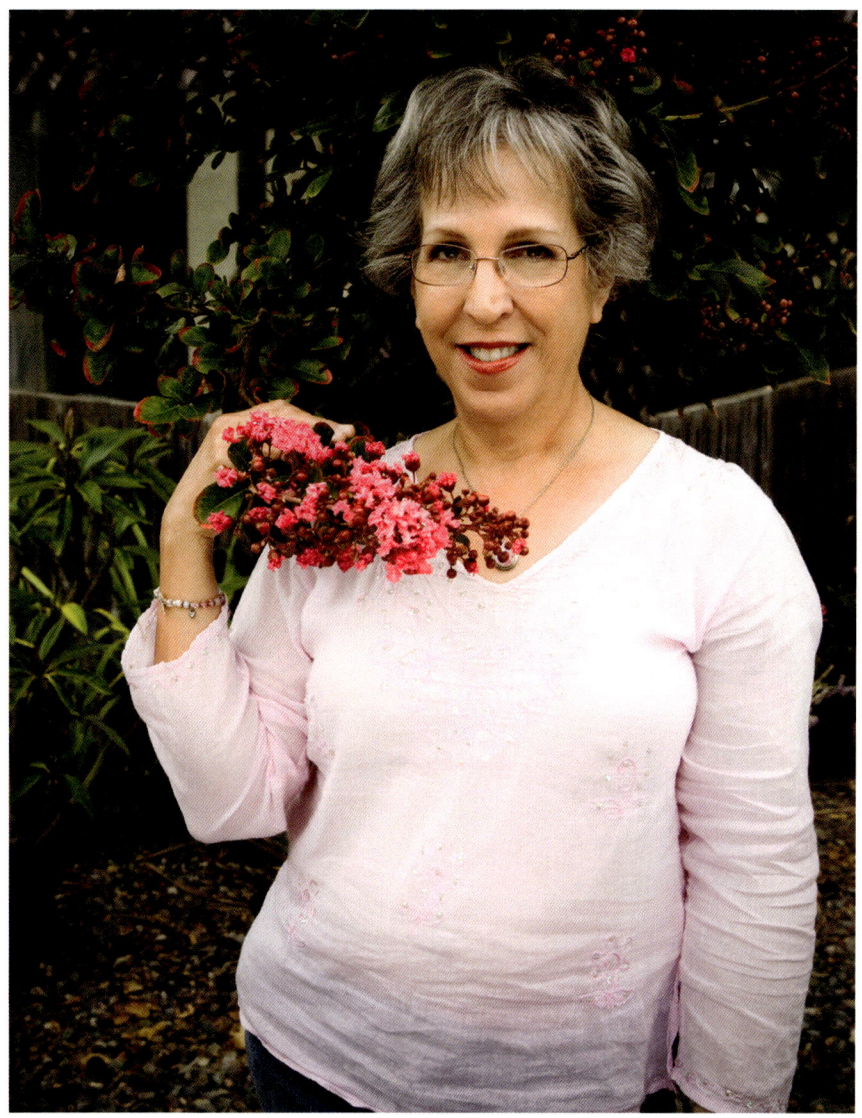

was happening to me I, discovered that 4 of the 12 women present that night were breast cancer survivors. Moreover, all of the women in the group signed up to take me to chemo appointments and sat with me the whole time. One of the survivors was also an oncology nurse herself and she went out of her way to help me after surgery even staying with me through a bad night at the emergency room after surgery complications.

Because of all of this support from ladies at my church in the book club, I was much better able to deal with the whole cancer "thing". Today I am a founding member of our parish Cancer Support Ministry because I feel that this is my new mission as a survivor. I continue to workout at least 4 times per week, work full time, and enjoy times with my friends at the theater or dinner. My husband died in 2006 but my children still have me here. For this I am truly grateful every day.

Perhaps the greatest quote I can share is from my darling nana who said the following when asked how she did it at age 90: "I wake up in the morning, put my feet on the ground, and say **'Thanks be to God'!!"**

> *Another amazing resource… a group of women in my book club… I discovered that 4 of the 12 women present that night were breast cancer survivors.*

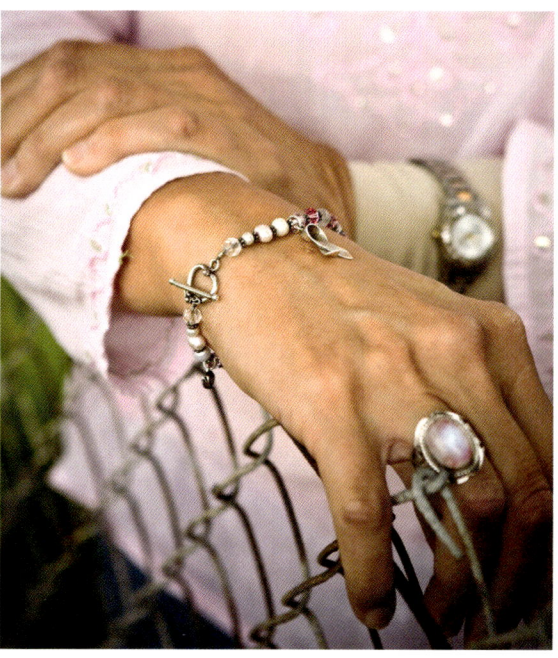

Photography courtesy of Sarah Soto

NOTE FROM SARAH SOTO
Photographer

Thanks Tom! I don't know if she mentioned it in her story, but that tree with the pink blossoms she's holding is the tree she and her late husband planted. It ONLY blooms on their anniversary. Isn't that incredible? So many great stories in that backyard…

Gail

"3-Time Survivor"

My name is Gail Bishop and I was diagnosed with breast cancer in 2000. Looking forward to the five-year cancer-free milestone, IT (the cancer) returned in 2004 and once again in 2008. I believe in the power of prayer, maintaining a good attitude, and lot's of laughter to keep me going. This disease has not stopped me from doing anything that I want to do!

Beginning in 2000 and continuing for almost 5 years I underwent treatments of: chemo, radiation, and Tamoxifen. When I first was diagnosed I was not scared, nor did I think I was dying. I had been praying for God to use me and to let me know what was my purpose in life; I viewed my diagnosis as a response. I told my pastor and Sunday school class to pray for me as I was going through something I knew nothing about. I ask them to pray that I would use this experience in a manner that I could serve God.

As I was going through my treatments it seems like calls started coming, telling me a friend, a relative, or someone they knew had breast cancer and would I talk with them. I would give each person a call and we would talk. After our conversation, they would tell me how I had helped them and was inspired about what I said to them.

Not knowing anything about breast cancer, I started going to support group meetings. Going to support group meetings and from other resources, I was told that African American women were diagnosed less with breast cancer but had a higher rate of dying from breast cancer. Just hearing about that and the lack of resources available to women in my community made me want to know what I could do to make a difference.

Then it just happened, I heard about a conference that was coming up October 2001, in Houston, Texas, sponsored by an African American Breast Cancer Survivorship Organization. Fortunately, I was able to attend. I learned so much at that conference; I was so inspired that when I returned home I started a chapter in San Francisco.

Even though I was going through chemo I did not hesitate to try to help others. My community needed education to learn about this disease. It was not about me, but about helping those that felt like they did not have a chance. I wanted everyone to know that it was time for us (my community) to Stop the Silence. It was a challenge to let women know that it was ok to talk about having a diagnosis of breast cancer and to let them know that they were just as much of a woman as any woman who had both of their breasts.

After doing my chemo and being on Tamoxifen for almost five years the cancer returned, this time to the lungs. I did not have to do chemo or radiation this time. My treatment was done orally. The side effects of oral chemo were not as bad. This time I was very angry, I did not understand why the cancer came back. But I did not give up. As I mentioned before, I trust and believe in God. It was something I had to go through so that I would let women know that if their cancer does come back— with God and all the great new technology—you can live.

> **I was told that African American women were diagnosed less with breast cancer but had a higher rate of dying from breast cancer.**

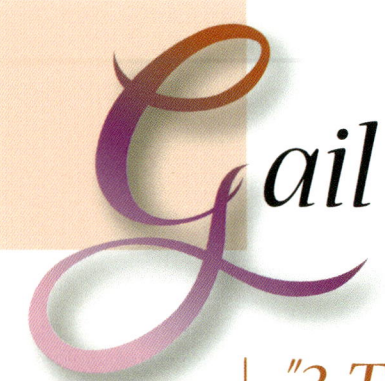

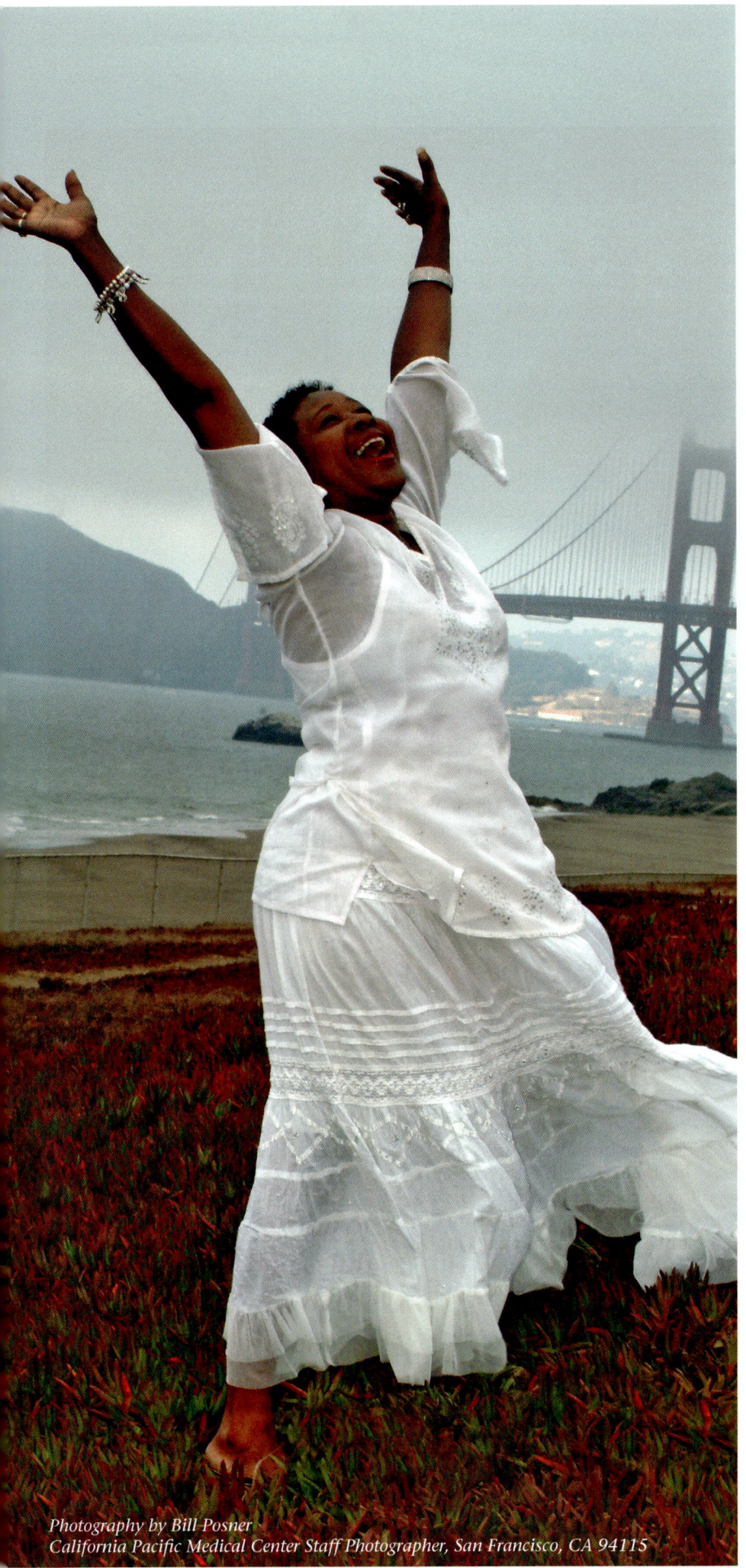

Photography by Bill Posner
California Pacific Medical Center Staff Photographer, San Francisco, CA 94115

I refused to let this disease stop me from living. I had really got involved in getting more information and resources. For the past 11 years, our San Francisco Chapter of the Sisters Network has had: health fairs, health summits, workshops, Gift for Life Block Walk Health Fairs, and the Pink Women Campaign. We have doctors and professionals to come out to our community to talk with us. Educating us on topics like: triple negative tumors, clinical trials, latest technology and medication.

> *"I may have cancer but it does not have me."*

In 2004 the tumors in the lungs were very small and were stable until 2008 when two of the tumors grew and moved to the liver. Again I was upset. But again, I refused to let the cancer get me down. I continued to fight for others and myself. It was then that I started saying:

"I may have cancer but it does not have me."

I continued going to conferences all over the United States and learned more so I could come back to let the community know. It was during this period that I became acquainted with clinical trials. We as African American women need to do more clinical trials. We do not do enough clinical trials for the doctors to really know how to treat us. Most of the clinical trials are done on white women with no African American women involved. After I was informed and learned more about clinical trials, my prayer was: Lord, if I have a reoccurrence I must do a clinical trial. Well, be careful for what you pray for. In April 2008, the cancer returned. I did do the clinical trial. February 14, 2011, my doctor told me that I am cancer free.

I am a firm believer you have to be very positive, in my case trust God and your doctors, and the treatments will work. Have patience, faith, laugh, and live everyday like it is your last day of your life. I have been off chemo now for almost 5 months and I am back in the swing of things. I'm feeling good, working out, going to conferences, workshops and family functions.

I want to take the opportunity to say thank you to all those who have been a support to me: My children Mandisa and Latisa, my grandchildren Richard, Melvin, Ronnell, Elysse, Michaela and Tutankhamun (Tut).

Tut is my youngest grandson, he was my medication during the last chemo treatments. I had to take care of him while I was doing chemo. He is a very active baby that kept me moving. There was no way I could lie down and be sick. That little boy stayed busy and into everything. He will be 3 years old June 30th. He is now going to preschool. Thank God for preschools.

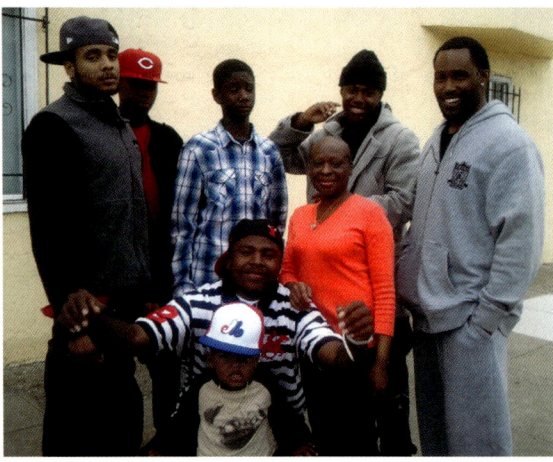

I would like to thank Tim Therman, the special man in my life who stuck by me, my sisters, brothers, family members and friends. My Sunday school class, Pastor Mervin J. Remond, Sr. and wife Valerie Redmond, my church family—Claire Caldwell, Kathy Hamilton, Evelyn Fisher, Pally Cottonham, Lucille Ackinson, Sisters Network SF Chapter and Sisters Network Inc and all other chapters. Also, Joe and Maxine Moore. Last but not least my doctor, Dr. Kathleen Grant. The best on planet Earth to me!

The Emotional Stages of Breast Cancer During Diagnosis, Treatment and Survival

by Pam Stephan
Reprinted from *About.com Guide*

Breast cancer is a life-threatening disease that requires rigorous treatment. If you have been diagnosed with breast cancer, you, your family and friends will be experiencing waves of emotion. Just as your diagnosis may differ from those of other breast cancer patients, your emotional experience may also differ. Knowing what other survivors have experienced and getting help early in the process can be helpful in navigating your way through this experience.

You may not have all of these emotions, but it's normal to have a range of emotions as you progress through treatment. Here are some emotional states that are similar to Kübler-Ross's Five Stages of Grief.

Emotions at Your Diagnosis:

Denial and Shock – "This can't be true."

Anger, Rage – "This isn't fair." "Why wasn't I protected from this?" "Why me?"

Stress and Depression – "My life is already busy, I can't stop to deal with this." "I feel so sad." "Why should I get treatment? I'll die anyway."

Grief and Fear – "I'm going to die, but I don't want to." "I'm going to lose part of my body." [health, attractiveness] "I will never feel safe again."

Acceptance, Adjustment – "Okay, it's true. I've got breast cancer, but I don't have to like it or let it define who I am."

Fight and Hope – "I'm going to fight for my life! I'm getting all the help and support that's out there for me."

Tina

"No Return Policy"

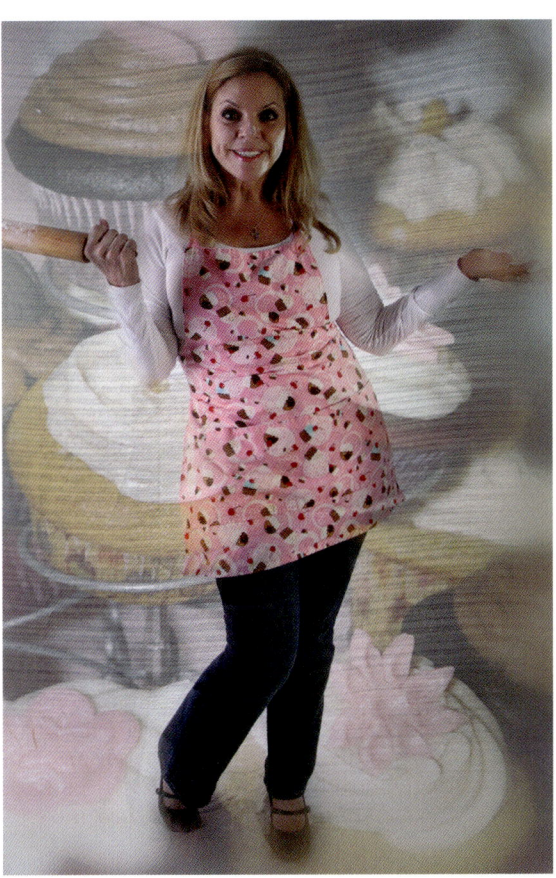

Photography by Joanna Herr

It was 7 years ago that my life changed. What was important to me then is quite different now. It was May 2004 when I was diagnosed with breast cancer, I was 46 years old. You never know what kind of curve ball life will throw at you, or when. Who knew that a simple visit to a new doctor due to new insurance would begin such an incredible journey in my life.

When all the tests were done I was given the news that not only did I have Lobular Carcinoma in Situ (LCIS), but the lumpectomy also showed a very special bonus of DCIS in Situ along with Atypical Hyperplasia. This was a gift that I really wish I could have taken back to the store, but there was a no return policy.

> …would I choose to be angry, frustrated, scared, depressed, positive, hopeful, full of faith, or whatever other emotion that might hit me.

39

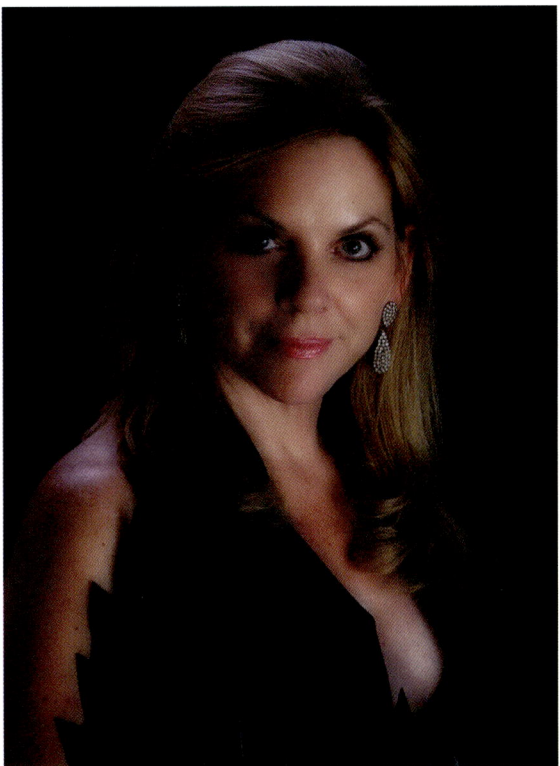

Photography by Joanna Herr

I immediately had to decide which way I was going to go on this; would I choose to be angry, frustrated, scared, depressed, positive, hopeful, full of faith, or whatever other emotion that might hit me. Now it wouldn't be truthful of me to say that I didn't go through a little bit of all of them, but overall I choose to have a very positive outlook shared with faith in God. Immediately I got to work on what to do, what my choices were, developing questions, and the worst part, telling my loved ones. I decided on a double mastectomy with reconstructive surgery. I had always wanted a breast reduction and lift, but come on, this was a heck of a way to get it.

The biggest change was learning not to sweat the small stuff, to just let things go. It definitely made me more aware of how important it is for all of us to show more love and compassion to everyone! But I only have control of my behaviors so it had to start with me. When the 2x4 hit's you upside the head and says wake up and pay attention to life as it can be taken away from you in a moment, you realize that there are much bigger things in life than you. Things like spending quality time with your friends and family, to be there as a mentor to others going through this, to volunteer time to help others. I'm happy to say that I am getting married this October to an incredible man that loves me just the way I am, inside and out! I'm blessed and continue to be grateful that I'm here today to give back.

Survivors Park

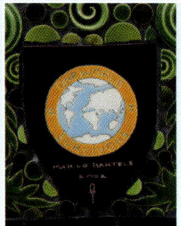

Cancer Survivors Parks promote survivorship and provide common sense information that will guide and support the patient through his or her cancer journey. There are currently 24 parks located throughout the USA and Canada.

Cancer Survivors Park is a small, quiet grassy spread next to San Diego Bay. The park has a large display, with life-size human figures, traveling through a maze of cancer treatments and success. Also at the display is a water fall.

Nearby is a walkway and large gazebo where people can contemplate the scenery and read the encouraging writings on the plaques.

Cancer Survivors Park was created for those who have been diagnosed with cancer, but is open to the entire public. The park is meant to be a quiet place, and not a place for large gatherings. The park is connected to Spanish Landing Park, a larger recreational park for picnics and other activities.

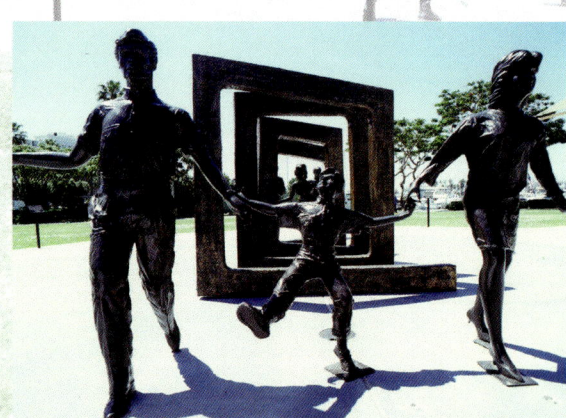

cancer patients, their families and friends. The idea of the Cancer Survivors Park was conceived to help emphasize the Foundation's key message: death and cancer are not synonymous.

Its Inspiration

Inspired by Richard and Annette Bloch Richard was diagnosed with terminal lung cancer in 1978, and told he had three months to live. He refused to accept this prognosis. After two years of aggressive treatment—he was cured. During his battle, Richard made a promise to himself: if he survived, he would devote his life to helping others fight cancer.

Richard and Annette established the R&A Bloch Cancer Foundation to help people diagnosed with cancer have the best chance of beating it as early as possible. The Foundation runs programs to inspire and educate

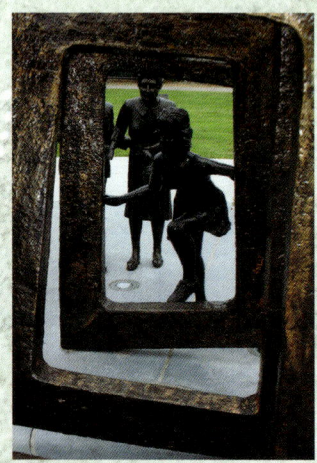

In the late 1980's, Richard fought and beat colon cancer. He died of heart failure on July 21, 2004 at the age of 78 survived by his wife Annette, daughters Linda, Barbara and Nancy and ten grandchildren.

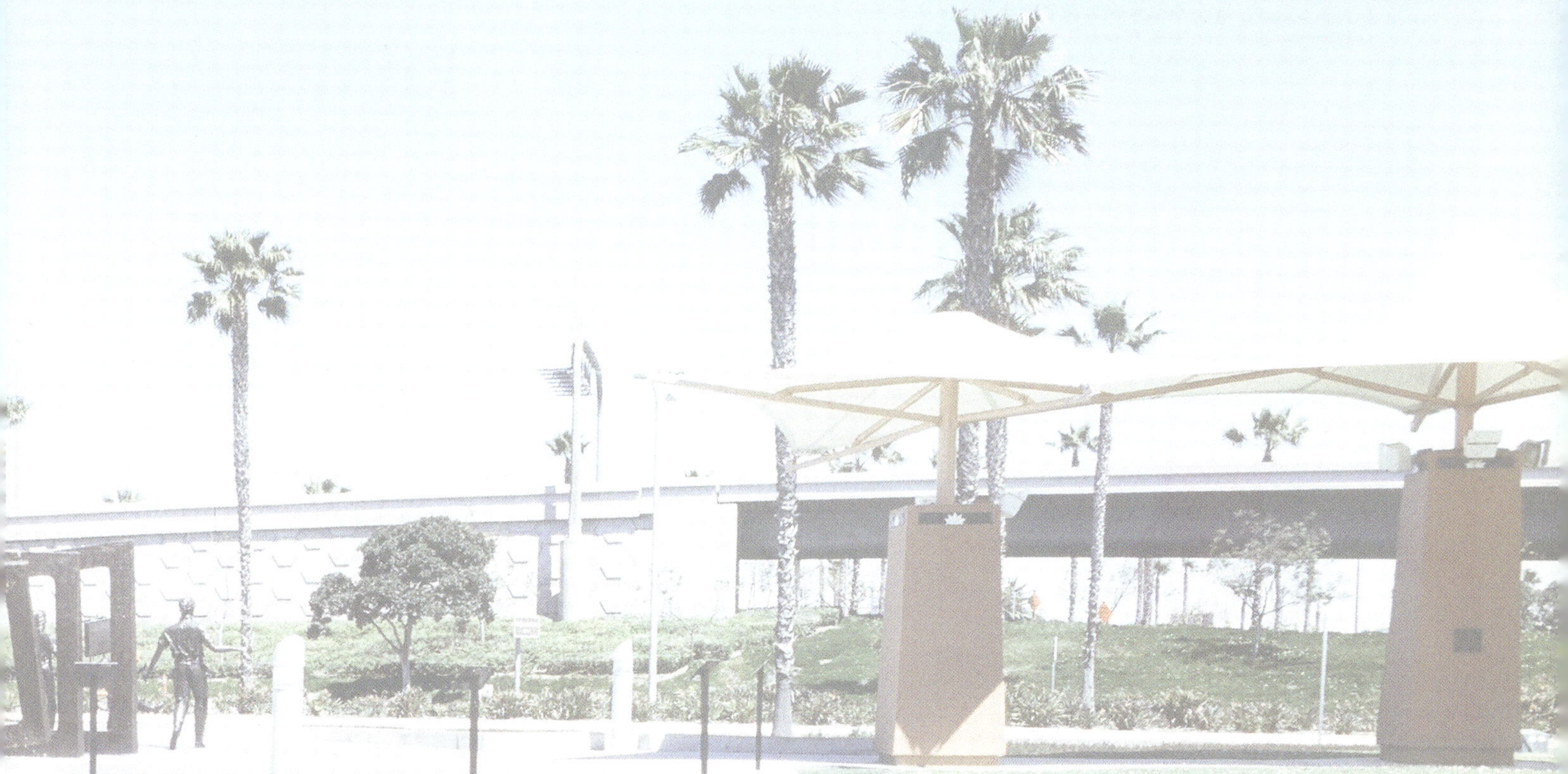

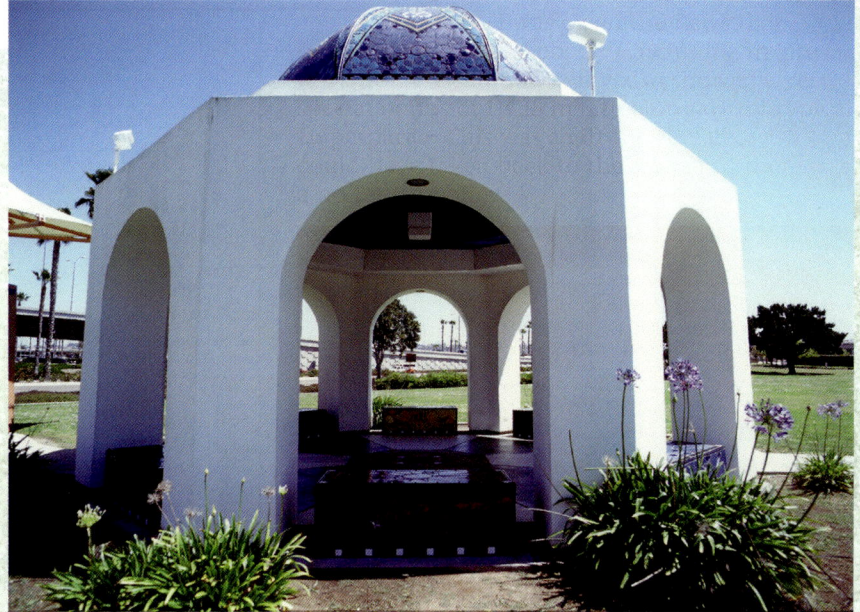

Photographs courtesy of
James K. Lemen

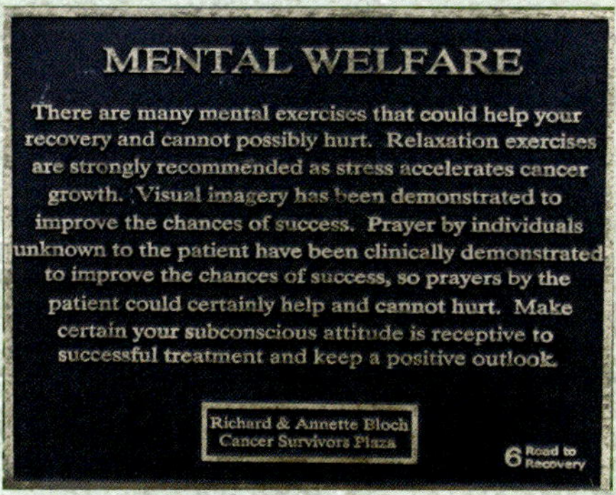

"Cancer...There's Hope"

The park has two fundamental elements that are common to the Bloch's Cancer Survivors Parks in other cities. The first of these is a major sculpture created by the renowned artist Victor Salmones. This sculpture is located in "Road to Recovery Plaza," the central focal point of the park. It consists of eight life-size figures passing through a maze depicting cancer treatments and success. People can walk among the figures, touch them, walk through the maze and generally visualize themselves being helped.

The second fundamental element in the park is a "Positive Mental Attitude Walk." This is covered walk way that people can stroll through while meditating and reading fourteen informational bronze plaques that provide inspiration and specific suggestions for fighting cancer.

Park Location

Survivors Park is located at the Eastern end of Spanish Landing off North Harbor Dr. in San Diego.

www.survivorsparksd.com

Sue

"Cancer and the Husband"

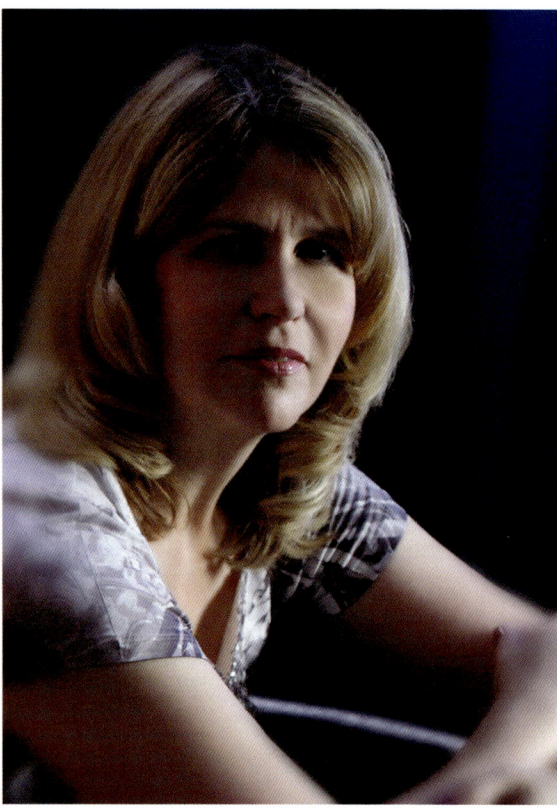
Photography by Joanna Herr

My name is Sue LaVoie and I'm 51 years old. On December 17, 2002, at the age of 43, I was diagnosed with Breast Cancer. On January 3, 2003, I had a lumpectomy and 3 days later received a call from my surgeon that I would need additional surgery to remove lymph nodes as the margins were not good. Two weeks later I had 3 lymph nodes removed, followed by 7 weeks of radiation and 5 years of Tamoxifen. My doctors told me I was lucky that my lump was small and close enough to the surface that it could be felt because they could not see it with a mammogram.

My first reaction to my diagnosis was fear as a friend of mine had just lost her 5 year battle two months prior. Then I worried about my kids. Who was going to take care of them, get them to their sporting events, band practice, and help with homework? My daughter was a junior in high school and I was afraid that I wouldn't see her graduate. My son was an eighth grader, very smart, and needed his mom.

I couldn't believe that I had cancer. I was very active, running 7 miles at least 5 days a week, had no family history of Breast Cancer and I had never smoked. I have four sisters, two older and two younger, but I was the one with cancer. My sisters and my dad were very supportive, but they all lived in another state. My husband was very unsupportive and blamed me, and told me it was my fault I got cancer. He was always angry at me and the kids, and I became very depressed. He even told my dad and sister that they could not stay at my home when they came down from Oregon to be with me for my second surgery.

Dealing with my unhealthy home environment and being exhausted all the time brought me into a deep depression. At this point I felt that life didn't really matter any more. I thought a lot about just ending it. I took an overdose as I felt it was my only way out. I spent a week in a hospital and was put on anti-depressants.

After leaving the hospital I became interested in learning all I could about Breast Cancer and I began attending support groups both for education and comfort.

I couldn't believe that I had cancer. I was very active, running 7 miles at least 5 days a week...

Nine months after my diagnosis a friend asked me to join her in the Avon Walk for Breast Cancer. I have raised money and walked this walk for the past seven years. I have met many wonderful women, all who have been touched by Breast Cancer in some way.

Since my experience with cancer I have become an active supporter of the Avon Walk for Breast Cancer, I am a "Breast Friends" mentor for the Long Beach Memorial Breast Center, raise money and walk for "Team Spirit", and have become very involved with A.W.O.L. (a way of life… after cancer).

Volunteering and helping other women who have Breast Cancer has been a very rewarding experience. I only wish I could quit my job and volunteer full-time.

When I'm not working, I enjoy walking, hiking, camping and spending as much time as I can with my kids and my grandson.

By the way, for those of you wondering what happened with me and my husband, read on. I found a group of women who had gone through what I had gone through with cancer. Some of these women had strong supportive husbands and others had husbands that

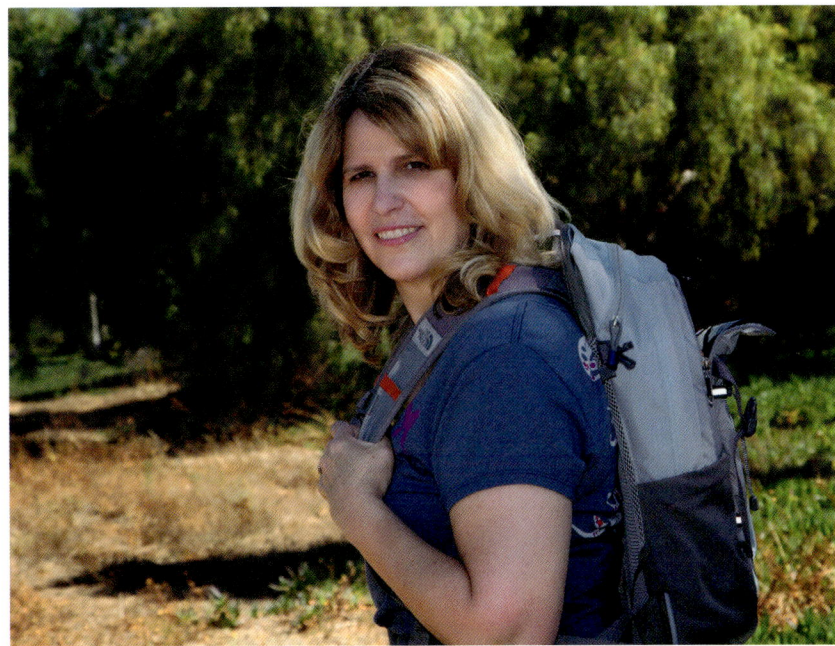

Photography by Joanna Herr

had left them. I started to realize that I matter and that there are people out there who care about me. I realized that I needed to be happy, so I saw a marriage counselor with my husband. My husband decided that our problems were all me and he quit seeing the counselor, so I left him. I didn't expect my husband to take it the way he did.

> **My husband decided that our problems were all me and he quit seeing the counselor, so I left him.**

Three months after I left, our marriage counselor called me and asked if I would consider coming back to counseling. Apparently, after I left my husband, he went back to the counselor on his own. Are you kidding me? We attended counseling for 10 months at which time I was asked by both the counselor and my husband if I would move back home. I eventually moved back home, and although things haven't always been good, it is better than it was before I left.

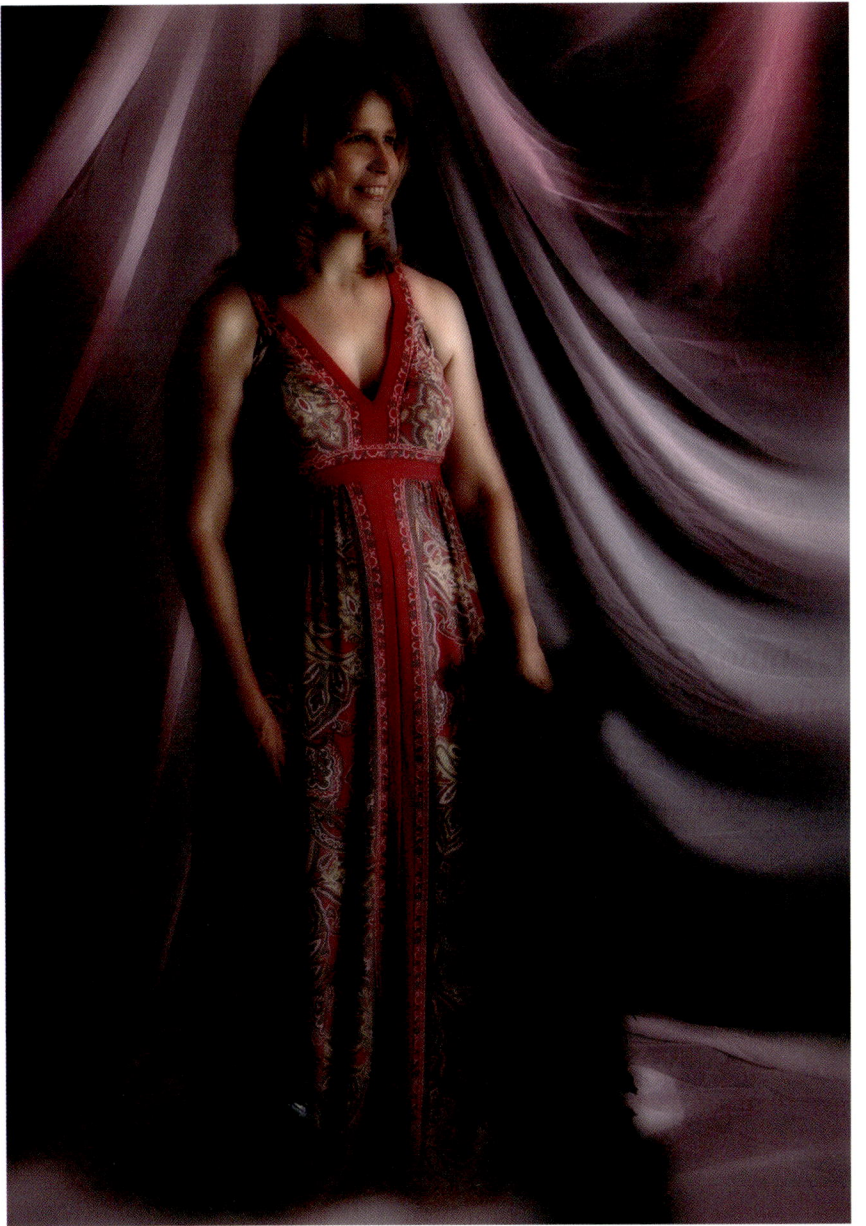

Photography by Joanna Herr

Virginia

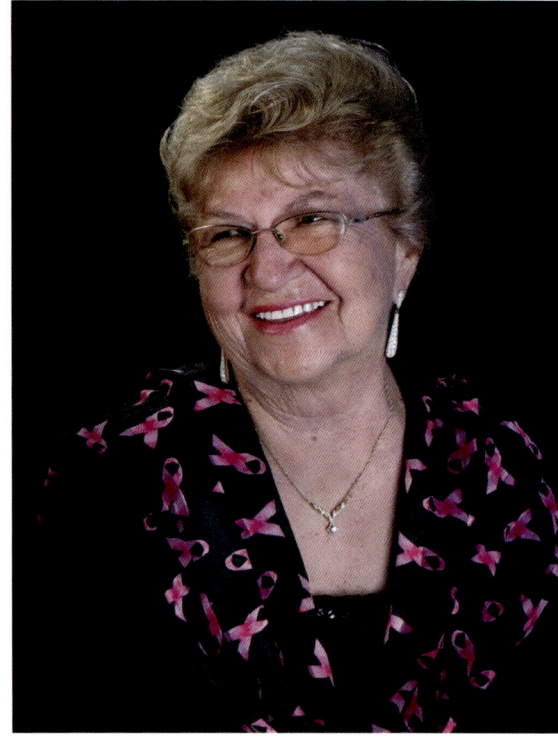

Photography by Joanna Herr

"The Angel Nurse"

March 2006, I went to the doctor's office to look into some minor back pain. An "Angel" in the office looked at my record and let me know that I was long overdue for a mammogram and insisted that we book one now. Good thing. It had been 7 years since my last one. It is amazing how time can slide by. I wish I could find that Angel Nurse. I owe her roses.

Of course they found something and an ultrasound and needle biopsy confirmed it. When given the bad news, my only comment was, "Where do we go from here?" I was 70 at the time. My Mom had told me that when you turn 70, ALL HELL BREAKS LOOSE. She was so right.

> ...she had much more extensive problems than I did, but she was so delightful to be around— a very happy person.

My first reaction, of course was fear, but my husband and family were so supportive. My surgery was scheduled for June 6, 2006. When I realized numerically it was 6-6-06 (needless to say I am superstitious), I requested an alternate date and my wonderful surgeon, Dr. Ryan at Kaiser Hospital was very understanding and rescheduled for one week later.

Surgery, June 15, 2006, a month to recover, then 25 radiation treatments, another month to heal, then in October something wonderful happened. I attended a 3-day retreat for breast cancer patients. That year, 2006, it was at a mountain resort in Big Bear, CA. I went and for 3 days everyone was pampered, cared for, massages, yoga, and taught self esteem and trusting again. They even had a talent show (in which I participated yodel). It was so wonderful and fun.

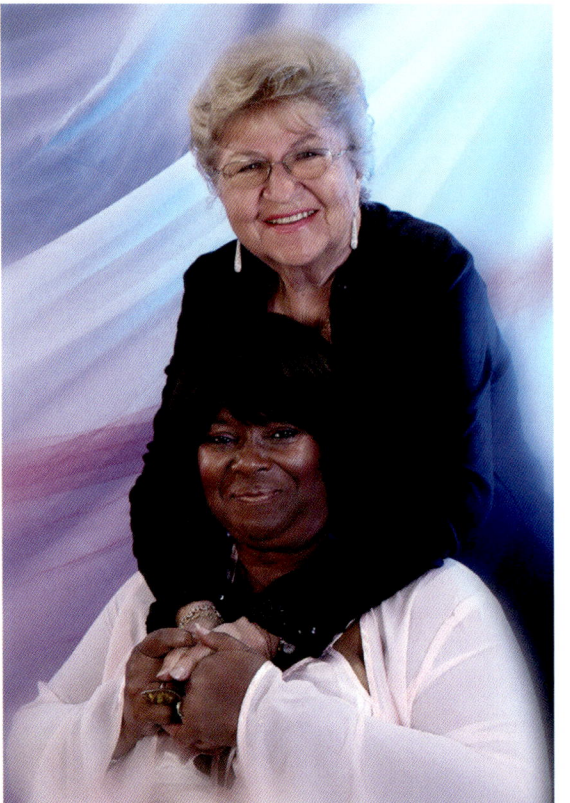

That is where I met my wonderful friend Shirley Rogers...she had much more extensive problems than I did, but she was so delightful to be around— a very happy person. I felt close to her from the very beginning and now 5 years later we are still close friends. We don't see each other as much as I would like since we live about 100 miles apart, but the heartfelt friendship is still there...she is my "sister." We are both here 5 years later by the Grace of God, the blessings of technology and some wonderful medical personnel.

Shirley

"To the Point..."

I was a 32 year old young woman with more life to live than pushing paper.

Out of this life, I had two bouts of Cancer. No, it is a good thing because from there I opened up my own business, I stayed positive and now I'm 56 and moving forward.

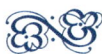

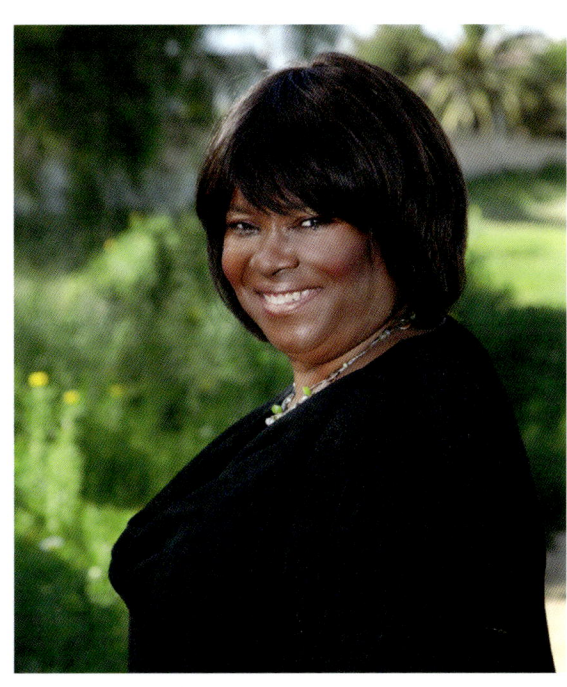

Photography by Joanna Herr

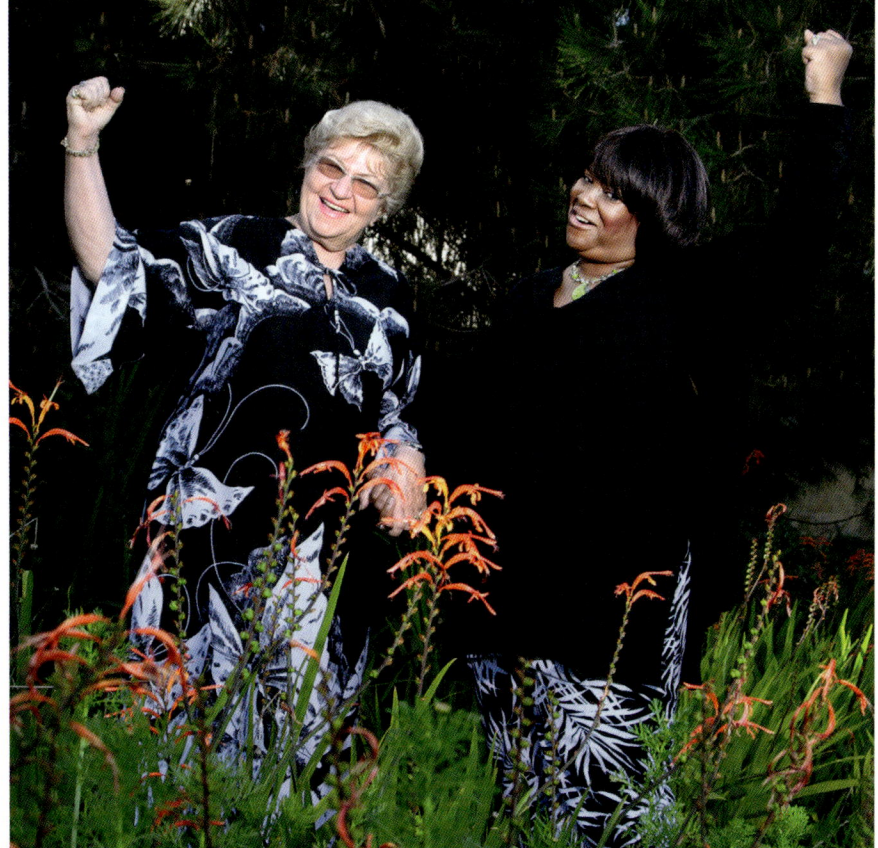

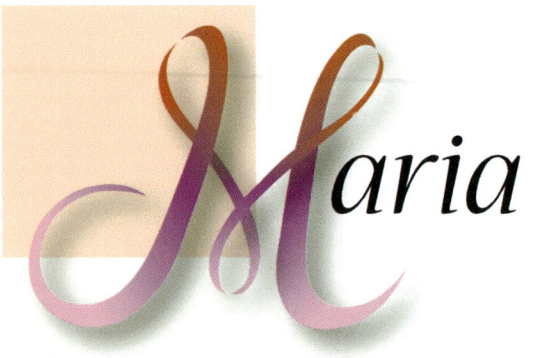

Maria

"Life's Biggest Disappointments Become God's Biggest Appointments."

My name is Maria Delis; I am a 44 year old single mom with a 13 year old son. I am a 2-year breast cancer survivor! I am so honored to share my story with you. It's been a road I never thought I would find myself on.

First, allow me to back track to Easter, April 12, 2009, just a little over a month before my diagnosis. I got engaged to a fabulous man that I had been dating 2 years. It's pretty incredible the way things happen in life. I was floating on cloud nine, but then "not-so-good stuff" happened. On Mother's Day, May 10th, I found a lump while doing a self-breast exam. Twelve days later I was diagnosed with Stage I breast cancer. As you can imagine, those words cut right straight through me. I felt like the doctor was talking to someone else in the room. I felt numb and didn't even cry right away. Then it all came crashing down. All I wanted to do was re-live that Easter Sunday over and over and tell myself that no one goes from the happiest day of their life to the saddest and scariest day ever!

Well I did. We began taking all the necessary steps to begin treatment. I found a wonderful team of doctors. We moved fast! I had surgery quickly. It was a conservative approach, lumpectomy and sentinel node biopsy. Once all the reports were in given my age and the aggressiveness (Grade 3 of 3) of the cancer, chemotherapy and radiation was the protocol recommended. After much thought, I knew I had to take a break from work during my treatment to heal, pray, and let God take over in my life.

This was going to be a big setback financially, as I am sure it is for so many other women. I have been on my own for 10 years. I have always been very responsible with my spending. I was taught: never live beyond your means, and have emergency money saved for the "rainy days", but I just didn't have enough to make it. One morning a dear friend of mine called with the names of a few organizations in Orange County that help women going through breast cancer with their financial and emotional needs. Talk about an angel! I immediately began to call them and obtain information, screening, and applications. These agencies are Breast Cancer Solutions, Breast Cancer Angels, and Beckstrand Foundation. My biggest piece of advice is go out and find these organizations in your area that can help with funds for living expenses. I was embraced with

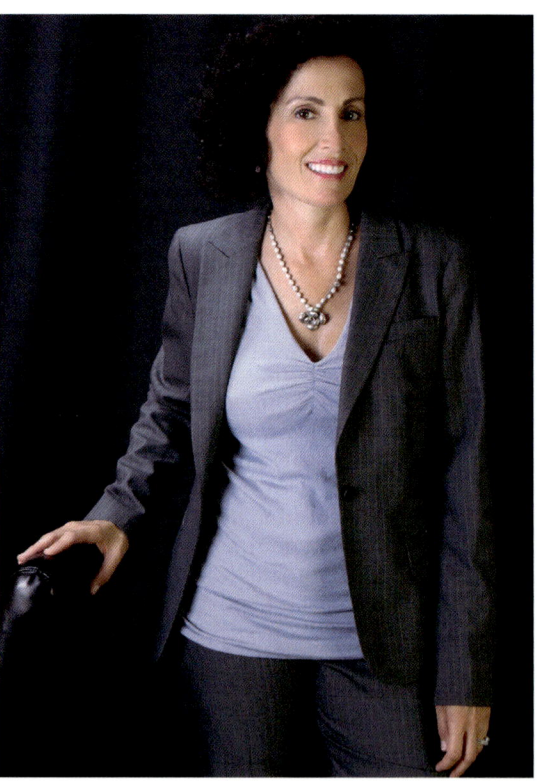

such kindness and support. It was quite touching to find these women so willing to help, listen to my story, and explain the process in which I could receive aid. Please contact them to get the help you need! They are incredible.

In May 2009, right before I was diagnosed, I was going through a major crossroads in my professional life. After being a dental hygienist for 23 years, I knew I wanted to do something that allowed me a little more flexibility and wasn't so hard on my body physically. Since my diagnosis and treat-

> *All I wanted to do was… tell myself that no one goes from the happiest day of their life to the saddest and scariest day ever!*

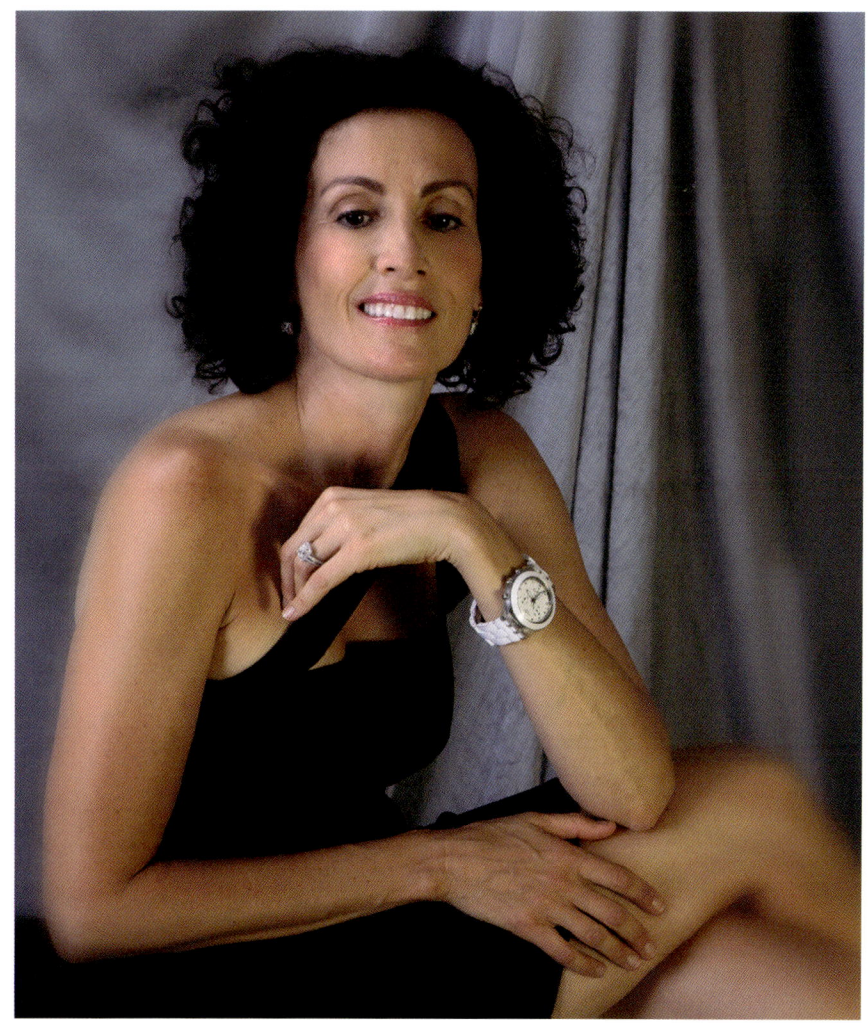

Photography by Joanna Herr

ment, it could not be clearer to me that God had another plan for my life. I have been doing quite a bit of self-development through retreats, meetings, readings, and prayer. At this point, I am still searching for the right profession that will allow me to use my gifts God has given. I pray daily the Lord will direct my path to help others and earn income as well.

> **Nutrition is key—high quality, low processed foods. Exercise…low impact, calming, meditative…**

In September 2010, on the road back, one of the most impactful and self-love retreats I attended on scholarship was A.W.O.L. I needed this retreat more than any other. I felt like I was a part of something bigger than breast cancer. I had allowed breast cancer to repress and define me. On that weekend, my life merged with other wonderful women who also forgot how to love themselves. The counselors took care of us, and enveloped us with love like I have never felt before. The preparation and all the details that went into making that weekend possible—totally unbelievable! We shared in professional workshops that gave us nothing to think about but ourselves. This is a very difficult thing for women to do in general. I felt alive again, beautiful, and special! I made some amazing friendships. In reflecting back on some moments that took place the last night was the highlight…the unveiling of the photo shoot…I was so proud of my picture! I was bouncing around so happy to show everyone. I had this confidence in me like I have never had. I guess one of the biggest challenges is how to keep that going on a day-to-day basis. Probably something I could use more of in my life is support groups. I don't make the time to be around other women who have gone through this on a regular basis. Get involved in local support groups!! This leads me to Survivorship…

In the past two years as a survivor, I have not had an easy path health-wise. I feel our medical profession has let us down with regards to Survivorship. I even heard a prominent breast surgeon from UCI say the same thing at a lecture. We go through treatment, and then we are never truly prepared for the complications that can arise from medications and such. The things I have learned: Nutrition is key—high quality, low processed foods. Exercise in a low impact, calming, meditative format; walking and yoga. Good sleep patterns. And ONE glass of red wine a day!! It has taken me some time to learn all this. I have an amazing Internist who practices holistic and conventional medicine. She never left a stone unturned. I was not feeling well for a long time and she kept uncovering issues. Because the chemo knocked out my white count, I am immuno-suppressed, so I have to follow a good routine. I was having terrible headaches, and after a brain MRI, they found a cyst removed in my sinus cavity. I had surgery. I developed adrenal exhaustion, which causes constant fatigue. I take supplements for that. I have had neck and lower back MRI's that show degenerative problems. Walking and core strengthening are essential.

It all sounds easy when I write this here, but I still struggle daily with all of it. I pull my strength from prayer and quiet time with the Lord. I know He has a big appointment for me to do wonderful things for His Kingdom here on Earth. I am grateful to be able to tell my story as I stand on the other side of cancer. I am honored to be featured in this great photo-journal publication. In June, I had another six month mammogram and all is clear. If my journey through cancer was to help just one person to know what is available to them, then my purpose is fulfilled. I want to help any way possible.

Please let me know what I can do for you, my Sister in Pink! God Be With You.

"I can do all things through Christ who strengthens me," Philippians 4:13

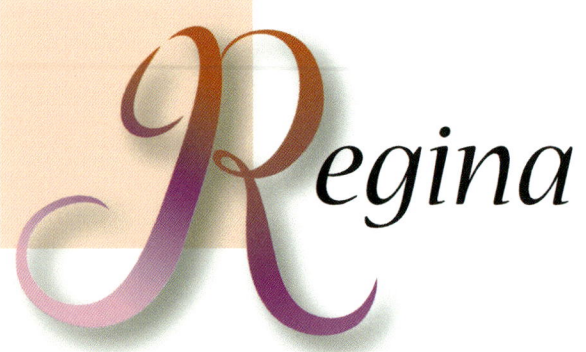

Regina

"Power to Be"

Regina E. Savage
Author/Motivational Speaker
12 Year Breast Cancer Survivor

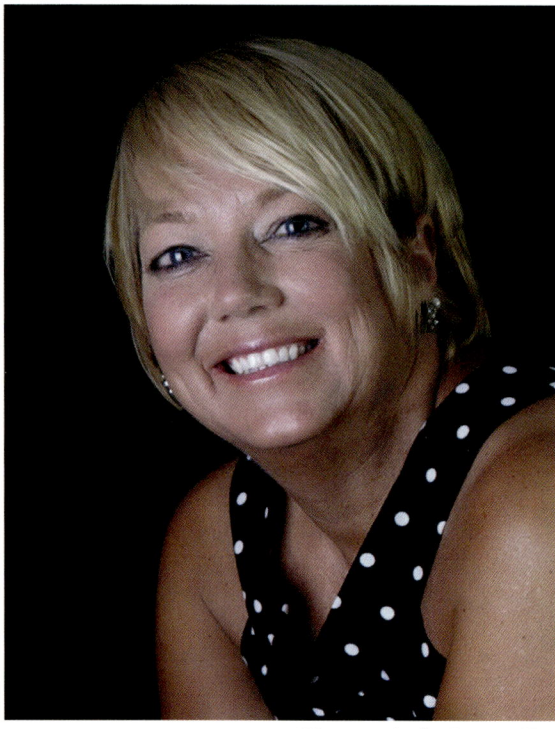

Photography by Joanna Herr

Twelve years ago, I was diagnosed with breast cancer and from that very first day I knew that life was never going to be the same. There I was, just an everyday gal like you, doing life. No one extraordinarily special, but loved by my family and friends. Doing fun things I liked to do and working at a job that I didn't particularly like but…hey, it paid well and the benefits were good. And I might add I had a little notoriety on my job… I was the first and only female hired as a street sweeper in the City of Long Beach. I take pride in that!!

And the job itself can have some interesting moments. You would be surprised at who you might see as you are driving by… Jessie James and Sandra Bullock, well you know, before the Academy Award. And there are some pretty funny situations that go on …like having a man come out to push his car out of the way, wrapped only in a towel only to have the towel fall, he kept pushing the car not realizing it, just so he would not get a ticket. But let me tell you it was pretty funny when he did. While others are sitting in an office I see the world go by, in real-time. Never a dull moment. But really try not to envy me.

There I was going through the treatment process, lab tests, surgeries, poke poke, slice slice, dab dab, stare stare, and poke poke some more. Man—could I be more invaded? I felt like I was the battle zone and the medical team was the Marines pouncing on me full guns blazing. Now mind you, I gave permission for it all to happen, but I think I was in a bit of a daze in the beginning. Then in a moment it hit me and suddenly I saw, "I need to fight this fight too!" While the professionals were fighting with medical tools I needed to fight with my mind. It was a sudden moment of clarity when I could see not only what I was fighting but why.

If there is one thing that I have learned from cancer, it is who I really am. The real me, the me that is capable of enduring and fighting through difficult things, the real me that wants to live and laugh and move forward. I never knew I had so much fight in me. Prior to having cancer I was outgoing, talkative, and adventurous but never really a go-getter. I was content to just cruise along in life.

> *It was a sudden moment of clarity when I could see not only what I was fighting but why.*

But now, I wanted to live. I was fighting for the Power to Be. To be here. To be with my family and friends. To create, to play, to contribute, to laugh and love. To be alive.

We all have the Power to Be. To be who we are, who we want to be, and move past this to live our lives fully and with enthusiasm. You can enjoy quiet walks on the beach or in a park or jump on the back of a Harley with your beau and ride off into the sunset.

No one said the journey of life would be easy… but come to think of it, I don't remember anyone really telling me how tough it could be either. Hmm, I suppose there might be a reason for that, but that can be left for another discussion.

For that matter the whole cancer thing pretty much sucks. But funny thing about bad things is that there can be redeeming factors that can come out of them. I know, bear with me on this one. But I do believe there is a lot of good that can come from cancer. I think it can help us to find ourselves and what we are meant to be doing, but I will explain that in just a moment.

> *When you think of it, someone had a sense of humor, because as if the fact that you have cancer is not bad enough… you lose your hair too.*

So for me there was bad, pretty bad, really bad, and The Worst. Losing my hair fell in the category of one of the Worst.

That was AHA moment. But before I had that moment I went through the sucky side of it. I had very long hair that I had never cut, and it was suggested several times, by nurses and my counselor, to cut it before it fell out to make it a bit easier. But I thought, how could I cut it, have that trauma, and then lose it? It would be like going through the trauma twice. Well, eventually I cut it short first and then later shaved it off when it was really falling out mainly because when I was driving down the road with my window down and my back seat of the car looked like I had a big shaggy dog!

When you think of it, someone had a sense of humor, because as if the fact that you have cancer is not bad enough ….you lose your hair too. And I have to say, I had pretty cool hair. I liked my hair. I think my hair liked being on me. Saying goodbye to it was not easy. It was like breaking up with someone you really were attached to, literally and very fond of. After all, we had been together for 36 years. It was such a devastating break up. It is not so much you lose your hair, it will grow back, it is more that you just cannot hide from the disease, and you become totally unrecognizable, even to yourself. That is the part that I thought was a bit unbearable. Even on days when you are going through treatment, but you are feeling pretty good, boom you look in the mirror and you think who the heck is that staring back at me? So for this, I decided I needed a sense of humor!

Because with my hair gone the world knew my dilemma, the world knew my personal details and that is what bothered me, I could not hide from this monster I was battling. This exposed me to other people's reactions and opinions. No HIPPA rules here. No privacy protection like in the Doctor's office or the hospital. And this exposure made me have to deal with it as well, no more ignoring it, I had cancer. Most of the time people were respectful, but I had to deal with looks and comments that I would have preferred to avoid.

So, in the midst of all these issues I decided the best way for me to deal with this was to draw my different emotions on the bathroom mirror in the form of hair, so when I looked in the mirror, even though I was as bald as could be, I would see hair surrounding my face. I used those special mirror makeovers to help me deal with my disease and my emotions.

For example, Sandra Dee was one of my drawings because she was the symbol of pretty and cute. I am so perky, I am ready to drive the world nuts! Hair or no hair. These were the good days, when I was feeling good, ready for a milkshake and to tackle the world, diagnoses or not!

But as I moved through the treatment process something changed in me. I had so many wonderful people who helped me and supported me, I was so loved by my Mom who has gone to every Doctor's appointment with me since day one, and I made friends in the support groups that stayed with me every step of the way.

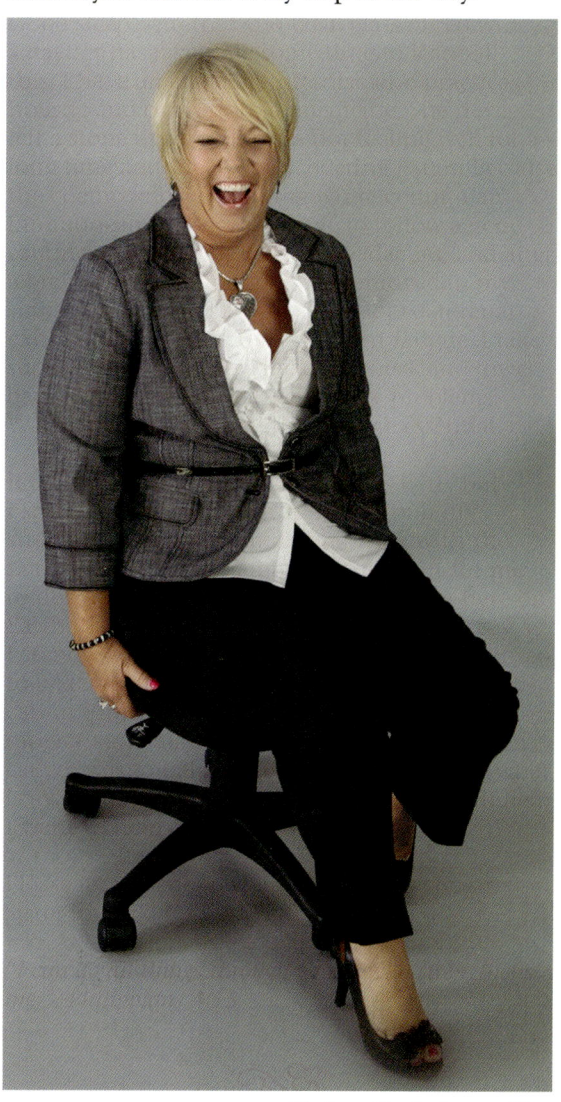

Photography by Joanna Herr

And this made me want to give back, I wanted to help others.

I realized I had the Power to give to others. To help cancer survivors, as I had been helped, to deal with the challenge of going through this disease and these emotions. I want them to find humor, to laugh, to hold their head up and fight the good fight. And at the end of the day, find pride in themselves for fighting a battle, and taking a journey they never asked for, but survived.

I started a Cancer Survivor Dragon Boat Team. This is a team of women who paddle in a large 20-person boat and compete in competitions. I would never have considered doing this before cancer, let alone starting a team for others. I would have never considered paddling, and paddling in races…who knew I could do that and encourage others as well. You see I like the outdoors and the thought of having a support group of sorts, outside in the fresh air, with women who had gone through what I had gone through…perfect! We could do this and we did. We have raced around the states, Canada, and even raced as the US Team in China! What an experience it has been! And we supported each other all the way, it was remarkable.

You see this is some of the good that can come from cancer as I mentioned earlier. Cancer opened the door for me to go for the gusto, to start over and to live my life.

One very special moment of giving back was when I had the honor of working as a counselor for a retreat for women cancer survivors. One of the gals in my group was having a very difficult time with the loss of her hair. It was then that I shared for the first time what I did to cope with the situation. How I found my sense of humor and expressed it on the mirror. How I found a way to laugh through the sadness and uncertainty.

When I shared what I had done, and we drew some hair on the mirror, there was a whole new look on her face and the others in my group. As if it just took a load off their minds to think that they could actually find humor in this daunting situation.

Their reaction was so strong for me, that it convinced me to write my book, *"Mirror Makeovers & Savvy Insights for the Everyday Gal Surviving Cancer & Baldness with a Sense of Humor,"* to help as many other women as possible and I could only hope that their faces lit up as much as these gals at a time when they needed it most. And I am proud to say that not only is the book helping but it has won two awards this year; Independent Publisher's Editor's Choice Highlighted Title (March 2011) and Independent Publisher's 2011 Living Now Gold Medal Award honoring books for a better living.

Cancer is not funny, but let's face it, sometimes when we are at wits end, a sense of humor is all we have and the ability to laugh at ourselves can only make us stronger.

Now keep in mind, when going through this process, not all days can be Sandra Dee days. Let's face it sometimes those perky days would be few and far between. So, I would get up, give it some thought as to how I was feeling, which generally did not take long with chemo brain, and I usually had to write it down so I would remember it, but then when I figured it out, I would draw my emotions on the mirror, and move through my day knowing that I was honoring myself and my emotions.

And some days I would feel a bit like this…

Now we all know her—yep, it's Medusa! It is a really bad hair day! On Medusa days, you're simply mad at the world and that's okay! We all deserve to feel this way; just remember not to stay in this place. Be mad, grit your teeth, scream, and turn the whole world or anyone who gets in your way into stone.

But then we move on to the next day, or maybe moment, depends on the hot flashes, when we need to pick ourselves up, brush ourselves off

> *I shared what I had done… As if it just took a load off their minds to think that they could actually find humor in this daunting situation.*

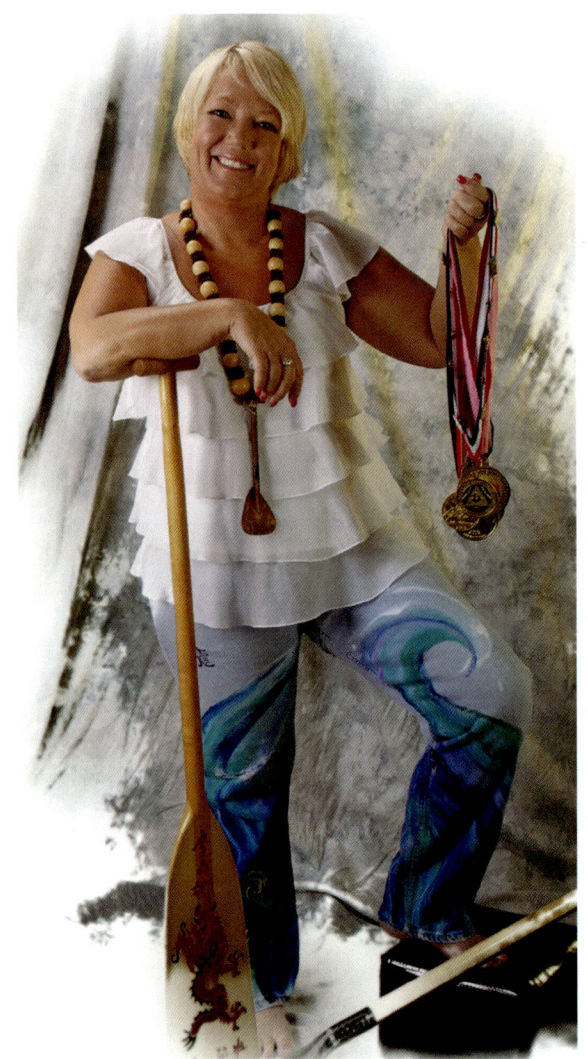

Photography by Joanna Herr

and get back into the adventure of life. Those are the Biker Girl days.

No one messes with this girl. She knows what she wants and she goin' for it. In style. You're not messing around anymore! Draw your helmet and act like one of those badass gals on the back of a Harley, nobody messes with them.

Look in the mirror and know that you own the world! You are kicking cancer in the ass, and if someone doesn't like it they'd better get out of your way!! You can do this.

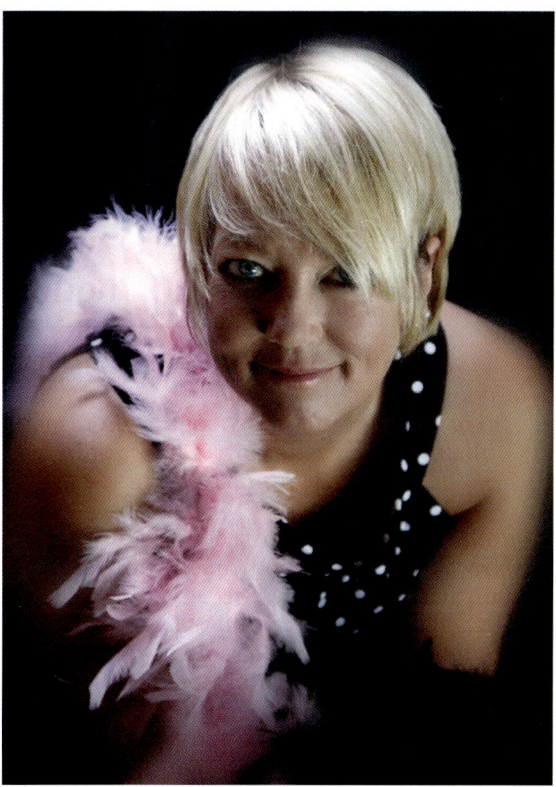

> *It is not about our appearances on the outside, it is how we feel on the inside! It is us knowing, feeling and having the power to see that we can kick this thing!*

It is not about our appearances on the outside, it is how we feel on the inside! It is us knowing, feeling and having the power to see that we can kick this thing! That we can use our strength, our sense of self and our power to envision a life moving forward, being strong and taking that Road to Recovery.

Who'd a thought that sharing this exercise would be the beginning of me becoming an author, a director and writer of a music video! In order to do this, I had to use my Power, the power in myself to be, to see and the power to want to give back, just like the song in my music video made by cancer survivors for cancer survivors with the KT Tunstall song, "Suddenly I See". The chorus is "Suddenly I See, why the hell it means so much to me," and it is so true.

And this is exactly what happened. I took that exercise, I encouraged others to draw their emotions on the mirror. The impact I saw on the women I shared it made me want to bring that joy, laughter and hope to other women.

Now this did not happen overnight, I had to learn to deal with my own emotions first, to honor what I was feeling and to move through it. That does not always come easy sometimes, but when you get there, when you learn to honor how you are feeling, address it, and deal with it, then you can get through it. After all, with a cancer diagnoses comes a lot of emotions; am I going to get through this, am I going to survive, what about my family, my friends, the dog, and then there is getting through the journey after the disease. It is just overwhelming at times. But that is why God made us women!! We are tough, we can get through things and we can move forward. After all we have the babies, we really wear the pants in the family and we are the ones with the hot flashes…we can get through anything.

So all the emotions I went through, I call the "Everyday Gals of Cancer," these are really our emotions and who we are or who we want to be on any given day. Because we are everyday gals and using our emotions make us realize that we are still the same beautiful gals we have always been, even with a different appearance on the outside, and some new and improved work on the body, inside and out, who we truly are can never be taken away from us! We can all deal with our emotions, use our Power to see and get through to the person we really want to be!

Now that I have told you some of my story of how I learned about myself, and found myself through this journey, 12 years to be exact and my advice is this, don't hide who you are, or how you are feeling. Take this journey, whether you are going through it now or have been through it and are on the other side and honor you! Find the good that can come from cancer and if you feel like Medusa, draw her on the mirror, and don't erase it. Take all of this, these emotions, this journey and find your Power to Be; to be who you truly are, life is uncertain for all of us, discover you now and enjoy it. Find you're Power to give; and give back; even the littlest of jesters can change a world and someone in it. And find your Power to see, to live your life, to see yourself healthy, happy and doing what it is you want to do, and see this all Cancer Free!

Groups & Links

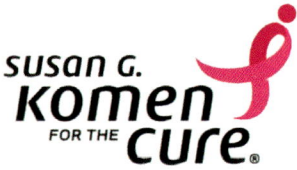

Susan G. Komen fought breast cancer with her heart, body and soul. Throughout her diagnosis, treatments, and endless days in the hospital, she spent her time thinking of ways to make life better for other women battling breast cancer instead of worrying about her own situation.

That concern for others continued even as Susan neared the end of her fight. Moved by Susan's compassion for others and committed to making a difference, Nancy G. Brinker promised her sister that she would do everything in her power to end breast cancer forever. That promise is now Susan G. Komen for the Cure®. As the world's largest grassroots network of breast cancer survivors and activists, we're working together to save lives, empower people, ensure quality care for all and energize science to find the cures.

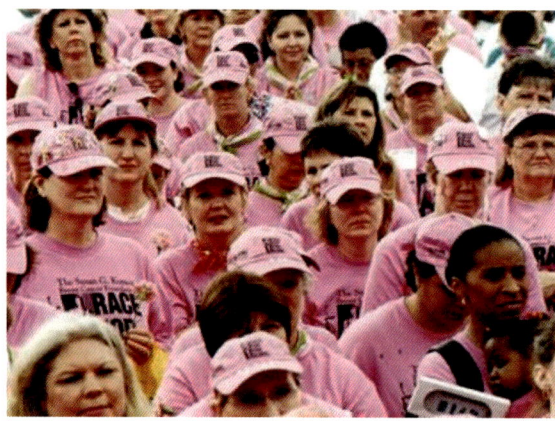

Thanks to events like the Susan G. Komen Race for the Cure® and the Susan G. Komen 3-Day for the Cure®, and generous contributions from our partners, sponsors and fellow supporters, we have become the largest source of nonprofit funds dedicated to the fight against breast cancer in the world.

ww5.komen.org

Breast Cancer RX

A breast cancer resources site for chemotherapy, mammograms and mastectomy procedures.

www.breastcancerrx.com

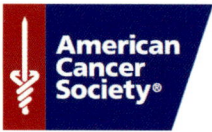 Saving lives by helping people stay well, get well, find cures, & fight back.

www.cancer.org

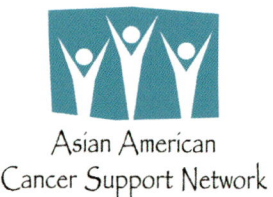 The Asian American Cancer Support Network provides an educational, supportive, and diverse network of resources for Asian Americans affected by cancer.

www.aacsn.org

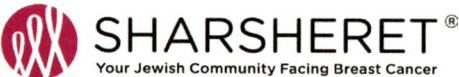

Sharsheret is a national not-for-profit organization supporting young Jewish women and their families facing breast cancer. Our mission is to offer a community of support to women, of all Jewish backgrounds, diagnosed with breast cancer or at increased genetic risk, by fostering culturally-relevant individualized connections with networks of peers, health professionals, and related resources.

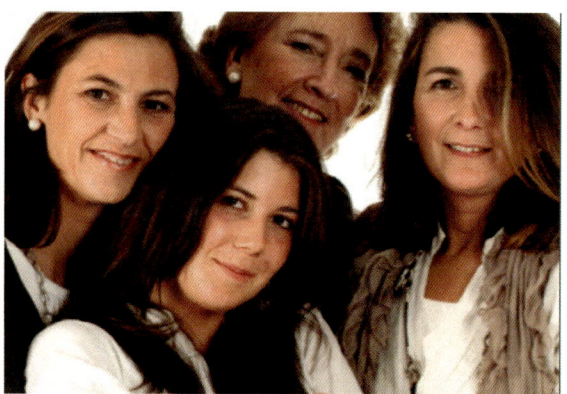

We understand what it's like to be a young Jewish woman facing breast cancer or ovarian cancer. We offer confidential, culturally-relevant support for you and your family, specific to your situation. We will help you connect to our community in the ways that feel most comfortable to you, taking into consideration your stage of diagnosis or treatment, as well as your connection to Judaism. Whether you are concerned about genetics, dating, fertility, parenting, your career, managing side effects from treatment, or preparing for the holidays, we will connect you to the services that best meet your particular needs. Think of Sharsheret as your personal gateway to the resources and connections you may need over time.

www.sharsheret.org

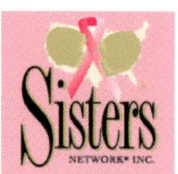 Sisters Network® Inc. is committed to increasing local and national attention to the devastating impact that breast cancer has in the African American community.

www.sistersnetworkinc.org

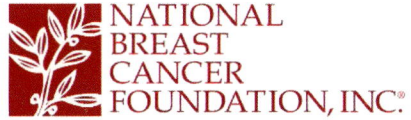

NBCF (National Breast Cancer Foundation) is committed to spreading knowledge and fostering hope in the fight against breast cancer. By funding free mammograms for women who could otherwise not afford them and supporting research programs in leading facilities across the country, NBCF helps inspire the courage needed to win this monumental battle. Be a part of the solution and discover how to help.

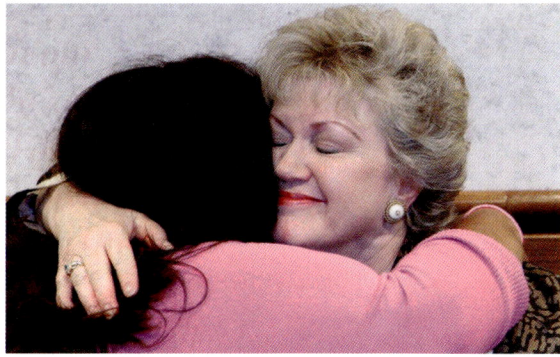

www.nationalbreastcancer.org

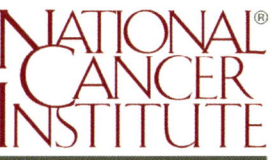 Coordinates the National Cancer Program, which conducts and supports research, training, health information dissemination, and other programs as to the cause, diagnosis, prevention, and treatment of cancer, rehabilitation from cancer, and the continuing care of cancer patients and the families of cancer patients.

www.cancer.gov

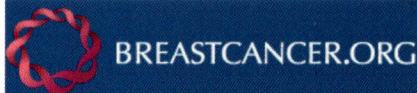

Breastcancer.org is a non-profit organization dedicated to providing information and community to those touched by this disease.

www.breastcancer.org

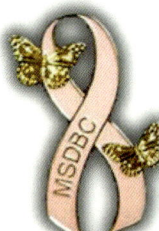 MSDBC is a national nonprofit co-founded by Charmayne Dierker, a mother and her daughter, Lillie Shockney. Free support services are provided, which are designed to help mothers who have daughters battling breast cancer. Over 10,000 women have already been helped!

http://mothersdaughters.org

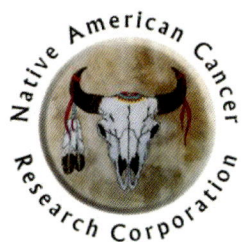 We are dedicated to helping improve the lives of Native American cancer patients and survivors. We seek to reduce Native American cancer incidence and mortality, and to increase survival from cancer among Native Americans.

http://natamcancer.org

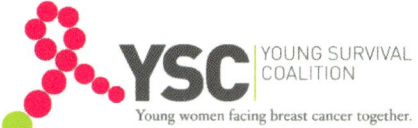

Young Survival Coalition (YSC) is the premier global organization dedicated to the critical issues unique to young women who are diagnosed with breast cancer. YSC offers resources, connections and outreach so women feel supported, empowered and hopeful.

YSC helps young women stand strong against the many unique challenges our population faces. Unlike post-menopausal women with breast cancer, we must deal with higher mortality rates, fertility issues and the possibility and ramifications of early menopause.

In YSC's network of young women, however, those challenges can look more like opportunities to accomplish shared goals. YSC works with its members to:

- *Serve as a community of support for young women with breast cancer.*
- *Advocate for more studies about young women and breast cancer; and*
- *Educate young women about the importance of breast self-awareness and knowledge;*

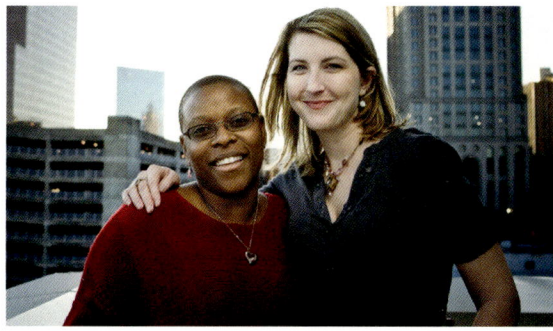

Through it all, YSC helps women find meaning, comfort and hope during one of the most challenging experiences of their lives.

www.youngsurvival.org

From Chrysalis to Wings

Mission Statement:

To provide support for and on behalf of children and adults who suffer emotionally with malformation of the body caused by birth defects or disfiguration due to illness or trauma. We pride ourselves in developing supportive and therapeutic solutions for those who experience psychological and emotional problems due to these issues.

Home of

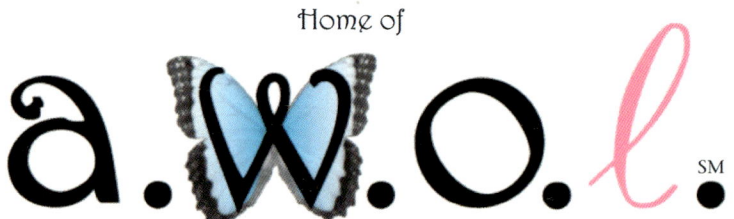

(A Way of Life...after breast cancer)

A.W.O.L. (A Way of Life...after breast cancer) founded by **Executive Director, Dr. Francine Zorehkey, LMFT,** of **From Chrysalis To Wings** and **Creative Director, Joanna Herr of Herr Photography, Inc.** is a program specifically designed for women who have or have had breast cancer. The central purpose of A.W.O.L. is to provide each woman with the support needed to cope with her illness and to improve the quality of her life, which includes an emphasis towards issues of **body image that can sometimes be minimized** by self, clinicians, family, and even people in the support system due to the life threatening factor of breast cancer. Dealing with these issues is essential to someone whose sense of self is highly based on how she looks on the outside.

As part of **A.W.O.L., From Chrysalis to Wings** conducts two yearly retreats to help breast cancer survivors tap into their grief and loss as a result of breast cancer diagnosis, the treatment, the loss of a breast and the altered body image. The retreats also give an opportunity to deal with guilt feelings, the anger and the "why me" question and provides an opportunity to express gratitude for their survival, and to remove the stigma of the disease. Retreats are held at a camp where a beautiful nature setting and a loving nurturing environment can be provided. In short, the 3-day (Thursday evening through Sunday morning) retreat is designed to help improve the quality of life and well-being of the survivors.

While all women suffer with anxiety about their breast cancer diagnosis and the invasive treatment, one quarter of women will also suffer from depression in the first or second year following a mastectomy. Some will work through the anxiety and depression, while others won't, and this may interfere with treatment and reduce a chance of full recovery.

For more information about project **A.W.O.L.**, please call **(949) 916-6851**.

www.chrysalistowings.com